T0257580

Tropical Medicine

Tropical Medicine

Edited by **Charline Ryler**

FOSTER
ACADEMICS

New Jersey

Published by Foster Academics,
61 Van Reypen Street,
Jersey City, NJ 07306, USA
www.fosteracademics.com

Tropical Medicine
Edited by Charline Ryler

International Standard Book Number: 978-1-63242-410-5 (Hardback)

Printed in the United States of America.

Contents

Preface

Tropical medicine has surfaced and retained its position as a significant discipline for the analysis of diseases native in the tropic, specifically those diseases which have infectious etiology and the emergence and reemergence of several tropical pathologies have currently provoked the interest of numerous fields of the analysis of tropical medicine, inclusive of novel infectious agents. Information based on evidence along with ordered updates are required. This book provides up-to-date information on various diseases and conditions of interest in the field. It encompasses pathologies caused by viruses, parasites and bacteria as well as tropical non-infectious conditions. The book not only discusses epidemiological aspects, but also preventive, genetic, therapeutic, social, bioinformatics, diagnostic, and molecular ones. This book serves as a great source of information with a broad geographical perspective.

This book is a result of research of several months to collate the most relevant data in the field.

When I was approached with the idea of this book and the proposal to edit it, I was overwhelmed. It gave me an opportunity to reach out to all those who share a common interest with me in this field. I had 3 main parameters for editing this text:

1. Accuracy – The data and information provided in this book should be up-to-date and valuable to the readers.

2. Structure – The data must be presented in a structured format for easy understanding and better grasping of the readers.

3. Universal Approach – This book not only targets students but also experts and innovators in the field, thus my aim was to present topics which are of use to all.

Thus, it took me a couple of months to finish the editing of this book.

I would like to make a special mention of my publisher who considered me worthy of this opportunity and also supported me throughout the editing process. I would also like to thank the editing team at the back-end who extended their help whenever required.

Editor

Part 1

Tropical Diseases Due to Bacteria and Viruses

Molecular Characterization of Dengue Virus Circulating in Manaus, the Capital City of the State of Amazonas, Brazil

Regina Maria Pinto de Figueiredo
Foundation for Tropical Medicine Dr. Hector Vieira Dourado (FMT/HVD)
Brazil

1. Introduction

The term dengue, of Spanish origin, was used to describe joint pain from an illness that attacked the British during the epidemic that affected the Spanish West Indies from 1927-1928. Dengue was brought to the American continent to the Old World during the colonization in the late eighteenth century. However, it is not possible to say according to the historical record if the outbreaks were caused by dengue virus, as its symptoms are similar to those of several other infections, especially yellow fever (Holmes et al., 1998). The etiology of dengue has been credited to the miasma theory, bacterial or protozoan infection and finally to an ultramicroscopic agent. Similarly, transmission has been considered by respiratory airway and finally, by mosquitoes.

The isolation of dengue virus (DENV) occurred in the 1940s during the epidemics of Nagasaki (1943) and Osaka (1944). The first known strain is coined DENV Mochizuki (Kimura & Hotta, 1944). In 1945, the Hawaii strain was isolated, and that same year other DENVs showing antigenic characteristics of different serotypes were isolated in New Guinea. The first two strains were designated serotype 1 and serotype 2. In 1956, other strains designated as serotype 3 and 4 were isolated. Thus, four dengue serotypes are known to date: DENV-1, DENV-2, DENV-3 and DENV-4 (Martinez Torres, 1990).

Genetic variation within each serotype was first demonstrated by serological techniques. Subsequently analysis of the viral genome showed that DENV-1and DENV-2 can be classified as having five genotypes or subtypes each while DENV-3 and DENV-4having four and two respectively (Rico-Hesse, 1990, Lanciotti et al., 1994). Recently, Rico-Hesse et al (2003) reviewed the classification of DENV genotypes by the analysis and comparison of the nucleotide sequence of the complete E gene of various strains. As a result it was defined thatDENV-2 and DENV-3 have four genotypes while DENV-1 and DENV-4 have five and three genotypes respectively (Cunha & Nogueira, 2005).

1.1 Etiology

Dengue Fever, a vector-borne disease, is the most important arboviral disease worldwide. Dengue viruses (DENVs) belong to the genus *Flavivirus*, family *Flaviviridae*. These are single-stranded positive-sense RNA viruses. DENV are grouped into four antigenically related but distinct serotypes named DENV-1, 2, 3 and 4.The four serotypes of DENV are diverse and not phylogenetically related but strongly related to flavivirus transmitted by mosquitoes. It is reported that these viruses have emerged about 1000 years ago from a monkey virus and its transmission to humans occurred in the last 320 years. Some studies indicated its origin in Africa and others in Asia (Weaver et al., 2004).

1.2 Clinical characteristics

Dengue has two main clinical forms: classic dengue fever (DF) and dengue hemorrhagic fever (DHF) with or without shock (PAN AMERICAN HEALTH ORGANIZATION, 1994). The symptoms of DF are headache, retro-orbital pain, breaking bones sensation, muscles or joints pain, rash and leucopenia. Dengue hemorrhagic fever is characterized by high fever, hemorrhagic phenomena often with hepatomegaly and, in severe cases, signs of circulatory failure. Patients with DHF may develop hypovolemic shock resulting from plasma leakage. This clinical manifestation is called dengue shock syndrome (DSS) and can be fatal (WORLD HEALTH ORGANIZATION, 2001).

1.3 Transmission

The dengue virus is transmitted to humans through the bite of hematophagous Diptera, the mosquito *Aedes aegypti*. In the Americas, *A. aegypti* is one of the most efficient vectors of Arboviruses and is highly anthropophilic thriving in close proximity to humans and adapts very well indoors, generally in humid environment (WORLD HEALTH ORGANIZATION, 2001).

Once contracted the virus, the mosquito remains infected during its entire life and may transmit the virus to individuals during blood meals. The infected *A.aegypti* females may also transmit the virus to the next generation of mosquitoes by transovarial. Although very seldom, this means of transmission is of great epidemiological significance demonstrating that the vector play an important role in the persistence of the virus in the environment and act as reservoirs (WORLD HEALTH ORGANIZATION, 2001; Castro et al., 2004; Joshi et al., 2006). Human beings are the main host and the virus replicates in the blood stream. Uninfected mosquitoes can contract the virus during blood meals from an infected individual. The virus multiplies in the cells of the mosquito during a period of 8 to 10 days. After this period, the vector is able to transmit the virus to humans again. In humans, the incubation period of dengue fever ranges from 2 to 7 days. Laboratory experiments showed that the mosquito *A. aegypti* may be infected simultaneously by different arboviruses and is also capable of transmitting them simultaneously (Araújo et al., 2006). According Wenming et al. (2005) it is possible that mosquitoes infected with DENV-2 and DENV-3 can transmit both in areas where two or more serotypes circulate. The poor environmental conditions of urban centers, the humidity and temperature as in Brazil associated with resistance of eggs of *A. aegypti* for long periods of desiccation favor the proliferation of mosquitoes and contribute to the spread of DENV. Dengue is currently considered the most important arbovirus and is a public health problem in tropical and subtropical countries (Guzman et al. 2006; WORLD HEALTH ORGANIZATION, 2001).

1.4 Dengue in Manaus

Infection by dengue virus in Brazil has increased significantly over the last decade, particularly after 1994, as a consequence of the spread of *A.aegypti*. The following serotypes,

DENV-1, DENV-2 and DENV-3 were common in most Brazilian cities. The DENV-4, co-circulating with DENV-1,was detected during the first epidemic reported in Brazil in Boa Vista - Roraima in 1981-1982 (Osanai, 1984).

In early 1998, the Laboratory of Arbovirology at the Foundation for Tropical Medicine Dr. Hector Vieira Gold (FMT/HVD) in Manaus in the state of Amazonas, started a program of monitoring and diagnosing of viral diseases transmitted by arthropods (arboviruses) to determine their etiological agents. The diagnosis was made by serologic studies using the MAC-ELISA test for detection of IgM antibodies. Sera samples from 8557 patients suspected of dengue were analyzed and 40% of the sera were ELISA positive for dengue virus. The DENV-1 was considered responsible for this epidemic (Figueiredo et al., 2004). In 2001, DENV-1 and DENV-2 were isolated in the State of Amazons and dengue hemorrhagic fever cases were registered (Figueiredo et al., 2002). In 2003, DENV-3 was isolated for the first time in the state of Amazonas from a patient coming from the state of Bahia (Figueiredo et al., 2003).

A variety of acute febrile diseases with and without hemorrhagic manifestations were diagnosed as dengue in Manaus in March 1998 by detection of specific IgM antibodies. Mayaro (MAYV) and *Oropouche* (OROV) viruses were also diagnosed. Infections with rubella and parvovirus were also observed (Figueiredo et al., 2004).

In 2008, DENV-4 was first identified in Manaus (Figueiredo et al., 2008). The Amazon is situated in the Northern Region of Brazil, bordered to the north with the State of Roraima, Venezuela and Colombia. Serotype DENV-4 was endemic to Venezuela and Colombia and this may have influenced the detection of this serotype in the Amazon due to its proximity to these countries (Figueiredo, 2008). The four serotypes of dengue and cases of DENV-3/DENV-4 co-infection are shown in Figure 1.

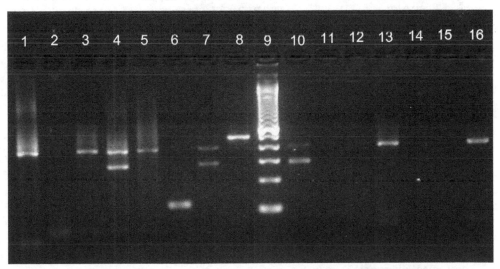

Fig. 1. Agarose gel electrophoresis. Lanes 1,3, 13, 16: DENV-4; Lane 4,7 and 10: DENV-3/DENV-4; Lane 6: DENV-2, Lane 8: DENV-1; Lane 9: DNA size standards 100Kb;

Nucleotide sequence analysis of DENV-4 present in the State of Amazonas showed to be of genotype I which is only present in the Asian continent and never described in the

Americas (De Melo et al., 2009). The introduction of this virus in Manaus is probably due to the fact that this is a city with eco-tourism development, and possess an Industrial Center (Free Zone of Manaus), with over 450 factories of large, medium and small size (PORTAL AMAZÔNIA) and many of them are of Asian origin (Figueiredo, 2008). It is possible that the virus has been introduced from an Asian-infected visitor or vector *A.aegypti*-infected.

1.5 Co-infection

Natural co-infection with dengue virus can occur in highly endemic areas where several serotypes have been transmitted for many years. Cases of simultaneous infection by more than one species of arboviruses in mosquito or human host were reported (Meyers& Carey, 1967; Gubler et al., 1985). In Brazil, one case of co-infection by DENV-1 and DENV-2 was reported in the patient with classic dengue fever (DF) from Southeastern region through immunofluorescence and RT-PCR (Santos et al., 2003). Another case of co-infection by DENV-2 and DENV-3, was observed in 2005 in the Northeastern region from a patient with DF (Araújo et al., 2006). Simultaneous infection by different strains of dengue virus in mosquitoes and humans underscores the potential for recombination (Santos et al., 2003). Although recombination is rarely recorded in positive-stranded RNA viruses (Lai, 1992), recombination occurrence in picornavirus, coronavirus, and alphavirus have been suggested. The latter viruses are also transmitted by mosquitoes (Hahn et al., 1998.Variations in dengue virus and the occurrence of co-infections with different DENV serotype may lead to genetic exchange between strains increasing the likelihood of recombination (Kuno, 1997).

During an outbreak of dengue in São José do Rio Preto, State of São Paulo, 365 samples were positives to DENV-3, 5 samples were to DENV-2, and 8 to Saint Louis encephalitis flavivirus (SLEV). Among the positive samples, one co-infection was detected for DENV-2 and DENV-3. Co-infection of each distint DENV serotype or other flavivirus during dengue outbreaks seems to be common (Terzian et al., 2010).

2. Laboratory diagnosis

2.1 Isolation of virus

The two basic methods for establishing a laboratory diagnosis of dengue fever are: the detection of viruses (egg, culture), or detection of IgM antibodies anti-dengue (serology). Blood samples for viral isolation should be collected within five days from the onset of symptoms. Serum is obtained by centrifugation and stored at -70°C.The inoculation of clinical specimens in adult mosquitoes or larvae in the culture technique is more sensitive for the detection of DENV. In laboratories where colonized mosquitoes are not available, samples can be inoculated in any mosquito cell lines available such as C6/36 (*Aedes albopictus* clone) that has a high sensitivity to DENV and other arboviruses.

2.2 Serological diagnosis

Sera should be collected from patients from the sixth day of illness and stored at -20°C. The MAC-ELISA is an antibody-capture assay of IgM from sera of patients suspected of DF. Briefy, the plate is sensitized with an anti-human IgM, and after various steps of the assay (blocking, dilution, washing, incubation overnight with the pool of antigen (DENV-1,

DENV-2 and DENV-3), the presence of specific IgM antibodies to dengue in the patient serum is shown by color change of the substrate that undergo enzymatic action of the conjugate. The color intensity is directly proportional to the amount of IgM antibodies contained in serum (Kuno et al., 1987).

2.3 Polymerase chain reaction (PCR) coupled with reverse transcription(RT-PCR)
The technique of PCR can be used to detect the presence of the DENV. Viral RNA is extracted using commercial kits. The RNA is reverse transcribed to cDNA in a first step. Then specific primers for DENV nucleotide sequence are used for the amplification of targeted sequence so as to detect a small amount of RNA molecules of DENV. This method is fast and rapid compared to cell culture. Reverse transcription and PCR technique was shown for the first time as a powerful technique for the detection of the DENV during convalescence, when the antibodies would limit its detection (WORLD HEALTH ORGANIZATION, 2001).

However, this method should still be considered an experimental approach. Is implementation on a large scale awaits further experiments. Moreover, a consensus on the adequate preparation of samples and for determining the sequences of bases in oligonucleotides capable of detecting all or most circulating genotypes of dengue need to be reached (WORLD HEALTH ORGANIZATION, 2001).

2.4 Virological diagnosis
The technique used to isolate DENV is continuous cell lines of mosquito cells C6/36 (*Aedes albopictus* clone) (Igarashi, 1978), grown in 25 cm flask with growth medium L-15 plus 5% of fetal bovine serum. To 1.5 mL of theL-15 plus 5% of fetal bovine serum containing the C6/36 cells in disposable falcon tubes (15 mL), 70 µl of serum from patients suspected of DF in acute phase was added and incubated at 28° C for two week. Culture media is changed two times per week and incubated. After 10 days of incubation, immunofluorescence (IF) technique is used for the identification of serotypes of dengue.

3. Discussion

In Brazil, first cases of DHF occurred after the introduction of DENV-2 in the State of Rio de Janeiro. The cases of DHF by DENV-2 occurred after an epidemic by DENV-1 in Rio de Janeiro four years ago (Dias et al. 1991; Zagne et al., 1994). The same pattern was seen in Cuba during the 1981 epidemic with sequential infection by two serotypes (DENV-1 and DENV-2), and an interval of six months to five years or so (Kouri et al., 1986).The dynamics of epidemic of dengue in the Amazon is similar to that of other regions of Brazil and America. In Manaus – Amazonas, the first cases of dengue were registered in March 1998 by serological studies during the first epidemic of dengue (Figueiredo et al., 2004). In 2001, it was possible to identify the DENV-1 as the causative agent of that epidemic (Figueiredo et al., 2002). That same year, cases of dengue hemorrhagic fever were registered in the State of Amazonas, with the viral isolation of DENV-2 (Figueiredo et al., 2002). In 2002, DENV3 was first isolated from a patient coming from Bahia. Since then, DENV-3 was diagnosed by viral isolation from several patients with DF (Figueiredo et al., 2003).The virus DENV-4 was detected during the first epidemic reported in Brazil in Boa Vista-Roraima in 1981-1982. At that time the DENV-1 was also found (Osanai, 1984). Since then, no isolate of DENV-4 was recorded anywhere else in the country until later in the year 2008 DENV-4 was isolated in Manaus from patients with DF (Figueiredo et al., 2008).

The DENV-4 present in the State of Amazonas and analyzed by nucleotide sequence was shown to belong to genotype I, only present in the Asian continent and never described in the Americas (De Melo et al., 2009).

Dengue fever in uncomplicated cases of co-infection has also been observed by other authors, contradicting the hypothesis that simultaneous infection with dengue virus permits the emergence of a more severe disease (Santos et al., 2003; Araújo et al.,2006). In areas where more than one serotype are transmitted at the same time, clinical cases caused by more than one serotype of dengue fever can be common (Lorono et al., 1999). The high rate of cases occurring during epidemics can result in many infections with multiple serotypes in humans (both clinical and subclinical), and also provide opportunity for mosquitoes to become infected with two or more serotypes (Gubler et al., 1985; Burke et al., 1988). This suggests that co-infection by multiple dengue serotypes may influence the clinical expression of disease and it was initially considered as an explanation for the emergence of DHF (Hammon, 1973).The Amazon is situated in the Northern Region of Brazil, bordered to the north with the State of Roraima, Venezuela and Colombia to the east with the State of Pará, the southeast by the State of Mato Grosso, to the south with the State of Rondônia and southwest with the State of Acre and Peru (Viverde Tourism). The proximity to other countries where endemic DENV-4 is observed as in Venezuela and Colombia may have influenced the detection of this serotype first in the Amazon. Besides the geographical location, being today a city with eco-tourism development, and the Industrial Pole of Manaus, with over 450 factories of large, medium and small size (PORTAL AMAZON), which attracts investors from around the world. Manaus receives many people from these and other states and countries.

It is important to remember that the DENV-3 was first detected in Manaus from a patient coming from Salvador-Bahia (Figueiredo et al., 2003).The analysis of the region the C/prM of the DENV-3 in this study belonged to genotype III strains. All DENV-3 isolated in the Amazon were very close to the Indian strain GWL-60 (N°acessoAY770512) and the Brazilian strain BR-74 886 (N access AY679147). Subtype III is related to outbreaks of DHF in India (Dash et al., 2006). In Brazil, the prevalence of DENV-3 two years after its introduction in 2000 was associated with major epidemics in terms of more severe clinical manifestations, and the number of deaths (Nogueira et al., 2005). Twenty-two isolates were classified as DENV-3 subtype III (Miagostovich et al., 2002). The similarity of these strains to other represented by the same genotype III ranged from 96% to 98% and 98-99% for sequences nucleotides and amino acids, respectively. These data demonstrate that this virus is circulating around the world, again indicating high potential for distribution, adaptation in in various geographic areas of the world. This subtype has been implicated in outbreaks of DHF in Asia, Africa and the Americas, and has high potential to cause a pandemic of dengue (Messer et al., 2003).

4. Conclusions

The emergence of dengue virus in Manaus follows the same pattern as to what occurs in other Brazilian cities. Every two to three years there are new outbreaks of dengue and the emergence of new serotypes followed by cases of dengue hemorrhagic. The emergence of DENV-4 in 2008 did not just caused a major epidemic with severe and fatal cases. Other serotypes were also observed. It is possible due to   competition between with other serotypes, DENV-4 took some time to become established and the population might have been protected by antibodies obtained in heterologous infections by heterologous serotypes. The viral strain should be studied in detail since it is an Asian genotype that has been associated with DHF in the Asian continent.

- In relation to the DENV-2 which appears in 2011 with very high frequency, Manaus already has the DENV-2 genotype II for some time and often associated with cases of hemorrhagic dengue fever in other regions.
- Another important point is the co-infections with DENV-3 and DENV-4 in patients with DF. Most of them are associated with mild DF.
- Considering the large number of samples negative for dengue fever in our study, and to take into account the occurrence of other viruses, clinically similar to dengue fever, and the possibilities available to new viruses emerging or reemerging as Manaus is surrounded by the Amazon rainforest and also a large urban center that welcomes visitors from around the world, other viruses need to be investigated.

5. Recognition

Laboratory of Virology at the Foundation for Tropical Medicine Dr. Hector Vieira Gold (FMT/HVD); Dr. RajendranathRamasawmy for review of the manuscript; ConselhoNacional de DesenvolvimentoCientífico e Tecnológico (CNPq) for financial support.

6. References

Araújo et al. Concurrent infection with dengue virus type-2 and DENV-3 in apatient from Ceará, Brazil.*MemInstOswaldo Cruz*, Rio de Janeiro, 2006. 101(8): 925-928.

Burke DS, Nisalak A, Johnson De, Scott RM, 1988. A prospective study of dengue infections in Bangkok.Am J TropMed Hyg, 1988,38:172– 180.

Castro, M.G.; Nogueira, R.M.; Schatzmayr, H.G.; Miagostovich, M.P.; Lourenco-De-Oliveira, R. Dengue vírus detection by using reverse transcriptionpolymerase chain reaction in saliva and progeny of experimentally infected *Aedesalbopictus* from Brazil. *MemInstOswaldo Cruz*, 2004.99: 809-814.

Cunha, R.V. & Nogueira, R.M. Dengue E Dengue Hemorrágico. In: *Dinâmica das doençasInfecciosas e Parasitarias*, 2005. p.1767-1781.

Dash, P.K. et al. Reemergence of dengue vírus type-3 (subtype-III) in Índia.Implications for increased incidence of DHF & DSS.*Virology Journal*, 2006.

De Melo FL, Romano CM, De Andrade Zanotto PM. Introduction of Dengue virus 4 (DENV-4) genotype I in Brazil from Asia?PLoSNeglTrop Dis. 2009; 3(4):390.

Dias, M.; Zagne, S.M.O.; Pacheco, M.; Stavola, M.S.; Costa, A.J.L. Dengue hemorrágicoemNiterói.*Revista da SociedadeBrasileira de Medicina Tropical*, 1991. 24 (2): 122.

Figueiredo, R.M.P.; Bastos, M.S.; Lima, M.L.; Almeida, T.C.; Alecrim, W.D. Dinâmica da sorologia e isolamento viral na epidemia de dengue em Manaus (1998-2001). In:

Resumos do XXXVIII Congresso da Sociedade Brasileira de Medicina Tropical, 2002.

Figueiredo, R.M.P; Silva, M.N.R.; Almeida, T.C.; Lopes, H.C.; Bastos, M.S. Diagnóstico virológico de dengue em pacientes com quadro febril não diferenciado. In: Resumos do XXXIX Congresso da Sociedade Brasileira de Medicina Tropical, 2003.

Figueiredo, R.M.P.; Thatcher, B.D.; Lima, M.L.; Almeida, T.C.; Alecrim, W.D.; Guerra, M.V.F. Doençasexantemáticas e primeiraepidemia de dengue ocorridaem Manaus, Amazonas no período de 1998 -1999. *Revista da SociedadeBrasileira de Medicina Tropical,*2004.37: 476-479.

Figueiredo RMP. Caracterização molecular e epidemiológica dos vírus dengue no Estado do Amazonas, Brasil. Tese – Universidade Federal do Amazonas-UFAM, Manaus-Amazonas, 2008.

Figueiredo RM, Naveca FG, Bastos SM, Melo MN,Viana SS, Mourão MP, Costa Ca,Farias IP. Dengue virus type 4, Manaus, Brazil. Emerg Infect Dis. 2008; 14: 667–669.

Gubler, D.J.; Kuno, G.; Sather, G. E. & Waterman, S.H. A case of natural concurrent human infection with two dengue viruses. Amer. J. trop. Med. Hyg., 34: 170-173, 1985.

Guzmán, M.G.; Garcia, G.; Kouri, G. El dengue y el dengue hemorragico: prioridades de investigacion. *Rev PanamSaludPublica*. 2006. 19(3): 204-215.

Hahn, C.S.; Lustig, S.; Strauss, E.G. and Strauss, J.H. Western equine encephalitis virus is a recombination virus. *Proc. Natl. Acad. Sci.* USA, 1998. 85: 5997-6001.

Hammon WM. Dengue hemorrhagic fever - do we know its cause? Am J Trop Med Hyg, 1973, 22: 82–91.

Holmes, E.C.;Bartley, L.M.; Garnet, G.P. The emergence of dengue past, present and future. In: KRAUSE, R. M. Emerging infectors, London: Academic Press, 1998. p. 301-25.

Igarashi, A. Isolation of SinghsAedesalbopictus cell clone sensitive to dengue andchikungunya viruses.*Journal of General Virology*, 1978. 40: 531-544.

Joshi, V.; Sharma, R.C.; Sharma, Y.; Adha, S.; Sharma, K.; Singh, H.; Purohit, A.; Singhi, M. Importance of socioeconomic status and tree holes i distribution of *Aedes* mosquitoes (Diptera:Culicidae) in Jodhpur, Rajasthan, India. *J. Med Entomol, 2006*. 43: 330-336.

Kimura, R.; Hotta, S.On the inoculation of dengue virus into mice.Nippon Igakka, 1994.bp.629-633.

Kourí, G.P.; Guzman, M.G; Bravo, J. Dengue hemorrágicoem Cuba.Crônica de umaepidemia.*Boletin de la Oficina Sanitaria Panamericana*, 1986.100: 322- 329.

Kuno, G.; Gomez, I.; Gubler, D.J. Detecting artificial antidengueIgM immune complexes using an enzyme-linked immunosorbent assay.*American Journal of Tropical Medicine andHygiene*, 1987.36: 153-159.

Kuno, G. Factors Influencing The Transmission Of Dengue Viruses.Pp. 61-88 In D.J. Gubler And G. Kuno, Eds. Dengue And Dengue Hemorrhagic Fever. CAB International, Wallingford, U.K, 1997.

Lai, M.M.C. Rna recombination in animal and plant virases.*Microbiol. Rev.,*1992. 56: 61-79.

Lanciotti, R.S.; Lewis, J.G.; Gubler, D.J.; Trent, D.W. Molecular evolution and epidemiology of dengue 3 viruses.*J Gen Virol*, 1994. 75: 65-75.

Lorono PM, Cropp CB, Farfan AJ, Vorndam AV, Rodriguez-Ângulo EM, Rosado-Paredes Ep, Flores-Flores Lf, Beaty Bj, And Gubler DJ. Common occurrence of concurrent infections by multiple dengue virus serotypes. American Journal Tropical Medicine and Hygiene, 61(5), 1999, pp. 725–730.

Martinez-Torres, M.E. Dengue hemorrágicoemcrianças: editorial. Havana: 1990. p.180.

Messer, WB, Gubler, D.J.; Harris, E.; Sivananthan K.; De Silva Am; Emergence and global spread of a dengue serotype 3, subtype III virus. Emerg Infect Dis, 2003. 9: 800-9.

Meyers, R.M. & Carey, D.E. Concurrent isolation from patient of two arboviruses,chikungunya and dengue type 2. Science, 1967. 157: 1307-1308.

Miagostovich et al. Genetic characterization of dengue vírus type 3 isolates in the State of Rio de Janeiro, 2001. Brazillian Journal of Medical and Biological Research, 2002. 35:869-872.

Nogueira, R.M.; Schatzma,Y.R.H.G.; Filippis, A.M.B.; Santos, F.V.; Cunha, R.V.; Coelho, J.O.; Souza, L.J.; Guimarães, F.R.; Araújo, E.S.M.; De Simone, T.S.; Baran, M.; Teixeira, G.; Miagostovich, M.P. Dengue virus type 3, Brazil, 2002. Emerg Infect Dis, 2005. 11: 1376-1381.

Osanai, C.H. Aepidemia de Dengue em Boa Vista, território Federal de Roraima, 1981-1982. Dissertaçao – Escola Nacional de SaúdePública, Rio de Janeiro, 1984.

Pan American Health Organization. Dengue and Dengue Haemorragic fever in the Americas: Guidelines for prevention and control. Washington: 1994.

Portal Amazon Zona Franca de Manaus Disponível no site www.manausonline.com.

Rico - Hesse, R. Molecular evolution and distribution of dengue viruses type 1 and 2 in nature. Virology, 1990. 174: 479-493.

Rico-Hesse, R. Microevolution and virulence of dengue viruses.AdvVir Res, 2003.59: 315-341.

Santos, C.L.S.; Bastos, M.A.A.; Sallum, M.A.M. & Rocco, I.M. Molecular characterization of dengue virases type 1 and 2 isolated from a concurrent human infection. Rev. Inst. Med. Trop. S. Paulo, 2003.45 (1): 11-16.

Terzian ACB, Mondini A, Bronzoni RVM, Drumond BP, Ferro BP ,Cabrera Sem, Figueiredo LTM, Chiaravalloti-Neto F, Nogueira ML . Detection of Saint Louis Encephalitis Virus in Dengue-Suspected Cases During a Dengue 3 Outbreak.Vector Borne and Zoonotic Diseases, 2010. Doi:10.1089/vbz.2009.0200.

Viverde Tourism -Informações cientificas da Amazônia. Disponível no site www.viverde.com.br

Zagne, S.M.O. et al. Dengue Haemorragic fever in the state of Rio de Janeiro, Brazil: a study 113 of 56 confirmed cases. Transactions of the Royal Society of Tropical Medicine and Hygiene, 1994.88: 677-679.

Weaver, S.C.; Barret, A.D.T. Transmission cycles, host range, evolution and emergence of arboviraldisease.Nat Rev Microbiol., 2004. 2: 789-801.

Wenming, P.; Man, Y.; Baochang, F.; Yongqiang, D.; Tao, J.; Hongyuan, D. Simultaneous infection with dengue 2 and 3 viruses in a Chinese patient return from Sri Lanka. JClinVirol, 2005. 32: 194-198.

World Health Organization.Dengue Haemorrhagic Fever: Diagnosis, Treatment, Prevention
    and Control, 2 nd ed., Geneva: WHO, 1997.

2

Genetic Diversity of Dengue Virus and Associated Clinical Severity During Periodic Epidemics in South East Asia

E. Khan, R. Hasan, J. Mehraj and S. Mahmood
Department of Pathology and Microbilogy
Aga Khan University, Stadium Road, Karachi
Pakistan

1. Introduction

The geographic distribution and genetic diversity of dengue virus is deeply rooted in Asia suggesting its origin from this region, with first reported out-break of DHF from Philippine in 1953 (Halstead, 1980). One of the characteristics notable in Asian regions, where the disease is endemic is that dengue hemorrhagic fever outbreaks occur in repetitive cycles of 3-5 years, (Ferguson et al, 1999). The incidence of disease and its severity varies across different dengue virus serotypes and also between primary and secondary infections of same serotypes(Vaughn DW et al).

Due to lack of in-vivo study models, there is little information about factors contributing to disease severity and its variation across dengue virus genotypes and the cyclical nature of dengue outbreaks. It is however critical to study these factors particularly in the South East Asian region where incidence of dengue cases is thought to be associated with variables such as water, sanitation, population density and rate of literacy as opposed to developed countries where ambient temperature, moisture and rainfall perhaps plays the major role. A better understanding of disease epidemiology and pathogenesis will help identify optimum control measures in the region. It will also develop systems for predicting the outcome of mass vaccination when the vaccine becomes available in this region.

The chapter has been divided in three parts: the first part will discuss the historical evolution of the dengue virus in the region its spatial and temporal distribution. It will also look at the effects of covariates such as poverty, water supply, sanitation and global warming on expansion of the dengue endemic regions. .

The second part of the chapter will focus on the genetic evolution of the viral isolates circulating in the region. Phylogenetic studies of dengue viruses have uncovered genetic variation within each serotypes, these variations have been organized in discrete clusters on dendograms. Analyses of such studies have broadened our horizon to relate the mutational changes with disease evolution and factors like seasonality and incidence variability. This part of chapter will focus on the common mutational variations that have been reported so far and how these relate with the disease dynamics in the endemic region.

In the third and final part of the chapter an attempt has been made to relate the mutational changes of dengue genotypes with disease severity. Vast array of literature has been published investigating relationship of genetic variation with disease severity. The structure of virus E- protein that confers the viral infectivity and host immune response of the virus (E.Descloux,2009) remains the focus of such studies. Sequence variation at different loci such as CprM, E/NS1, preM/E, C/prM/M and untranslated regions etc. have been investigated for its association with disease severity. This part of chapter will throw some light on our current understanding of disease severity and it relation with genetic variation.

2. Historical background of dengue virus in South East Asian

Geographically South East Asia comprises of land south of China to east of India extending as far as to the north of Australia. Although geographically the region is well defined, the list of countries included in this region varies due to political reasons. For the purpose of this review W.H.O based definition has been used. In addition status of dengue virus in further south of the region; including countries like Pakistan and Bangladesh have also been included to encompass the broader spectrum of the region.

2.1 Dengue vector evolution

Evidences suggest that vectors *Ades aegypti* and *Ades albopictus* originated from darker sylvan forms found in African tropical forests. It is believed to have reached New World from West Africa via slave ships during the 17th century (Gubler, D.J.1998). *Adesaegypti* was introduced into the coastal cities of South East Asia from East Africa around nineteenth century via the shipping industry. With the eruption of World War II it became deeply entrenched in many cities (Gubler, D.J.1998). The mitochondrial genetic diversity studies have revealed circulation of two distinct clusters of *Ades aegypti* in South East Asia one with strains from French Polynesia, Guinea and Brazil while the other cluster is of strains that migrated from Europa Island in Mozambique and Amazonia (Mousson et al 2005). In contrast; *A. albopictus* is known to be native to South East Asia. It has spread within past few decades to various countries primarily due to introduction of trade of used tyres worldwide. Using ecological niche modeling Benedict and co-workers have predicted the risk of global invasion by *Ades albopitus* secondary to cargo trade and increasing air travel. Although temperate and humid climates are prerequisites for the optimum survival of both the vectors but *A. albopictus* is known to better acclimatize to the cold and dry weather due to its ability of efficient egg diapause during the extreme conditions, thus favoring its survival in the regions with exotic temperature ranges (Benedict, M.Q, *et al* 2007).

2.2 Factors leading to disease spread in SEA

The factors responsible for the insurmountable expansions of dengue in the region are complex and thought to be intricately linked with vector-host-virus triad, socioeconomic stresses and climatic variations. There are excellent reviews that discuss the impact of these factors in details (Aiken, S.R. 1978, Kendall, C. et al 1991, Halstead, S.B. 1966). Only salient factors in context of SEA will be discussed here. The distribution of DHF outbreaks in SEA correlates with emergence of mosquito A. aegypti in South East Asian countries perhaps due to displacement of indigenous A. albpictus in the region. This is considered to be associated with uncontrolled urbanization leading to shanty towns with inadequate pipe water supply and poor sanitation.

A. *albopictus* is semi domestic species that breeds on natural and man-made breeding sights; it feeds on variety of animals, birds and man. The A. aegypti on the other hand is more acclimatized to urban set-up, once established the density of this mosquito is directly proportional to density of human population and artificial breeding sites (Merril S.A *et al* 2005), it feeds almost exclusively on humans. Moreover A. aegypti is considered to be more competent vector for dengue virus. Genetic traits that determines successful midgut infection by DEN virus have been mapped on several loci on A. aegypti chromosomes (Benedict, M.Q, *et al* 2007) indicating that vector competence is genetically determined.

The extent to which these mosquitoes compete with each other in the environment is not clear, nonetheless the balance of two species in the region is important, and the socioeconomic factors in SEA appear to be displacing *A.albopictus* in favour of *A.aegypti* leaving the population more susceptible. The poor socioeconomic conditions are major contributing factor to sustained vector activity with severe form of disease in the South East Asia. The breeding habitats of A.aegypti have been strongly associated with squatter settlements, inadequate piped water supply and sewage facilities (Halstead, S.B. 1966). In addition, there are impacts of higher environmental temperature in the region. High temperature is inversely related to the mosquito gonotropic cycle and viral extrinsic incubation period; this increases the egg laying episodes resulting in more blood meals and increased risk for viral transmission. In addition shorten extrinsic viral incubation period culminate to increase virus load at time of inoculation (Focks D.A. et al 1993). These effects have been proven for dengue vectors in simulation studies conducted by (Cox J et al 2001) and it has been projected that increase in global temperature would increase the length of transmission season in temperate regions.

2.3 Dengue fever and dengue hemorrhagic fever

The word dengue is believed to have originated from Swahili language "*ki denga pepo*", which describes sudden cramp like seizure. The clinical symptoms suggestive of dengue virus infection can be traced back to Chinese Chin Dynasty (265-420 AD) where disease was considered as water poison and was known to be associated with water and insects (anonymous 2006).

Emergence of the disease in the new world can be traced back to the transmigration of the vector in the 17th century. There are reports that suggest possible epidemics of dengue like illness in three major continents (Asia, Africa and North America) as early as 1779 and 1780, within Asia Batavia (now known as Jakarta) was affected by this outbreak (Halstead,S.B. 1966). By early nineteenth century Dengue fever was known to be endemic in the rural areas of South East Asia probably due to the indigenous vector *A.albopictus*. It manifested as self limiting disease to which native population developed immunity at early age. With the advent of *A. aegypti* at Asian ports, the disease spread to the main inland cities and towns. It is assumed that unlike rural population, the urban populations of South East Asia remained susceptible to dengue virus and were then infected by newly imported vector. Dengue epidemics progressively became less frequent as urban population became immune to the disease, until 1953 when a new form of dengue fever was reported from Thailand and Manila, where children suffered from fever followed by bleeding diathesis; the disease was then called as *Philippine Fever* (Aiken, S.R. 1978). By 1960's the hemorrhagic form of disease had spread to Malaysia, Vietnam, Sri Lanka, Singapore and Indonesia (Halstead, S.B. 1966). The disease epidemiology extended and outbreaks of dengue hemorrhagic fever (DHF) were reported from India 1988) French Polynesia (1990), Pakistan (1992) and Bangladesh (2000).Until recently, DHF was considered to be disease of childhood, especially in South

East Asia where mean age of cases under fifteen, and the modal age of five or slightly higher was reported from countries such as Thailand, Philippines and Malaysia, however, recent reports are now documenting increasing number of DHF and DSS in adult population as well (Khan E et al 2007). The precise cause of DHF/DSS remains elusive despite enormous research in this area. Evidences suggest interplay of multiple factors such as host genetic make-up with unique immune response and viral virulence may play a role in determining the severity of the disease.

2.4 Pathogenesis of severe dengue disease

There are two form of Severe disease, namely dengue shock syndrome (DSS) and DHF without shock. It is proposed that devastating coagulation derangements due to host immune response leads to heamorrhage and shock in severe cases. The concept of original antibody sin leading to immune enhancement is considered to be the main reason whereby infection with one type of dengue virus sensitizes an individual and that subsequent infection with different virus type elicits a hypersensitivity reaction (secondary infection). Various studies have been conducted to show the association of elevated cytokines in patients presenting with DHF and DSS. Elevated serum levels of cytokine and chemokines such as IL-2, IL-8, IL-6, IL-10, IL-13, TNF and INF-γ have been found to be significantly associated with patients presenting with DHF and DSS in clinical setting (Azeredo et al., 2001; Hung, et al., 2004, Clyde. K. et al., 2006). It has been proposed that the pro-inflammatory cytokines released by the cross reactive memory T-cellls, induce plasma leakage by its effects on the endothelial cells (Eva.H. et al 2004; Aviruntanan et al., 1998). In fact in-vitro studies have rendered endothelial cell monolayers permeable by the application of chemokine such as IL-1β (Cardier et al.,2005). In vitro-and in-vivo models of studies also suggest role of decreased nitric oxide levels and its relation with IL-10 and raised viral load (Simmons et al., 2007). There is evidence that suggests relation of increased expression of certain cytokines such as IL-1β, TNF-γ, and IL-6 with elevated NO production (Guzik et al., 2003).

With the advances in genomic and bioinformatics tools the scope of genetic studies has greatly expanded particularly in depth data on genomic changes and its association with disease epidemiology, seasonality and severity has been made available. Growing availability of comparative genome sequence data has provided important insights into the molecular evolution of dengue virus. Evidence strongly suggests appearance of new strains correlating with DHF/DSS epidemics. Despite the wealth of genomic data now available the exact cause and effect of viral virulence and clade changes is yet to be proven, however it is quite evident that different serotypes and viral linage is continually changing with local extinction and emergence of new clade and that the introduction of new clade in the region translates in form of outbreaks of DHF and DSS.

3. Distribution of dengue virus serotypes in SEA

Dengue like other RNA viruses is prone to genetic mutations as it replicates using RNA-Polymerase; enzyme that lacks proof reading mechanism. The mutation rates in the order of 10^{-3} has been reported for dengue (ElodieDes et al 2009) in different host settings. Such mutations often result in variants that become targets of selection; an outcome of underlying genotype and its environment. Despite these facts dengue virus do not evolve as fast as other RNA viruses. The only **macro evolutionary** divergence is perhaps the radiations in its four serotypes in its primate host (sylvatic strains) around one thousand years ago (ElodieDes et al 2009). There after genetic mutation in the envelope protein and receptor binding domains resulted in its emergence as infectious pathogen in human population. The divergent forms of these sylvatic strains are often found to be circulating in human habitat, suggesting that enzootic cycles with some spill over in the surrounding human population. This has been shown in Malaysian populations settled near forest and marshy habitats (Wang, E. et al., 2000). The phylogenetic studies conducted based on envelope gene sequences of basal portion of sylvatic linage, DENV 1,-2,-4 of Malaysian descent suggest that endemic /epidemic strains of these viruses diverged from sylvatic ancestors more than 1000 years ago (Wang, E. et al., 2000). Thereafter, only micro evolutionary change within dengue serotypes have taken place, these changes have nevertheless resulted in substantial genetic diversity with emergence of endemic and epidemic strains in different parts of the region.

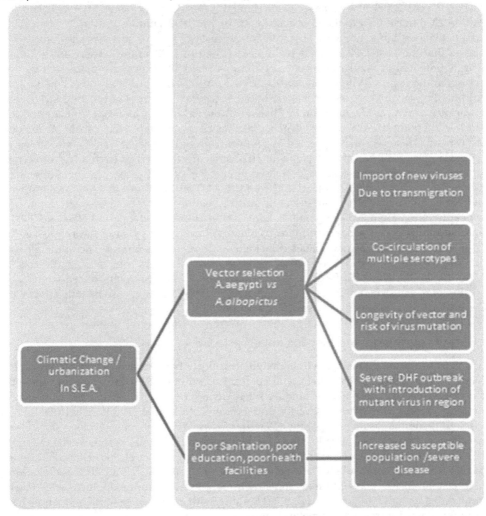

Fig. 1. The effects of climatic and social change on vector evolution and disease severity

DEN-3 viruses have undergone independent evolution which has resulted in emergence of four genetic subtypes of which subtype I-III circulate in the South East Asian Region. Subtype I comprises of viruses from Indonesia, Malaysia and the Philippines; subtype II of viruses from Thailand and subtype III includes viruses from Sri Lanka India and Pakistan. The genetic evolution in these subtypes is primarily reported mutations in the prM/M and E structural protein genes. In spite of these mutations, the genomic region has retained greater than 95% amino acid sequence similarity (Lanciotti, R.S et al.,1994), suggesting that these are highly conserved regions responsible for protein architecture and / or biological function.

Phylogenetic studies suggest that there are regional foci of virus extinction and selection, one such region is Thailand where the indigenous DEN-3 virus circulating up to 1992 disappeared and was replaced by two new lineages perhaps from a common ancestor (Wittke, V. et al. 2002). The sequence of all Thai DEN-3 isolates recovered after 1992 had T at position 2370 in contrast to the C at this site in the pre-1992 samples(Wittke, V. et al. 2002), and nucleotides difference was observed in at least 45 sites of total 96 sites studied. It appears that the post-1992 strains have replaced the pre-1992 strains). These studies point towards potential of regular extinctions of strains of DEN-3 virus and replacement by new variants in the region (Wittke, V. et al. 2002). Natural selection and / or genetic bottle neck could be the plausible causes for this variation. Since the extinction of pre 1992 strains and appearance of new epidemic strain in Thailand occurred during inter-epidemic period it is therefore hypothesized that the genetic bottleneck is perhaps the cause of regional replacement. This is further supported by studies from India reporting shift and dominance of the dengue virus serotype-3 (subtype III) replacing the earlier circulating serotype-2 (subtype IV) with emergence of increased incidence of DHF and DSS in subsequent outbreaks (Dash, P.K.et al. 2006). Strains from the 2005 outbreak in Karachi (Pakistan) were found to be similar to those from Indian strains of dengue serotype 3, and were responsible for deadly outbreak in 2005-06 (Jamil. B. et al. 2007). Thus over the period 1989 and 2000, a new clades of DENV-3 genotype III viruses have replaced older genotype and clades in this region and emergence of new clades coincided with severe epidemics. The epidemiologic data suggests that the DEN-3 virus responsible for recent epidemic outbreaks in Mozambiques, Gutamealla, Pakistan and SriLanka may have been introduced from India, and changing age structure of dengue patients from 1996–2005 may also be indicative of the selected virus moving into new areas(Kanakaratne, N. et al.2009).

4. Genetic evolution and disease severity in SEA

The micro evolutionary change within dengue serotypes has resulted in substantial genetic diversity with emergence of endemic and epidemic genotypes. With current advances in the field of genetic and molecular techniques scientists are now trying to decipher relation of changing clades with disease severity and epidemic potential. With the availability of complete genomic sequence of the Dengue virus different genetic loci have been investigated to find this relationship. Envelope –gene (E-gene) sequence is the most frequently investigated locus, (Wittke,V.et al., 2002;-Thu, H.M. et al.,2004;Islam, M.A.et al., 2006,27) followed by capsuler C-prM gene (Kukreti, H. 2008;,Dash, P.K. 2006;,Kanakaratne, N. 2009;Jamil B,2007). In addition non-structural (NS) viral proteins such as NS1 and untranslated genomic region 3'-UTR, 5' UTR along with complete genomic sequences have been investigated to relate the genetic changes with the disease severity (Mangada, M.N. et al., 1997;Zhou,Y.et al.,2006;Islam, M.A.et al.,2006. Despite the wealth of genomic data available the exact cause and effect of viral virulence and clade changes is yet to be proven, however, viral linage is continually changing with local extinction and emergence of new clade. The introduction of new clade in the region translates in form of outbreaks of DHF and DSS. In order to analyze if there is a selection of specific clade in South East Asia that is circulating in the region and causing DHF outbreaks we conducted a meta-analysis. Studies conducted from 1950 to 2009 in South East Asian region that have investigated association of disease severity with specific sequence mutations in the dengue virus genome were retrieved. The objective was to analyze association of disease severity with the specific genomic mutation in the clade circulating and causing periodic epidemics in South East Asia. Since DENV-2 and DENV-3 are more common in this region our study was focused on these two genotypes only. Objectives of the metaanalysis were to identify association of specific genetic mutation in DENV-2 and DENV-3 with clinical severity seen during periodic epidemics in South East Asia. The specific review question was:Is clinical severity of dengue in the South East Asian region associated with emergence of specific mutations in genomes of DENV-2 and DENV-3 genotypes? We hypothesized that there is changing pattern of dengue virus genotypes in South East Asia and these mutations are associated with clinical severity of the disease.

4.1 Methods
4.1.1 Literature search
The literature search was performed from February 2010 to June 2010. Data sources include Medline via Pubmed (1950-February 2010), Cochrane data base of systematic reviews, Google scholar and experts in the field. Secondary references and review articles were scanned for thematic review. Hand search of the journal was also carried out. However, unpublished and ongoing studies could not be explored. Terminologies i.e. dengue type 1-4,

Author's name	Why excluded?
Araujo J.M.G. *et al,* (2009)	Conducted in Brazil, (also include dengue strains from regions other than South east Asia) but country of origin of these isolates was not clear, Sequences were selected from gene bank.
Lanciotti RS.*et al,* (1994)	Conducted in USA, origin of isolates not clear (also include dengue strains from other geographical regions other than South east Asia) The DEN-3 viruses used in this study were obtained from the collection at the Division of Vector-Borne Infectious Diseases, Centers for Disease Control and Prevention, Fort Collins, Colo., U.S.A.
Soundravally R, *et al* (2007)	Focused on host factors as cause of disease severity rather than on virus gene mutations
Soundravally R., *et al* (2008 a)	Focused on host factors as cause of disease severity rather than on virus gene mutations
Soundravally R., *et al,* (2008b)	Focused on host factors as cause of disease severity rather than on virus gene mutations
Gibbons RV. *et al,* (2007)	Does not give sequence analysis in detail

Table 1. Features of the excluded studies

dengue fever, dengue hemorrhagic fever, genetic variation, sequence analysis, south East Asia were used individually as well as in various combinations. Two independent reviewers; reviewed the titles, abstracts and full text articles and selected potentially relevant studies based on inclusion criteria established prior to the literature search. Discrepancy between the reviewers were sought to reach on consensus in consultation with third reviewer. Those potentially irrelevant studies that were ultimately excluded are listed together with the reason for exclusion in Table 1.

4.1.2 Inclusion criteria
Studies which reported dengue virus genotype (mutation / sequencing of viral genetic material) and clinical features of dengue fever patients were included.

4.1.3 Design of the studies
All type of observational studies i.e. case report, case series, surveys and descriptive cross-sectional studies which were focusing on genotype and clinical presentation of dengue patients were included in the review. *Population:* Population includes patients of dengue fever of all age groups. No age and sex restriction were applied. *Outcome of interest:* Difference in nucleotide and protein sequences were analyzed and compared according to geographical origin, the sampling period and the clinical presentation. Clinical severity of the disease is defined as presence of DF, DHF or DSS. *Language:* Only articles in English language were included in the review.

4.1.4 Exclusion criteria
All those studies focusing on dengue vector control, clinical trials on vaccines, clinical trials on drugs, pure prevalence or incidence, unusual case report or case series without genotype and studies conducted in countries other than south East Asian region were excluded.

4.1.5 Data extraction
Data extraction of the included studies was done by using structured data extraction form specifically made for the review. Data was extracted for country of origin, year of publication, clarification of objectives, type of study, its duration and setting, results on both genotype and clinical severity etc.

4.1.6 Data synthesis
A narrative data synthesis was carried out to show result summary of all included studies which include description of clinical features and genotype of dengue virus. However, meta-analysis could not be performed due to non availability of required data i.e. measure of strength of association. Hence, pooled effect of genetic variation on clinical severities among dengue patients could not be provided.

4.1.7 Quality assessment
According to Cochrane Collaboration's recommendation, the quality of included studies have been assessed by using criterion which asses the quality of studies by focusing on study type, sample size calculation, clarity of objective, selection of cases, and internal validity of selected studies.

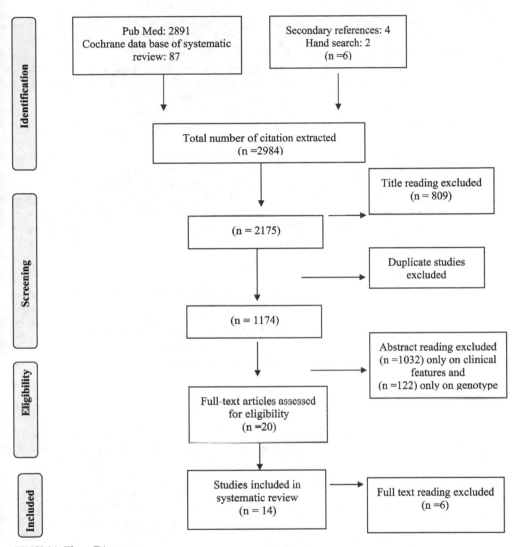

PRISMA Flow Diagram

Fourteen studies were finally selected based on inclusion criteria i.e., association of dengue genotype and clinical severity of the diseases in the patients and were conducted in different countries of South East Asia. Setting of these studies were; Thailand 6 (Zhang, C. et al 2006, Rico-Hesse R. et al. 1998, Wittke,V.et al.,2002), Myanmar (Thu H.M. et al.,2004), India (Kukreti, H. et al.,2008;Dash, P.K.et al.,2006), Bangladesh (Islam, M.A.et al.,2006), Sri Lanka (Kanakaratne, N. et al.,2009), Taiwan (King, C.C. et al.,2008) and Pakistan (Jamil B, et al 2007). These studies were published from 1997 to 2009. Since the focus of our study was on DEN-2 and DEN3 viruses 12 studies out of these 14 were finally included in this study

4.1.8 Study sample characteristics

Eight studies were conducted in the hospital settings (Zhang, C. et al 2006, Rico-Hesse R. et al. 1998, Wittke,V.et al.,2002, Kukreti, H. et al.,2008;Dash, P.K.et al.,2006, Islam, M.A.et al.,2006, al,Kanakaratne, N. et al.,2009), three in the community (Zhou Y, et al 2006, Dash PK, et al 2006, Kanakaratne, N. et al.,2009), where as data was extracted from laboratory records in two studies (Jamil B, et al, 2007, King, C.C. et al.,2008) and dengue virus strain were taken from frozen stock of clinical serum samples in two (18, 21).

Age ranges for dengue patients in these studies varied from 1 year to 70 years. The total numbers of dengue patients were 7663 in these studies. Characteristics of the studies included in this review have been summarized in table 2. A total of 285 virus isolates were subjected to genotyping/ sequence analysis in these studies. All four genotypes were studied in three studies (Zhou Y, et al 2006,Jarman RG, et al 2008, Rico-Hesse R. et al. 1998); only DEN 3 in five studies (Wittke,V.et al.,2002, Kukreti, H. et al.,2008; Islam, M.A.et al.,2006), only DEN 2 in three studies (Zhou Y, et al 2006,Mangada MNM et al 1997, Zhang, C. et al 2006), only DEN 4 in one studies (KlungthongC, et al, 2004), whereas DEN 1 and DEN 3 in one study (Kukerti H, et al 2008) and DEN 1, DEN 2 and DEN 3 studied in one study (Jarman RG et al 2008).

4.1.9 Clinical definition

Dengue case was defined on the bases of presence of IgM, IgG, or fourfold or greater rise in hemagglutination inhibiting (HI) antibody titer against dengue virus, and presence of dengue virus specific nucleic acids in RT-PCR. Clinical severity was defined as presence of hemorrhagic manifestation and DHF related symptoms such as thrombocytopenia, skin rash, gum bleeding, gastrointestinal bleeding, hemorrhagic sclera, epistaxis, edema and ascitis. Where as other studies simply defined as presence of DF, DHF grade I, II and III and DSS as per WHO criteria.

5. Nucleotide sequencing and phylogenetic analysis

Envelope –gene (E-gene) sequence was most frequently investigated loci, nine studies were focused on this region followed by C-prM gene, in three studies both genetic loci studied in one study (9) and one study included NS1 along with PrM and E loci. The 3'-UTR, 5' and 3' UTR and complete genomic sequences were studied in one each

Homology search and comparisons of most obtained sequences were performed using commercially available software systems such as DNASIS, DNAStar, 3' –UTR secondary structures were estimated using MFOLD package, while nucleotide sequence alignments (Phylogenetic analysis) were performed using CLUSTAL X, MEGA version, and maximum likely hood methods available e.g. PAUP PROGRM

The quality of included studies was assessed by using criterion which asses the quality of studies by focusing on study type, sample size calculation, clarity of objective, selection of cases, and internal validity of selected studies. From total of 16 points scale, individual score on quality assessment criteria was as follows 8.5 (Rico-Hesse R. et al. 1998), 7.0 (Zhou Y, et al 2006,Jarman RG, et al 2008, Jamil B, et al, 2007), 10.5 (Dash PK, et al 2006, Kukreti, H. et al.,2008), 5.0 (Wittke,V.et al.,2002), 6.5 (Zhang, C. et al 2006,), 10 (Zhou Y, et al 2006, Mangada MNM et al 1997), 7.5 (Wittke,V.et al.,2002, Jarman RG, et al 2008, King, C.C. et al.,2008), 12(KlungthongC, et al, 2004). Since most of the severe DHF outbreaks in SEA have been associated with DEN-2 and DEN-3, mutational changes and its relation to disease severity of these two serotypes will be discussed here in detail.

5.1 Mutations observed
5.1.1 E-gene mutations
In case of DEN-2 virus, maximum numbers of viral isolates have been analyzed in studies from Thailand. The E-NS1 region of 77 different variants of DEN-2 studied using Maximum Parsimony analysis of 240 nucleotide sequence, showed 11 of 240 nucleotide variation; 4.6% divergence but did not reveal significant segregation of virus according to geographic location (Rico-Hesse R. et al. 1998). Similarly, Phylogenetic analysis of 120 E gene of DEN-2 by another group from Thailand has confirmed existence of six genotypes of this virus; however evolutionary relationships among the genotypes is difficult to determine (Zhang, C. et al 2006). In terms of dengue pathogenesis these studies failed to show segregation of DF versus DHF-associated viruses on the evolutionary tree. There are no clear-cut evolutionary divergence or branching of DF versus DHF isolates, suggesting that nucleotides from this region of the genome encode amino acids that are apparently not under immune selection (Rico-Hesse R. et al. 1998 and Zhang, C. et al 2006,).

DEN-3 has replaced DEN-2 as most frequently isolated virus in Thailand since late 1980's (Wittke,V.et al.,2002). The evolutionary history of Thai DEN-3 viruses, has been studied by comparative analysis of the nucleotide sequence of E protein genes of currently prevailing isolates with those from all previously published E gene sequences of DEN-3 virus available in Gen Bank (Wittke,V et al. 200218), this study has shown E-gene of DEN-3 to be relatively conserved at amino acid level, however, four amino acid changes have been identified within genotype II of Thai strains. The amino acid changes observed at positions (E172 I-V) and (E479 A-V) are the only difference found between pre and post-1992 viruses. Similarly, there is little evidence to support in-situ evolution among the virus samples that were studied over prolong period ranging from days to months in a selected community in Thailand(Jarman, R.G.et al.,2008) very few mutational changes were noted, and association of these mutations with disease severity could not be delineated either. Analysis by E-sequence of eight DEN-3 strains from Bangladesh (2002 out-break strains) were found to be very closely related to Thai isolates that caused out-break in 1998 in Thailand. The multiple alignment of amino acid (aa) sequence revealed that Bangladeshi isolates and Thai isolates shared common aa changes at position E127 (I-V), suggesting that 2002 outbreak in Bangladesh was due to introduction of Thai isolates (Islam, M.A.et al.,2006), however the statistical association of aa changes with disease severity could not be delineated. In case of Sri Lankan DEN-3, type III is the most frequent strain with two distinct clades IIIA and IIIB linked to mild and severe disease epidemics on the island respectively (Kanakaratne, N. et al.,2009). Phylogenetic studies of E-NS1 junction of DEN-2 isolates from Sri Lanka has categorized the isolates into 4 genotypes designated as Malaysian/Indian subcontinent, Southeast Asian, American, and West African (Sylvatic) and Sri Lankan isolates are closely related to Indian / Malaysian genotype.

5.2 C-prM mutations
The phylogenetic analysis of 433 base pair region (nucleotides 180−612) of the DEN-3 *CprM* gene junction showed that sequences of Delhi isolates (2006 outbreak) were closely related to sequences from Guatemala (1998) and presented a nucleotide identity of 95.9−98.2% (mean 97.05%). On comparison of Delhi 2006 sequences with other Indian sequences from years 2003, 2004, and 2005, mean sequence divergence of 2.85%, 2.15%, and 1.6%, respectively, were observed (Kukreti, H. et al.,2008. Common amino acid mutations observed in 2006 DENV-3 sequences are given in table 3. Similar study performed on DEN-3 isolates of 2003-04 outbreaks in New Delhi, found them to be closely related and belonged to subtype III from Sri Lanka (Dash, P.K.et al.,2006). Moreover, Phylogenetic analysis of C/PrM/M region of

DEN-3 isolates from Pakistan (2004-05 outbreak isolates) also showed sequence homology with 2003-04 New Delhi outbreak strains suggesting that circulation of common isolates of DEN-3 subtype III in the region . There was no clear statistical association of disease severity

DENV-Protein	Geographical Origin	year	aa change (positions)	Relation to Disease severity	Ref
Envelope (E) Den 3	Thailand	2002	E124 (P-S) E132 (H-T) E172 (I-V) E479 (V-A)	Could not be ascertained	(Rico-Hesse R *et al*)
Envelope (E) Den 3	Thailand	2008	Phylogenetic analysis= multiple genetic variants (mutational positions not mentioned)	Could not be ascertained	(Jarman RG)
DEN 3 E region	Taiwan	2008	E301 (L to T)		(King, C.C. et al.,2008)
Envelope (E) Den 3	Bangladesh	2005/6	E81 (I-T) E140 (I-T) E127 (I-V)	Distinct clade causing epidemic outbreak	(Islam, M.A.et al.,2006)
Den 3 C-preM/E	Srilanka	2003-06	Phylogenetic analysis= multiple genetic variants (mutational positions not mentioned)	2 distinct clades linked to mild (IIIA) and severe (IIIB) disease epidemics	(Kanaka-ratne et al)
CprM Den 3	India	2005/6	CprM88 (I-V) CprM 121(A-A) CprM127 (I-P) CprM122 (G-G) CprM55 (A-L) CprM 128(V-G)	No association of any particular variant with serious dengue disease	(Kukreti H)
C-prM	India	2006	C-prM108(M-I) C-prM112(T-A)	may be attributed to increased incidence of DHF & DSS in India	(Dash PK)
CprM Den 3	Pakistan	2005-2006	C-prM	Similar to New Delhi strain 2004	Jamil B, et al
DEN 3 prM region	Taiwan	2008	CprM 55 (L-H) PrM 57 (T-A)	No association with disease severity could be determined	(King CC)

Table 2. Genetic Characteristics and relation to disease severity in patients with DEN-3 infections reports from South East Asian Region

with specific serotype, as viruses isolated from DHF patients fell at different locations on the phylogenetic tree (Kukreti, H. et al.,2008;Dash, P.K.et al.,2006).

Using maximum likelihood and Bayesian approaches, phylogenetic analysis of Taiwan's indigenous DENV-3 isolated from 1994 and 1998 dengue/DHF epidemics were found to be of three different genotypes –I, II and III each associated with DEN-3 circulating in Indonesia, Thailand and Sri Lanka, respectively(King, C.C. et al.,2008). The authors of this study analyzed complete nucleotide sequence of DEN-3 for its mutation and its relation with regional evolution. The highest level of nucleotide sequence diversity, and the positive selection site was detected at position 178 of the NS1 gene.Although the authors have identified the NS 1 gene as the positive selection site and the envelope protein site for purifying selection pressure, however direct association of these changes with disease severity was not determined. Study from Bangkok Thailand performed sequence analysis on E/NS-1 region of Thai isolates to determine if viral strains from less severe DENV infections had distinct evolutionary nucleotide pattern then those with more severe form (Rico-Hesse R. et al.,1998). This study found that two distinct genotypes were identifiable from both DF and DHF cases, suggesting its evolution from common progenitor that perhaps shares the potential to cause severe disease.

DENV-Protein	Geographical Origin	year	aa change (positions)	Relation to Disease severity	Ref
E/NS1 (77 DEN-2 virus strains studied)	Thailand	1998 from 1980	11 nucleotides (4.6% divergence) between Strain PUO-218-280. 22 nt or 9.2% divergence PUO-218-D80141	No specific association with disease severity	(Klungthong C)
E/NS1 junction Den 2	Srilanka	2003-06	239-nt (from positions 2311–2550)	Could not be ascertained	(Kanaka-ratne et al)
3′ and 5′ UTR Den 2	Thailand	1996-97	5′ NCR homologus 3′ UTR trinucleotide change 297± 299 (two transversions and one transition)	Trinucleotide change may alter the functional characteristic of Secondary structure	(Mangada MNM)
Den 2 E /C/NS2A	Thailand	2006	approx 10^{-3} substitutions	no apparent association	(Zhang C)
3′-UTR	Thailand	1973 to 2003	Variable secondary structures were detected	No clear association	(Zhou Y)

Table 3. Genetic Characteristics and relation to disease severity in patients with DEN-2 infections reports from South East Asian Region

5.3 Untranslated Region (UTR) mutations

The 3' UTR region is thought to play a pivotal role in the DENV biology; it contains several conserved regions as well as 3' long Stable Hair Pin structure which is conserved among all the members of the family *Flaviviridae*. It has been proposed that this structure interacts with viral and host nucleic acid and protein factors to form a complex to regulate transcription and replication (Zhou, Y. et al.,2006. Therefore it appears to play a significant role in the efficiency of RNA- translation, and virus ability to cause infection, hence the role of 3-UTR in determining the severity of dengue disease seems plausible. The literature reviewed under this study did show considerable intra-serotype diversity at 3-UTR region with greatest variability seen in DEN-4 followed by DEN-1.

A comparative analysis of 3' UTR conducted for DENV isolates from Bangkok, Thailand compared Thai sequences with 61 globally sampled isolates of DENV taken from patients with varying disease severity. Although some genetic variations were found both within and among the serotypes notably at 3' Long Hairpin Stable structure, however these mutations did not show consistent association with the clinical outcome of the DENV infection (Zhou, Y. et al.,2006). Study focusing on terminal 3' 5'UTR sequences of four DEN-2 from Thailand 1998 outbreak strains, showed complete homology for sequences at 5' UTR (highly conserved region) when compared with the prototype virus New Guinea C strain

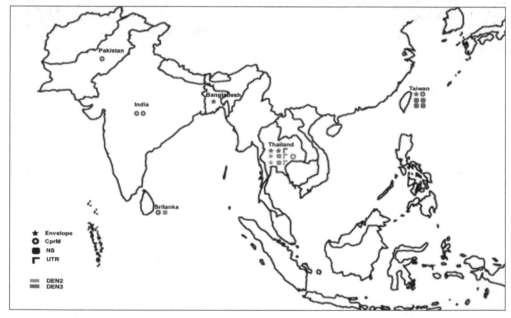

Fig. 2. The Geographical distribution of mutations in DEN-2 and DEN-3 viruses detected at different genomic loci of isolates from South East Asia

6. Conclusion

Ades aegypti was introduced into the coastal cities of South East Asia from East Africa around nineteenth century via the shipping industry. With the eruption of World War II it deeply entrenched in many cities. The distribution of DHF outbreaks in SEA correlates with emergence of mosquito *A. egypti* in South East Asian countries due to uncontrolled urbanization leading to displacement of indigenous *A. albpictus* from the region.

Phylogenetic analysis suggests that there are foci of virus extinction and selection in South East Asian region, one such region is Thailand where the indigenous DEN-3 virus circulating up to 1992 has disappeared and replaced by two new lineages perhaps from a common ancestor. These studies point towards potential of regular extinctions of strains of dengue virus particularly DEN-3 virus and replacement by new variants in the region. Natural selection and / or genetic bottle neck are plausible causes for this variation. Since the extinction of pre 1992 strains and appearance of new epidemic strain in Thailand occurred during inter-epidemic period we therefore hypothesize that the genetic bottleneck is perhaps major cause of regional replacement. This is further supported by studies from India reporting shifting and dominance of the dengue virus serotype-3 (subtype III) replacing the earlier circulating serotype-2 (subtype IV) with emergence of increased incidence of DHF and DSS in subsequent outbreaks. Strains from the 2005 outbreak in Karachi (Pakistan) were found to be similar to those from Indian strains of dengue serotype 3, and were responsible for deadly outbreak in 2005-06.

Despite the growing genomic data base in the gene bank there are fundamental gaps in our understanding of epidemiological and evolutionary dynamics and its relation with disease severity. There are two possibilities that explain the association between clade replacement and increased viral virulence. The first is the possibility of these viruses to be better fit and therefore produce high viremia in infected humans, consequently with better transmission of virus by the vector. The other hypothesis to explain the possible virulence of emerging clades in the region is its improved ability to avoid neutralization by serotypes cross reactive antibodies (Kochel et al., 2005). Thus there is relative abundance of different serotypes and viral linage is continually changing in South East Asia. In face changing threshold of host immunity, periodic epidemics of DHF and DSS is due to local extinction and emergence of new clades. Over the period 1989 and 2000, a new genotype of DENV-1 and new clades of DENV-3 genotype III viruses have replaced older genotype and clades in this region and emergence of new clades coincided with severe epidemics.

Thus South East Asia displays greatest degree of genetic diversity, suggesting that it is the hub for the evolution of new epidemic strain. However, selection of specific clade and association of specific sequence variation with disease severity at various genomic levels reported in the literature reviewed in this study lacks strength of association i.e. reporting Relative Risk (RR)/ Odds Ratio (OR) limits our interpretation regarding causality or pin pointing specific clade with virus virulence, and therefore further studies are recommended.

7. Acknowledgment

This work was supported by University Research Council of the Aga Khan University, special thanks are extended to Mr. Faisal Malik for expert help in formatting of figures and tables

8. References

Aiken S R, Leigh C H, (1978),Dengue haemorrhagic fever in South East Asia.Transactions of the institute of British geaographers,New series ,Vol. 3, No. 4, (1978), pp.476-497

Annonymous.(2006) etymologia dengue. Emerg.Infec. Dis 2006; vol.12 (6) 893

Araújo JMG, Nogueira RMR, Schatzmayr HG, Zanotto PMA, Bello G. Phylogeography and evolutionary history of dengue virus type 3. Infection, Genetics and Evolution. 2009;9(4):716-25.

Benedict M Q, Levine R S, Hawley W A, Lounibos L P. (2007).Spread of the Tiger:Global risk of invasion by the mosquito Aedesalbopictus. Vector born zoonotic Dis. Vol .7, No. 1,(Jan 2008),pp.76-85.

Benedict, MQ., Levine, R.S., Hawley, W.A. and Lounibos, L.P. (2007). Spread of the Tiger: global risk of invasion by the Mosquito Aedesalbopictus. Vector Borne Zoonotic Dis. 2007 ; Vol.7(1): pp.76–85.

Cox J, Brown H E, Rico-Hesse R. (2011). Variation in vector competence for dengue viruses does not depend on mosquito midgut binding affinity. PLoS: Neglected Tropical Diseases, Vol. 5, No. 5, (May 2011)

Dash PK, Parida MM, Saxena P, Abhyankar A, Singh CP, Tewari KN, et al. Reemergence of dengue virus type-3 (subtype-III) in India: Implications for increased incidence of DHF & DSS. Virology Journal. 2006;3(1):55.

Desprès P, Frenkiel MP, Deubel V. Differences between cell membrane fusion activities of two dengue type-1 isolates reflect modifications of viral structure. Virology. 1993;196(1):209-19.

Downs SH, Black N. The feasibility of creating a checklist for the assessment of the methodological quality both of randomised and non-randomised studies of health care interventions.Journal of Epidemiology and Community Health. 1998;52(6):377.

ElodieDescloux, Van-Mai Cao-Lormeau, Claudine Roche, Lamballerie XD. Dengue 1 Diversity and Microevolution, French Polynesia 2001–2006: Connection with Epidemiology and Clinics. PLoSNegl Trop Dis. 2009;3(8).

Ferguson N, Anderson R, Gupta S.The effect of antibody-dependent enhancement on the transmission dynamics and persistence of multiple-strain pathogens.Proceedings of the National Academy of Sciences of the United States of America. 1999;96(2):790

Focks, D.A., Haile, D.C., Daniels, E., Moun, G.A., 1993. Dynamics life table model for aedes aegypti: Analysis of the literature and model development. J. Med. Entomol. 30, 1003–1018.

Gibbons RV, Kalanarooj S, Jarman RG, Nisalak A, Vaughn DW, Endy TP, et al. Analysis of repeat hospital admissions for dengue to estimate the frequency of third or fourth dengue infections resulting in admissions and dengue hemorrhagic fever, and serotype sequences. The American journal of tropical medicine and hygiene. 2007;77(5):910.

Gubler D J,Reiter P, Ebi K L, Yap W, Nasci R, Patz J A. (2001). Climate variability and change in the United States: Potential vector and rodent born diseases. Enviromental health perspectives, Vol.109, no.2, (May 2001), pp. 223- 233.

Gubler DJ. (1997). Dengue and dengue heamorrhagic fever fever: its history and resurgence as a global public health problem. In: Dengue and dengue heamorrhagic fever, D.J. Gubler, and G.Kuno, eds. (oxford, UK: CAB international) pp.1-22

Gubler DJ. (1998). Dengue and dengue heamorrhagic fever. ClinMicrobiol Rev 11:480-496

Halstead S B. (1966).Mosquito-borne haemorrhagic fevers of South and South-East Asia. Bulletin of world health organization , Vol. 35, No.1,(1966) ,pp.3-15

Halstead SB. Dengue haemorrhagic fever—a public health problem and a field for research. Bulletin of the World Health Organization. 1980;58(1):1.

Hawley WA, Pumpuni CB, Brady RH, Craig GB Jr. (1989).Overwintering survival of Aedesalbopictus(Diptera: Culicidae) eggs in Indiana. Journal of Medical Entomology, Vol. 26,No.2 (Mar 1989),pp122-129.

Henry A, Thongsripong P, Gonzalz I F, Ocampo N J, Dujardin J P. (2009). Wing shap of dengue vectors from around the world. Infection, Genetics and Evolution, Vol. 10, No. 2 (Mar 2010),pp. 207-214

Islam MA, Ahmed MU, Begum N, Chowdhury NA, Khan AH, Parquet MC, et al. Molecular characterization and clinical evaluation of dengue outbreak in 2002 in Bangladesh. Jpn J Infect Dis. 2006.

Jamil B, Hasan R, Zafar A, Bewley K, Chamberlain J, Mioulet V, et al. Dengue virus serotype 3, Karachi, Pakistan. Emerging Infectious Diseases. 2007.

Jarman RG, Holmes EC, Rodpradit P, Klungthong C, Gibbons RV, Nisalak A, et al. Microevolution of Dengue viruses circulating among primary school children in KamphaengPhet, Thailand. Journal of virology. 2008;82(11):5494.

Kanakaratne N, Wahala W, Messer WB, Tissera HA, Shahani A, Abeysinghe N, et al. Severe dengue epidemics in Sri Lanka, 2003–2006. Emerging infectious diseases. 2009;15(2):192.

Kendall C, Hudelson P, Leontsini E, Winch P, Lloyd L, Cruz F.(1991).Urbanization, Dengue, and the health transition: Anthropological contributions to international health. Medical anthropology quarterly , new series,contemprory issues of anthropology in international Health.Vol.5,No.3, (Sep.,1991),pp.257-268.

Khan E, Siddiqui J, Shakoor S, Mehraj V. et al. Dengue outbreak in Karachi, Pakistan 2006: experience at tertiary care center. Trans. R. Soc. Trop. Med. Hyg (2007) 101, 1114-1119

King CC, Chao DY, Chien LJ, Chang GJJ, Lin TH, Wu YC, et al. Comparative analysis of full genomic sequences among different genotypes of dengue virus type 3.Virology Journal. 2008;5(1):63.

Klungthong C, Zhang C, MammenJr MP, Ubol S, Holmes EC. The molecular epidemiology of dengue virus serotype 4 in Bangkok, Thailand. Virology. 2004;329(1):168-79.

Kukreti H, Chaudhary A, Rautela RS, Anand R, Mittal V, Chhabra M, et al. Emergence of an independent lineage of dengue virus type 1 (DENV-1) and its co-circulation with predominant DENV-3 during the 2006 dengue fever outbreak in Delhi. International journal of infectious diseases. 2008;12(5):542-9.

Lanciotti RS, Lewis JG, Gubler DJ, Trent DW.Molecular evolution and epidemiology of dengue-3 viruses.Journal of General Virology. 1994;75(1):65.

Mangada MNM, Igarashi A. Sequences of terminal non-coding regions from four dengue-2 viruses isolated from patients exhibiting different disease severities. Virus genes. 1997;14(1):5-12.

Merrill S A, Ramberg F B,Hagedorn H H.(2005). Phylogeography and population structure of Aedesaegypti in Arizona. The American journal of tropical medicine and hygeine, Vol. 72, No. 3, (2005), pp.304-310

Messer WB, Gubler DJ, Harris E, Sivananthan K, de Silva AM. Emergence and global spread of a dengue serotype 3, subtype III virus. Emerging infectious diseases. 2003;9(7):800-9.

Mousseon, L., Dauga, C., Garrigues, T., Schaffner, F., Vazeille, M. (2005).Phylogeography of
        Ades (Stegomyia) aegypti (L) and Ades (Stegomyia) albopictus (Skuse)
        (Diptera:Culicidae) based on mitochondrial DNA variations. Genet. Res. Camb.
        Vol. 86., pp. 1-11

Nagao Y, Svasti P, Tawatsin A, Thavara U. (2007). Geographical structure of dengue
        transmission and its determinants in thailand. Epidemiol.Infec, Vol.136 ,
        (2008),pp.843- 851.

Rico-Hesse R, Harrison LM, Nisalak A, Vaughn DW, Kalayanarooj S, Green S, et al.
        Molecular evolution of dengue type 2 virus in Thailand.The American journal of
        tropical medicine and hygiene. 1998;58(1):96.

Rico-Hesse R, Harrison LM, Salas RA, Tovar D, Nisalak A, Ramos C, et al. Origins of
        Dengue Type 2 Viruses Associated with Increased Pathogenicity in the Americas*
        1. Virology. 1997;230(2):244-51.

Riesenberg LA, Leitzsch J, Massucci JL, Jaeger J, Rosenfeld JC, Patow C, et al. Residents' and
        attending physicians' handoffs: a systematic review of the literature. Academic
        Medicine. 2009;84(12):1775.

Soundravally R, Hoti SL. Immunopathogenesis of dengue hemorrhagic fever and shock
        syndrome: role of TAP and HPA gene polymorphism. Human immunology.
        2007;68(12):973-9.

Soundravally R, Hoti SL. Polymorphisms of the TAP 1 and 2 gene may influence clinical
        outcome of primary dengue viral infection. Scandinavian journal of immunology.
        2008;67(6):618-25.

Soundravally R, Hoti SL. Significance of transporter associated with antigen processing 2
        (TAP2) gene polymorphisms in susceptibility to dengue viral infection. Journal of
        Clinical Immunology. 2008;28(3):256-62.

Thu HM, Lowry K, Myint TT, Shwe TN, Han AM, Khin KK, et al. Myanmar dengue
        outbreak associated with displacement of serotypes 2, 3, and 4 by dengue 1. Emerg
        Infect Dis. 2004;10(4):593-7.

Twidddy, S., Holmes, E. and Rambaut, A. (2003).Inferring the rate and time scale of dengue
        virus evolution.Mol.Biol.Evol. Vol:20, pp.122-129

Vaughn DW, Green S, Kalayanarooj S, Innis BL, Nimmannitya S, Suntayakorn S, et al.
        Dengue viremia titer, antibody response pattern, and virus serotype correlate with
        disease severity. The Journal of infectious diseases. 2000;181:2-9.

Wang,E., Ni,H.,Xu,R., Barrett, A.,Watowich,S., GublerD., and Weaver,S. (2000)Evolutionary
        relationships of endemic/epidemic and sylvatic dengue viruses. J.Virol. Vol(74):
        pp.3227-3234

Wittke V, Robb TE, Thu HM, Nisalak A, Nimmannitya S, Kalayanrooj S, et al. Extinction and
        rapid emergence of strains of dengue 3 virus during an interepidemic period.
        Virology. 2002;301(1):148-56.

Zhang C, MammenJr MP, Chinnawirotpisan P, Klungthong C, Rodpradit P, Nisalak A, et al.
        Structure and age of genetic diversity of dengue virus type 2 in Thailand. Journal of
        General Virology. 2006;87(4):873.

Zhou Y, MammenJr MP, Klungthong C, Chinnawirotpisan P, Vaughn DW, Nimmannitya S,
        et al. Comparative analysis reveals no consistent association between the secondary
        structure of the 3'-untranslated region of dengue viruses and disease syndrome.
        Journal of General Virology. 2006;87(9):2595.

3

The Re-Emergence of an Old Disease: Chikungunya Fever

Bordi Licia et al.*
Laboratory of Virology, National Institute for Infectious Diseases "L. Spallanzani", Rome
Italy

1. Introduction

Until recently, very few physicians in industrialized countries had heard the word "Chikungunya", and fewer knew how to spell it. Chikungunya, a viral infection transmitted by mosquitoes, derives its name from Makonde, a language spoken in south Tanzania, and means "that which bends up", referring to the posture of patients afflicted with severe joint paints characterizing this infection. Chikungunya virus (CHIKV) was first isolated in Tanzania in 1952 (Robinson, 1955) and has come to the world attention recently, when it caused a massive outbreak in the Indian Ocean region and India (Enserik, 2006). Since 1952, CHIKV has caused a number of epidemics, both in Africa and Southeast Asia, many of them having involved hundreds-of-thousands people. In 2005 the largest Chikungunya fever epidemic on record occurred. The most affected region was La Reunion Island, where CHIKV infected more than a third of the population and killed hundred of people. The 2005/2006 outbreak, started from Comoro Islands, rapidly spread to several countries in the Indian Ocean and India (Enserik, 2006; Mavalankar et al., 2007). Compared to earlier outbreaks, this episode was massive, occurred in highly medicalized areas such as La Reunion, and had very significant economic and social impact. More than 1000 imported CHIKV cases have been detected among European and American travellers returning from the affected areas since the beginning of the outbreak in the Indian Ocean region (Fusco et al., 2006; Taubiz et al., 2007), giving rise, in 2007, to the first autochthonous European outbreak in Italy (Charrel & de Lambellerie, 2008; Rezza et al., 2007). Since 2006, the Regional Office of the French Institute For Public Health Surveillance in the Indian Ocean has conducted epidemiological and biological surveillance for CHIKV infection. During the period December 2006-july 2009, no confirmed case was detected on Reunion Island and Mayotte, but new outbreak were reported in Madagascar. After few years of relative dormancy in Réunion Island, CHIKV transmission has restarted in 2009 and 2010, with one case imported in France (May 2010) (D'Ortenzio et al., 2010). This episode has refreshed the concerns about the possibility of renewed autochthonous transmission in Mediterranean countries.

* Meschi Silvia[1], Selleri Marina[1], Lalle Eleonora[1], Castilletti Concetta[1], Carletti Fabrizio[2], Di Caro Antonino[2] and Capobianchi Maria Rosaria[1]
[1]*Laboratory of Virology, National Institute for Infectious Diseases "L. Spallanzani", Rome, Italy*
[2]*Laboratory of Microbiology and Infectious Disease Biorepository, National Institute for Infectious Diseases "L. Spallanzani", Rome, Italy*

2. Microbiology

CHIKV is an alphavirus belonging to the *Togaviridae* family. Alphaviruses are small and spherical, with a 60-70 nm diameter capsid and a phospholipid envelope. The RNA single-strand of positive polarity encodes four non structural proteins (nsP1-4) and three structural proteins (C,E1,E2). Viral replication is initiated from the time of attachment of viral envelope to cellular host receptors (Strauss & Strauss, 1994). Endocitosis of the virus occurs, following which, delivery of the viral nucleocapsid into cytoplasm takes place. The replication cycle is considerably fast, taking around 4hours. Alphaviruses are sensitive to disseccation and to temperatures above 58°C (Khan et al., 2002; Strauss J.H. & StraussE.M., 1994). About 30 species of arthropod-borne viruses are included in the alphavirus genus, antigenically classified into 7 complexes. These viruses are widely distributed throughout the world, with the exception of Antarctica, and 7 of them cause a syndrome similar to Chikungunya fever, arthralgia and rash: Barmah Forest and Ross river viruses (Oceania), O'nyong-nyong and Semliki Forest viruses (Africa), Mayaro (South America), Sindbis and Sindbis-like (Africa, Asia, Scandinavia and Russia) (Taubiz et al., 2007).

3. Vector and reservoir

In Asia and the Indian Ocean region the main CHIKV vectors are *A. aegypti* and *A. albopictus*.(Jeandel et al. 2004 ; Zeller, 1998). A larger range of *Aedes* species *(A. furcifer, A. vittatus, A. fulgens, A. luteocephalus, A. dalzieli, A. vigilax, A. camptorhynchites)* transmit the virus in Africa, and *Culex annulirostris, Mansonia uniformis,* and anopheles mosquitoes have also occasionally been incriminated (Jupp P.G. et al., 1981; Jupp P.G. & McIntosh, 1990; Lam et al., 2001;). In India, the dominant carrier of Chikungunya virus is *A. aegypti*, which breeds mainly in stored fresh water in urban and semi-urban environments (Yergolkar, 2006). *A. albopictus* has a wide geographical distribution, is particularly resilient, and can survive in both rural and urban environments. The mosquito's eggs are highly resistant and can remain viable throughout the dry season, giving rise to larvae and adults the following rainy season. Originating from Asia, and initially sylvatic, *A. albopictus* has shown a remarkable capacity to adapt to human beings and to urbanisation, allowing it to supersede *A. aegypti* in many places, and to become a secondary but important vector of dengue and other arboviruses (Knudsen, 1995). *A. albopictus* is zoophilic and anthropophilic, is aggressive, silent, active all-day long, and has a lifespan longer than other mosquitoes (up to 8 weeks) and, in the last decades has expanded to several areas previously known to be *Aedes*-free (Charrel et al., 2007). It seems that most new introductions of *A. albopictus* have been caused by vegetative eggs contained in timber and tyres exported from Asia throughout the world. Other emerging events also contributed to the introduction of *A. albopictus* mosquitoes into previously unaffected areas, such as climate change and the increasing use of plastic containers in developing countries. Indeed, climate changes may have several effects on vector biology: increasing temperatures may improve survival at higher latitudes and altitudes, increase the growth rates of vector populations, and alter their seasonality; increased rainfall may have an effect on the larval habitat and population size, and finally an increase in humidity could favourably affect vector survival (Gubler et al., 2001). The use of plastic containers in developing countries, where they are usually not correctly disposed and remain in the environment for years, has also been linked with the spread of the mosquitoes: acting as rain-water receptacles, and being exposed to sunlight, they can become perfect "incubators" for mosquito eggs, where the ideal conditions of temperature and humidity are achieved easily and naturally.

Human beings serve as the Chikungunya virus reservoir during epidemic periods. In Africa some animals (monkeys, rodents, and birds) constitute the virus reservoir during not-epidemic periods, sustaining virus circulation in the environment in the absence of human cases. Outbreaks might occur in monkeys when herd immunity is low; the animals develop viraemia but no pronounced physical manifestations (Inoue et al., 2003; Wolfe et al., 2001). An animal reservoir has not been identified in Asia, where humans appear to be the only host.

4. Clinical manifestation

4.1 General features

After infection with Chikungunya virus, there is a silent incubation period lasting 2–4 days on average (range 1–12 days) (Lam et al., 2001). Clinical onset is abrupt, with high fever, headache, back pain, myalgia, and arthralgia; the latter can be intense, affecting mainly the extremities (ankles, wrists, phalanges) but also the large joints (Hochedez et al., 2006; Lam et al., 2001; Quatresous, 2006; Robinson, 1955; Saxena et al., 2006). Skin involvement present in about 40–50% of cases, and consists of (1) a pruriginous maculopapular rash predominating on the thorax, (2) facial oedema, or (3) in children, a bullous rash with pronounced sloughing, and (4) localised petechiae and gingivorrhagia (mainly in children) (Brighton et al., 1983; Fourie & Morrison, 1979). Radiological findings are normal, and biological markers of inflammation (erythrocyte sedimentation rate and C-reactive protein) are normal or moderately elevated (Fourie & Morrison, 1979; Kennedy et al., 1980). Iridocyclitis and retinitis are the most common ocular manifestations associated with Chikungunya fever; less frequent ocular lesions include episcleritis. All ocular manifestations have a benign course with complete resolution and preservation of vision. Retinitis shows gradual resolution over a period of 6 to 8 weeks (Mahendradas et al., 2008). CHIKV infection seems to elicit long-lasting protective immunity, and experiments performed using animal models have shown a partial cross-protection among CHIKV and other alphaviruses (Edelman et al., 2000; Hearn Jr. & Rainey, 1963).

4.2 Arthralgia

Erratic, relapsing, and incapacitating arthralgia is the hallmark of Chikungunya, although it rarely affects children. These manifestations are normally migratory and involve small joints of hands, wrists, ankles, and feet with pain on movement. Symptoms generally resolve within 7–10 days, except for joint stiffness and pain: up to 12% of patients still have chronic arthralgia three years after onset of the illness. Arthralgia experienced by CHIKF patients closely resembles the symptoms induced by other viruses like Ross River Virus (RRV) and Barmah Forest virus (BFV) (Jacups et al, 2008; Mahalingam et al., 2002). Such alphavirus-induced arthralgia mirrors rheumatoid arthritis, a condition which is characterised by severe joint pains due to inflammation and tissue destruction caused by inflammatory cytokines such as IL-1b, IL-6 and TNF-a (Barksby et al., 2007). It is thus plausible that CHIKV infection induces similar pro-inflammatory cytokines that cause arthralgia, explaining why joint pains are constant ailments of many patients infected with CHIKV even years after recovery from the initial febrile phase (Lakshmi et al., 2008). More recently, global analyses on the specific involvement of cytokines and chemokines have showed that IL-1b, IL-6, and RANTES were associated with disease severity (Ng et al.,

2009). Moreover, since high concentrations of these pro-inflammatory factors were found in the joints of humans afflicted with RRV-induced polyarthritis, they probably have a causative role in chronic joint and muscle pains that plague patients (Lidbury et al., 2008). The finding that aberrant Type I interferon signalling in mice led to severe forms of CHIKF (Couderc et al., 2008) further highlighted the important role cytokines play in the pathology of CHIKV infection.

4.3 Other pathologies

Chikungunya is not generally considered to be a life-threatening disease. Usually the clinical course is fairly mild, but fatal cases directly or indirectly linked to infection with CHIKV have been observed during the Indian-Ocean outbreak (Josseran et al., 2006). The main evidence of a mortality linked to Chikungunya fever epidemics has been obtained in La Reunion, Mauritius, and India by comparing expected and observed mortality data. In all cases, during the months when the epidemics were raging, the observed mortality significantly exceeded the expected one. In particular, in La Reunion the monthly crude death rates in February and March 2006 were 34.4%and 25.2% higher, respectively, than expected. These corresponded to 260 excess deaths (an increase of 18.4%) with a rough estimate of the case-fatality rate for Chikungunya fever of ≈1/1,000 cases. The case-fatality rate calculated on increased crude death rates in Mauritius and Ahmedabad, India, is substantially higher than that calculated in La Reunion: approximately 4.5% (15,760 confirmed or suspected cases and 743 excess deaths) and 4,9% (60,777confirmed or suspected cases and 2,944 excess deaths), respectively (Beesoon et al., 2008; Mavalankar et al., 2008). These differences may be attributed to many factors (greater disease severity, preexisting patient conditions, different patient management, or coincident excess deaths from other causes) but may also be due to a different efficacy of the surveillance systems for Chikungunya fever, that probably worked poorly in Mauritius and India, leading to underestimating the total number of cases (Fusco et al., 2010). The possible link between CHIKV infection and multiorgan failure is still under investigation.

Neurological complications such as meningo-encephalitis were reported in a few patients during the first Indian outbreak in 1973, and during the 2006 Indian outbreak (Chatterjee et al., 1965; Ravi, 2006). The possible mechanisms underlying these processes remain unknown. Studies performed on animal models showed that CHIKV-infected young mice had weakness and walking difficulties which could be due to necrosis and inflammation of skeletal muscles (Ziegler et al., 2008). CHIKV antigens and viral replication have been detected in human myogenic precursors such as satellite cells but not in muscle fibers (Ozden et al., 2007), suggesting that muscle satellite cells could be potential virus reservoirs. The pathologic symptoms of encephalitis owing to CHIKV infection as well as central nervous system (CNS) infections (Chatterjee & Sarkar, 1965) were expected, since *in vitro* experiments showed that the virus could infect and replicate for extended periods in mouse brain cells (Precious et al., 1974). More recently, it was found that mouse CNS tissues such as the choroid plexi could also be targets of CHIKV, lending more credence to the fact that CHIKV infections do affect CNS cells and tissues (Couderc et al., 2008). Work is currently underway by several research groups around the world to decipher this mechanism in CHIKV infections. Moreover, during the 2006 Indian-Ocean outbreak, rare cases of Guillain-Barré syndrome (GBS) associated with CHIKV infection have been described (Lebrun et al., 2009; Wielanek et al., 2007).

Other rare complications described after CHIKV infection are mild hemorrhage, myocarditis, hepatitis (Lemant et al., 2008) .

5. Diagnosis

Diagnosis of infection with CHIKV is based on molecular biology (RT-PCR) and serology methods. The first one is useful during the initial viraemic phase, at the onset of symptoms and normally for the following 5-10 days, when CHIKV RNA reaches very high levels (viral loads of 3.3 x 10^9 copies/ml) and can be detected (Carletti et al., 2007; Parola et al., 2006). Afterwards, the diagnosis is based on serological methods (ELISA, immunofluorescence, hemoagglutination inhibition (HI) and infectivity neutralization (Nt)).

IgM specific against CHIKV are detectable 2-3 days after the onset of symptoms by ELISA immunofluorescent assay and persists for several weeks, up to 3 months (Litzba et al, 2008; Sam & AbuBakar, 2006); rarely, IgM can be detected for longer periods, up to 1 year. IgG specific against CHIKV appear soon after IgM antibodies (2-3 days) and persists for years. Testing of a couple of sera collected in the acute and the convalescent phases of the disease is mandatory for the identification of recent infection using serology methods that cannot distinguish IgG Ab from IgM Ab (i.e. HI and Nt). It is also very useful to confirm results obtained with other methods, especially taking into account the although rare persistence of IgM antibodies. Viral isolation can be performed from serum of infected patient on insect or mammalian cell lines (i.e. C6/36 or Vero E6) during the early phase of the disease, when the viral load is very high and the immune response is still not detectable; however it is useful only for epidemiology or pathogenesis studies or for thorough molecular characterization (Fusco et al., 2010). The sensitivity and specificity of rapid bedside tests commercially available are poorly established, and the possibility of false-positive reactions resulting from cross-reactivity with dengue or other arboviruses such as o'nyong-nyong virus has to be considered (Blackburn et al., 1995). Serologically, chikungunya virus is most closely related to o'nyong-nyong virus and is a member of the Semliki Forest antigenic complex. Individual serological testing is not particularly useful, except when faced with atypical or severe forms, or in travellers returning from an epidemic zone (Pile et al., 1999).

6. Treatment

Currently, there are no available specific therapeutics against CHIKV. Treatment is purely symptomatic and can include rest, fluids, and medicines to relieve symptoms of fever and aching, such as ibuprofen, naproxen, acetaminophen, or paracetamol. Non-steroidal anti-inflammatory drugs (NSAIDs) are primarily used to treat inflammation but high doses, administrated to control arthralgia, could cause thrombocytopenia, gastrointestinal bleeding, nausea, vomiting and gastritis (Jain et al, 2008; Pialoux et al., 2007). Steroids have been occasionally used but their efficacy was not significant (Taubitz et al., 2007). Some time ago chloroquine, a drug useful for prophylaxis and treatment of malaria, showed promising results for treating chronic Chikungunya arthritis (Brighton, 1984), while a recent trial conducted on French Reunion Island proved that there is currently no justification for the use of chloroquine to treat acute chikungunya diseases (De Lamballerie et al., 2008). However, the usefulness of chloroquine in the treatment of Chikungunya infection deserves further investigation that could take advantage on the availability of a non-human primate animal model (Labadie et al., 2010). Ribavirin (200 mg twice a day for seven days) given to patients who continued to have crippling lower limb pains and arthritis for at least two weeks after a febrile episode, had a direct antiviral property against CHIKV, leading to faster resolution of joint and soft tissue manifestations (Ravichandran & Manian, 2008). Briolant and collegues screened various active antiviral compounds against viruses of the Alphavirus genus *in vitro* and demonstrated that 6-azauridinet was more effective against CHIKV, as compared to ribavirin. Moreover, the combination of IFN-alpha2b and ribavirin had synergistic antiviral effect on Chikungunya virus (Briolant et al., 2004).

It is widely recognized that passive vaccination is an appropriate preventive and therapeutic option for many viral infections in human, including those spread by viral vertical transmission, especially when no alternative therapy is available (Dessain et al., 2008). Human polyvalent immunoglobulins purified from plasma samples obtained from donors in the convalescent phase of CHIKV infection exhibited a high *in vitro* neutralizing activity and a powerful prophylactic and therapeutic efficacy against CHIKV infection *in vivo* in mouse models (Couderc et al., 2009). Due to the demonstrated efficacy of human anti-CHIKV antibodies in a mouse model, purified polyvalent CHIKIg (commercialized under the brand Tégéline) could be used in humans for prevention and treatment, especially in individuals at risk of severe CHIKV disease, such as neonates born to viraemic mothers and adults with underlying conditions. Polyclonal immune globulins present the advantage of a broad reactivity but the therapeutic intervention is limited, due to the short viremia in acute phase of CHIKV infection: thus the only benefit this treatment has to offer would be to help reducing viremia faster (Kam et al., 2009). As an alternative, more specific human monoclonal antibodies (MAbs) could be used. In a recent study two unique human mAbs, specific for the CHIKV envelope glicoproteins, strongly and specifically neutralized CHIKV infection *in vitro* (Warter et al., 2011).

7. Prevention

Although no licensed vaccines are currently available for CHIKV, potential vaccine candidates have been tested in humans and animals with varying success. Due to the easiness in preparation, the first developed vaccines were formulations of whole-virus grew on cells and inactivated either by formalin or tween-ether (Eckels et al., 1970; Harrison et al., 1967, 1971; White et al., 1972).

Further vaccines are focused on attenuated strains of CHIK obtained after serial passages in cells cultures (Edelman et al., 2000; Levitt et al., 1986). One of these promising candidates is TSI-GSD-218, a serially passaged and plaque-purified live CHIK vaccine, tested for safety and immunogenicity in human Phase II trials by the US Army Medical Research Institute (Edelman et al., 2000). Seroconversion was obtained in 98% of vaccinees volunteers by day 28 and neutralizing antibodies persisted in 85% of cases at one year after immunization. However transient arthralgia occurred in 8% of the volunteers. Some chimeric candidates vaccines were developed using either Venezuelan equine encephalitis (VEEV) attenuated vaccine strain TC-83, a naturally attenuated strain of eastern equine encephalitis virus (EEEV), or Sindbis virus (SV) as a backbone and the structural protein genes of CHIKV. Vaccinated mice were fully protected against disease and viraemia after CHIKV challenge (Wang et al., 2008). The maturity of reverse genetic technology has provided unprecedented opportunities for manipulation of the alphaviral genome to improve attenuation strategies. Thus, unlike traditional attenuation approaches that rely on cell culture passages, which typically result in attenuation that depends only on small numbers of attenuating point mutations, alternative genetic strategies such as viral chimeras offer the promise of more stable attenuation (Kennedy et al., 2011). In addition to the risk of reactogenicity, attenuation based on small numbers of mutations can also result in residual alphavirus infectivity for mosquito vectors. This risk, which was underscored by the isolation of the TC-83 VEEV vaccine strain from mosquitoes in Louisiana during an equine vaccination campaign designed to control the 1971 epidemic (Pedersen et al., 1972), is especially high when a vaccine that relies on a small number of point mutations is used in a nonendemic location that could support a local transmission cycle. In a recent study chimeric alphaviruses, encoded CHIKV-specific structural genes (but no structural or nonstructural proteins capable of interfering with development of cellular antiviral response) induced protective immune response against subsequent CHIKV challenge (Wang et al., 2011). More in detail, recombinant chikungunya virus vaccine, comprising a non-replicating complex adenovirus vector encoding the structural polyprotein cassette of chikungunya virus, consistently induced in mice high titres of anti-chikungunya virus antibodies that neutralised both an old Asian isolate and a Réunion Island isolate from the recent epidemic (Wang et al., 2011).

A novel CHIK vaccine candidate, CHIKV/IRES, was generated by manipulation of the structural protein expression of a wt-CHIKV strain via the EMCV IRES (Plante et al., 2011). In particular, the internal ribosome entry site (IRES) from encephalomyocarditis virus replaced the subgenomic promoter in a cDNA CHIKV clone, thus altering the levels and host-specific mechanism of structural protein gene expression. This vaccine candidate exhibited a high degree of murine attenuation that was not dependent on an intact interferon type I response, highly attenuated and efficacious after a single dose.

Another approach was the selective expression of CHIK viral structural proteins recently obtained by Akata and colleagues using virus-like particles (VLPs) *in vitro*, that resemble replication-competent alphaviruses (Akahata et al., 2010). Immunization of monkeys with these VLPs elicited neutralizing antibodies against envelope proteins from different CHIKV strains and obtained antibodies transferred into mice protective against subsequent lethal CHIKV challenge. The last frontier in the approach of CHIK vaccine design is the DNA vaccine strategy. An adaptive constant-current electroporation technique was used to immunize mice (Muthumani et al., 2008) and rhesus macaques (Mallilankaraman et al., 2011) with an intramuscular injection of plasmid coding for the CHIK-Capsid, E1 and E2. Vaccination induced robust antigen-specific cellular and humoral immune responses in either case.

To date a number of CHIKV vaccines have been developed, but none have been licensed. While a number of significant questions remain to be addressed related to vaccine validation, such as the most appropriate animal models (species, age, immune status), the dose and route of immunization, the potential interference from multiple vaccinations against different viruses, and last, the practical cost of the vaccine, since most of the epidemic geographical regions belong to the developing countries, there is real hope that a vaccine to prevent this disease will not be too long in arriving.

Since a vaccine is not available actually, protection against mosquito bites and vector control are the main preventive measures. Individual protection relies on the use of mosquito repellents and measures in order to limit skin exposure to mosquitoes. Bednets should be used during the night in hospitals and day-care facilities but *Aedes* mosquitoes are active all-day-long. Control of both adult and larval mosquito populations uses the same model as for dengue and has been relatively effective in many countries and settings. Breeding sites must be removed, destroyed, frequently emptied, and cleaned or treated with insecticides. Large-scale prevention campaigns using DDT have been effective against *A. aegypti* but not *A. albopictus*. Control of *A. aegypti* has rarely been achieved and never sustained (Reiter et al., 2006). Recent data show the different degrees of insecticide resistance in *A. albopictus* and *A. aegypti* (Cui et al., 2006). However, vector control is an endless, costly, and labour-intensive measure and is not always well accepted by local populations, whose cooperation is crucial. Control of CHIKV infection, other than use of drugs for treatment of disease, development of vaccines, individual protection from mosquitoes and vector control programs, also involves surveillance that is fundamental for early identification of cases and quarantine measurement. A model used in investigation of the transmission potential of CHIKV in Italy has proven useful to provide insight into the possible impact of future outbreaks in temperate climate regions and the effectiveness of the interventions performed during the outbreak (Poletti et al., 2011).

8. Geographic distribution and map

Chikungunya fever has an epidemiological pattern with both sporadic cases and epidemics in west Africa, from Senegal to Cameroun, and in many other African countries (Democratic Republic of Congo, Nigeria, Angola, Uganda, Guinea, Malawi, Central African Republic, Burundi, and South Africa). Moreover, many epidemics occurred in Asia (Burma, Thailand, Cambodia, Vietnam, India, Sri Lanka, Timor, Indonesia, and the Philippines) in the 1960s and in the 1990s (Jain et al., 2008; Pialoux et al., 2007).

Major epidemics appear and disappear cyclically, usually with an inter-epidemic period ranging from 7 to 20 years. The huge outbreak that increased concern about CHIKV started in Kenya in 2004, where the seroprevalence rates reached 75% in Lamu island (Pialoux et al., 2007), before reaching the Comores, Seychelles, and Mauritius islands. The virus reached La Reunion island, a French overseas district, in March–April 2005, probably as a result of importation of cases among immigrants from the Comores. The outbreak had two phases: after some thousands of cases which occurred in March-April 2005, very few cases were reported during the austral winter, while the second epidemic peak arose in the initial months of 2006. For the first time, a substantial number of deaths (254) were attributed, directly or indirectly, to CHIKV. From late 2005 onwards, hospitals in some Indian states found themselves swamped with patients complaining of fever and joint pain, which turned out to be Chikungunya fever (Fusco et al., 2010). The World Health Organization Regional Office for South-East Asia has reported that 151 districts in nine states/provinces of India have been affected by Chikungunya fever between February and October 2006 (Pialoux et al., 2007).

Several imported cases were reported in industrialized countries among travellers returning from endemic areas, mainly tourists and immigrants (Depoortere & Coulombier, 2006). In particular, many cases were detected in early 2006, when the outbreak involved the Indian Ocean islands. The Indian Ocean islands, India, and Malaysia are popular tourist destinations. According to the World Tourism Organization, an estimated 1 474 218 people travelled from Madagascar, Mauritius, Mayotte, Reunion, and the Seychelles to European countries in 2004 (Depoortere & Coulombier, 2006; Parola et al., 2006).

The European country with the highest number of imported cases was France, especially the south-eastern region of Provence-Alpes-Côte d'Azur, and Marseille in particular, home to a large Comorian community (Cordel et al., 2006; Hochedez et al., 2007). Other European countries that reported imported cases include Belgium, Bosnia, Czech Republic, Croatia,

Germany, Greece, Italy, Serbia, Spain, Switzerland, Norway, and the United Kingdom (Beltrame, A. 2007; Deporteere & Coulombier, 2006; Fusco, F.M. 2006; Pialoux et al., 2007; Taubitz et al., 2007). In 2006, CHIK fever cases have also been reported in traveller returning from known outbreak areas to Canada, the Caribbean (Martinique), and South America (French Guyana). During 2005-2006, 12 cases of CHIK fever were diagnosed serologically and virologically at CDC in travellers who arrived in the United States from areas known to be epidemic or endemic for CHIK fever, and 26 additional imported cases with onset in 2006 underscores the importance of recognizing such cases among travellers (CDC, 2006; CDC 2007).

Moreover, CHIKV gave rise in 2007 to the first autochthonous European outbreak in Italy, in the northern region of Emilia-Romagna (Rezza et al., 2007; Charrel et al., 2008).

In June 2007, an Indian citizen returned to Italy after a visit to relatives in Kerala, India, developed 2 episodes of fever. During the second febrile episode, he visited his cousin in Castiglione di Cervia. The cousin had an onset of symptoms, with fever and arthralgia, on July 4. This sequence of events started the first Chikungunya fever outbreak in a temperate country, that lasted approximately 2 months with a total 247 cases of Chikungunya fever occurred in the region (217 laboratory-confirmed, 30 suspected) (Fusco et al., 2010). A unique sequence of events seems to have contributed to the establishment of local transmission in Emilia-Romagna: the high concentration of competent vectors A. *albopictus* in the area at the time of arrival of the index case, the presence of a sufficient human population density and the temporal overlapping of arthropod activity (seasonal syncronicity) (Charrel et al., 2008; Rezza et al., 2007).

During 2008, cases of Chikungunya fever have been reported from many countries in Asia other than India, as well as active epidemics from Singapore, Sri Lanka, and Malaysia (Leo et al., 2009).

Since 2006, the Regional Office of the French Institute For Public Health Surveillance in the Indian Ocean has conducted epidemiological and biological surveillance for CHIKV infection. During the period December 2006-July 2009, no confirmed case was detected on Reunion Island and Mayotte, but new outbreaks were reported in Madagascar. After few years of relative dormancy in Réunion Island, in August 2009, a cluster of cases was identified on the western coast of Réunion Island (D'Ortenzio et al., 2009) and, subsequently, an outbreak of CHIKV infection was described on Réunion Island in 2010 (D'Ortenzio et al., 2011). Moreover, recent publications described cases of Chikungunya fever in tourist returning from Maldives, confirming the circulation of the virus by the end of 2009 (Pfeffer et al., 2010; Receveur et al., 2010)

These episodes have refreshed the concerns about the possibility of renewed autochthonous transmission in Mediterranean countries and highlight the need for surveillance in countries where emerging infections may be introduced by returning travellers. Travellers can serve as sentinel population providing information regarding the emergence or re-emergence of an infectious pathogen in a source region. Travellers can thus act as carriers who inadvertently ferry pathogens that can be used to map the location, dynamics and movement of pathogenic strains (Pistone et al, 2009). Thus, with the increase in intercontinental travel, travellers can provide insights into the level of the risk of transmission of infections in other geographical regions.

The geographic range of CHIKV is mainly in Africa and Asia (Fig. 1)

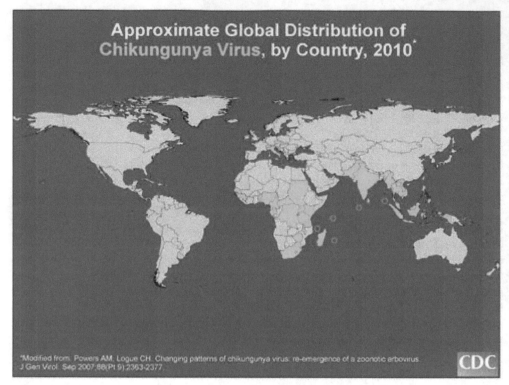

Fig. 1. Geographical distribution of CHIKV shown in the most recent map coming from the CDC's Traveler's Health website (http://wwwn.cdc.gov/travel/default.aspx).

9. Phylogenesis

Three lineages of CHIKV, with distinct genotypic and antigenic characteristics, have been identified. Isolates that caused the 2004-06 Indian Ocean outbreak form a distinct cluster within the large eastern and central Africa phylogenetic group, in addition to the Asian and west African phylogenetic groups (Powers et al., 2000; Schuffenecker et al., 2006). Phylogenetic analysis of CHIKV strains circulating in *A. Albopicus*-humans transmission cycles, obtained during outbreaks, have identified the independent acquisition of a common mutation in E1 glycoprotein (E1gp), namely A226V, in strains isolated from different geographic regions (Schuffenecker et al., 2006; de Lambellerie et al., 2008). This mutation, together with M269V, D284E mutations of E1 CHIKV glycoprotein have been described as molecular signatures of the Indian Ocean outbreak (Arankalle et al., 2007; Tsetsarkin et al., 2007; Vazeille at al., 2007). In particular, the A226V mutation, which was absent in the strains isolated during the initial phases of the outbreak in Réunion, appeared in >90% of the isolates after Dicember 2005. This change could be related to virus adaptation to the mosquito vector species. Together with the lack of herd immunity, this might explain the abrupt and escalating nature of the Reunion outbreak. Has been clearly demonstrated that the A226V mutation is able to increase viral fitness in the *Aedes albopictus* vector (Tsetsarkin et al., 2007; Vazeille et al., 2007), that, in turn, may expand the potential for CHIKV to diffuse to the Americas and Europe, due to the widespread distribution of this vector, in particular in Italy (Knudsen, 1995). In a previous paper we characterized 7 viral isolates (5 imported and 2 autochthonous cases), with respect to the molecular signatures of the Indian Ocean Outbreak in E1, particularly the A226V mutation. Imported cases included 3 returning from Mauritius in 2006 and 2 returning from India in 2006 and 2007, respectively; the autochthonous cases occurred during the 2007 Italian outbreak (Bordi et al., 2008). CHIKV sequences of a 1013 bp fragment of E1 gene (nucleotide positions 10145-11158, respect to the reference strain S27) have been analyzed (Fig.2).

All 7 isolates carried the M269V and D284E Indian Ocean signatures while the A226V mutation was present in all the isolates imported from Mauritius, in the autochthonous cases from the Italian outbreak and in the isolate imported from India in 2007, but was absent in the case imported from India in 2006.

Our findings indicated that, during 2006 and 2007, multiple strains have been imported to Italy from countries where explosive Chikungunya outbreaks were ongoing. All the strains isolated in Italy, both imported and autochthonous, displayed two molecular signatures of

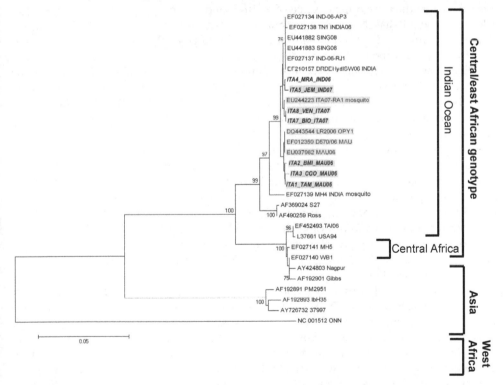

Fig. 2. Phylogenetic tree of CHIKV strains performed on partial E1 gene
CHIKV sequences of a 1013 bp fragment of E1 gene (nucleotide positions 10145-11158, respect to the reference strain S27) have been analyzed. The strains isolated from human cases in Italy are in bold (Bordi et al., Clin Infect Dis, 2008)

the Indian Ocean outbreak (M269V and D284E). Concerning the A226V mutation, this was present in all imported and autochthonous cases, with the exception of the isolate imported from the Indian subcontinent in 2006. The absence of this mutation in the isolate imported in 2006 from India was in agreement with published data (Arankalle et al., 2007), and with available GenBank sequence data, indicating that the virus strains circulating in India in 2006 lacked this mutation.

The presence of A226V in the isolate imported from India in July 2007 and in the isolates from the 2007 Italian outbreak (originating from a case imported from India) supports the view that the virus envelope sequence of strains from India changed over time, acquiring after 2006 the E1 mutation associated with enhanced fitness in *Aedes albopictus*. So it appears that the acquisition and fixation of the A226V mutation may be a common pathway of chikungunya explosion in epidemic areas, in a parallel interplay with the mosquito vector dynamics. Noteworthy, the outbreak in Singapore, where the A226V mutation was absent, has been rapidly controlled.

10. Immune-pathogenesis

Given the expanding geographic range of CHIKV and its potential to rapidly cause large scale epidemics, it has become important to understand the immune and pathogenic mechanisms active during CHIKV infections in order to guide the development of targeted and effective control and treatment strategies.

In a review the possible interactions of the immune system with the different stages of the CHIKV life cycle have been discussed (Kam et al., 2009). The first encounter of CHIKV with human host is intradermal inoculation by the mosquito: replication of the virus starts at the site of inoculation. Different resident cell types are present in this location, including keratinocytes, dermal dendritic cells (DCs), Langerhans cells (LCs), and dermal macrophages, cells involved in the innate immune response.

The innate immune response is the first barrier against viruses, being able to inhibit viral replication through cytolytic and non-cytolytic mechanisms. IFN system plays an important role in limiting virus spread at an early stage of infection. *In vitro* growth of all tested alphaviruses can be greatly suppressed by the antiviral effects of Interferon-α/β (IFN-α/β) when it is added to cells prior to infection, and, more specifically, CHIKV replication is significantly influenced by type I and II IFNs (Courderc et al., 2008; Schilte et al., 2010; Sourisseau et al., 2007). The finding that aberrant Type I interferon signalling in mice led to severe forms of CHIKF (Couderc et al., 2008) further highlighted important roles cytokines play in the pathology of CHIKV infection. Moreover, in a very recent study Wauquier and colleague demonstrated that CHIKV infection in humans elicit strong innate immunity involving the production of numerous proinflammatory mediators. Interestingly, high levels of Interferon IFN-α were consistently found. Production of interleukin (IL) 4, IL-10, and IFN-γ suggested the engagement of the adaptive immunity. This was confirmed by flow cytometry of circulating T lymphocytes that showed a CD8+ T lymphocyte response in the early stages of the disease, and a CD4+ T lymphocyte mediated response in the later stages (Wauquier et al., 2011).

It was already known that skin cell fibroblasts were susceptible to CHIKV infection (Sourisseau et al.,2007); recently has also been demonstrated that CHIKV antigens could be detected *in vivo* in the monocytes of acutely infected patients (Her et al, 2010). CHIKV interactions with monocytes, and with other blood leukocytes, induced a robust and rapid innate immune response with the production of specific chemokines and cytokines. In particular, high levels of IFN-α were rapidly produced after CHIKV incubation with monocytes. The identification of monocytes during the early phase of CHIKV infection *in vivo* is significant as infected monocyte/macrophage cells have been detected in the synovial tissues of chronically CHIKV-infected patients, and these cells may behave as the vehicles for virus dissemination. This may explain the persistence of joint symptoms despite the short duration of viraemia (Her et al., 2010).

Since the A226V mutation has been associated with enhanced replication and fitness of CHIKV in *A. albopictus* vector and has also been shown to modulate cholesterol requirement for infection of insect cells (Tsetsarkin et al., 2007), in a recent paper we investigated the possible involvement of A226V mutation in enhancing human pathogenesis in non vector hosts, by testing the replication competence in primate cell cultures of two isolates, differing for the presence or absence of this mutation (Bordi et al., 2011). We observed that the presence of A226V mutation did not influence the replication kinetics on primate cells. Moreover, the time course of appearance of cytopathic effect (CPE) and of cells immunostained with CHIKV-specific antiserum, was very similar for both the isolates, as well as the shape of the virus-positive multicellular foci, thus suggesting a similar mechanism of spread of the virus in the infected cell cultures.

In addition, we considered the possibility that the A226V mutation could be associated with partial resistance to the inhibitory action of IFN-α in classical experiments of inhibition of virus replication. Surprisingly, the A226V-carrying strain was more susceptible to the antiviral action of recombinant IFN-α. (Fig.3)

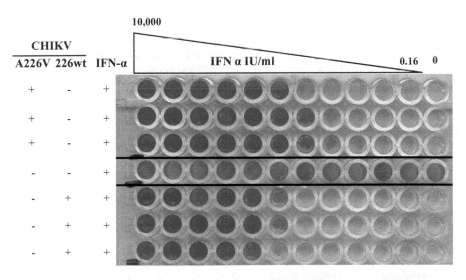

Fig. 3. Dose-dependent reduction of viral CPE by recombinant IFN-α.

In vitro experiments of inhibition of virus replication by recombinant IFN-α on Vero E6 cells showing a dose-dependent reduction of CPE for both isolates: the A226V, carrying isolate and the wt (Bordi et al., New Microbiol, 2011).

Overall, our result did not support the concept that A226V mutation confers a replicative advantage in primate cell cultures, neither supported the possibility that partial resistance to the inhibitory action of IFN-α could account for the explosive spread of the mutated strain in the human population in the countries where this mutation had occurred. However, the possibility that the interplay between the virus and the innate defence system may act at different levels of the virus/host interaction is to be taken into consideration, by exploring, for instance, other steps of the IFN response activation.

At the moment, understanding CHIKV immuno-biology is still in its infancy and there is a long way to go before answers related to the interaction between virus and host immunity will be obtained. These will certainly be important in designing novel antiviral control strategies against the spread of CHIKV infection.

11. References

Akahata W., Yang Z.Y., Andersen H., et al. A VLP vaccine for epidemic Chikungunya virus protects nonhuman primates against infection. Nat Med, 2010; 16: 334-338

Arankalle V.A., Shrivastava S., Cherian S., et al. Genetic divergence of Chikungunya viruses in India (1963-2006) with special reference to the 2005-2006 explosive epidemic. J Gen Virol, 2007; 88: 1967-1976

Barksby H.E., Lea S.R, Preshaw P.M., et al. The expanding family of interleukin-1 cytokines and their role in destructive inflammatory disorders. Clin Exp Immunol, 2007; 149: 217-225

Beesoon S., Funkhouser E., Kotea N., Spielman A., et al. Chikungunya fever, Mauritius, 2006. Emerg Infect Dis, 2008; 14: 337-338

Beltrame A., Angheben A., Bisoffi Z., et al. Imported Chikungunya infection, Italy. Emerg Infect Dis, 2007; 13: 1264-1266

Blackburn N.K., Besselaar T.G. & Gibson G. Antigenic relationship between chikungunya virus strains and o'nyong nyong virus using monoclonal antibodies. Res Virol, 1995; 146: 69–73

Bordi L., Carletti F., Castilletti C. et al. Presence of the A226V mutation in autochthonous and imported Italian chikungunya virus strains. Clin Infect Dis, 2008; 47: 428-429

Bordi L., Meschi S., Selleri M., et al. Chikungunya virus isolates with/without A226V mutation show different sensitivity to IFN-a, but similar replication kinetics in non human primate cells. New Microbiol, 2011; 34: 87-91

Brighton S.W., Prozesky O.W. & de la Harpe A.L. Chikungunya virus infection. A retrospective study of 107 cases. S Afr Med J, 1983; 63: 313–315

Brighton S.W. Chloroquine phosphate treatment of chronic Chikungunya arthritis: an open pilot study. S Afr Med J, 1984; 66: 217-218

Briolant S., Garin D., Scaramozzino N. et al. In vitro inhibition of Chikungunya and Semliki Forest viruses replication by antiviral compounds: synergistic effect of interferon-alpha and ribavirin combination. Antiviral Res, 2004; 61: 111-117

Carletti F., Bordi L., Chiappini R., et al. Rapid detection and quantification of Chikungunya virus by a one-step reverse transcription polymerase chain reaction real-time assay. Am J Trop Med Hyg, 2007; 77: 521-524.

Centers for Disease Control and Prevention (CDC).Chikungunya fever diagnosed among international travelers--United States, 2005-2006. MMWR Morb Mortal Wkly Rep., 2006; 55: 1040-2.

Centers for Disease Control and Prevention (CDC). Update: chikungunya fever diagnosed among international travelers--United States, 2006. MMWR Morb Mortal Wkly Rep., 2007; 56:276-7.

Charrel R.N., de Lamballerie X. & Raoult D. Chikungunya outbreaks--the globalization of vector-borne diseases. N Engl J Med, 2007; 356: 769-771

Charrel R. & de Lamballerie X. Chikungunya in north-eastern Italy: a consequence of seasonal synchronicity. Euro Surveill, 2008; 13: pii: 8003

Chatterjee S.N., Chakravarti S.K., Mitra A.C. et al. Virological investigation of cases with neurological complications during the outbreak of haemorrhagic fever in Calcutta. J Indian Med Assoc, 1965; 45: 314-316

Chatterjee S.N. & Sarkar J.K. Electron microscopic studies of suckling mouse brain cells infected with Chikungunya virus. Indian. J Exp Biol, 1965; 3: 227-234

Cordel H., Quatresous I., Paquet C. et al. Imported cases of chikungunya in metropolitan France, April 2005 - February 2006. Euro Surveill, 2006; 11: E060420.3

Couderc T., Chrétien F., Schilte C. et al. A mouse model for Chikungunya: young age and inefficient Type I interferon signalling are risk factors for severe disease. Plos Pathogen, 2008; 4: e29

Couderc T., Khandoudi N., Grandadam M. et al. Prophylaxis and therapy for Chikungunya virus infection. J Infect Dis, 2009; 200: 516-523

Cui F., Raymond M. & Qiao C.L. . Insecticide resistance in vector mosquitoes in China. Pest Manag Sci, 2006; 62: 1013-1022

D'Ortenzio E., Grandadam M., Balleydier E. et al. Sporadic cases of chikungunya, Reunion Island, August 2009. Euro Surveill, 2009; 14: pii: 19324

D'Ortenzio E., Grandadam M., Balleydier E. et al. A226V strains of Chikungunya virus, Réunion Island, 2010. Emerg Infect Dis, 2011; 17: 309-311

de Lambellerie X., Leroy E., Charrel R.N. et al. Chikungunya virus adapts to tiger mosquito via evolutionary convergence: a sign of things to come? Virol J, 2008; 5: 33

de Lamballerie X., Boisson V., Reynier J.C. et al. On chikungunya acute infection and chloroquine treatment. Vector Borne Zoonotic Dis, 2008; 8: 837-839

Depoortere E., & Coulombier D. Chikungunya risk assessment for Europe: recommendations for action. Euro Surveill, 2006; 11: E060511.2

Dessain S.K., Adekar S.P., & Berry J.D. Exploring the native human antibody repertoire to create antiviral therapeutics. Curr Top Microbiol Immunol, 2008; 317: 155–183

Eckels K.H. Harrison V.R. & Hetrick .FM. Chikungunya virus vaccine prepared by Tween-ether extraction. Appl Microbiol, 1970; 19: 321-325

Edelman R., Tacket C.O., Wasserman S.S. et al. Phase II safety and immunogenicity study of live Chikungunya virus vaccine TSI-GSD-218. Am J Trop Med Hyg, 2000; 62: 681-685

Enserink M. Infectious diseases. Massive outbreak draws fresh attention to little-known virus. Science, 2006; 311: 1085

Fourie E.D. & Morrison J.G. Rheumatoid arthritic syndrome after chikungunya fever. S Afr Med J, 1979; 56: 130–132

Fusco F.M., Puro V., Di Caro A. et al. Cases of Chikungunya fever in Italy in travellers returning from the Indian Ocean and risk of introduction of the disease to Italy. Infez Med, 2006; 14: 238-245

Fusco F.M. et al. (2010). Chikungunya fever, a re-emerging disease, In: *Tropical and Emerging Infectious Diseases*, Maltezou Helen C. and Achilleas Gikas, 93-110, ISBN: 978-81-308-0389-0

Gubler D.J., Reiter P., Ebi K.L. et al. Climate variability and change in the United States: potential impacts on vector- and rodent-borne diseases. Environ Health Perspect, 2001; 109 Suppl 2: 223-233

Harrison V.R., Binn L.N. & Randall R. Comparative immunogenicities of chikungunya vaccines prepared in avian and mammalian tissues. Am J Trop Med Hyg, 1967; 16: 786-791

Harrison V.R, Eckels K.H., Bartelloni P.J. et al. Production and evaluation of a formalin-killed Chikungunya vaccine. J Immunol, 1971; 107: 643-647

Hearn H.J. Jr. & Rainey C.T. Cross-protection in animals infected with Group A arboviruses. J Immunol, 1963; 90: 720-724

Her Z., Malleret B., Chan M. et al. Active Infection of Human Blood Monocytes by Chikungunya Virus Triggers an Innate Immune Response. J Immunol, 2010; 184: 5903-5913

Higgs S. The 2005–2006 chikungunya epidemic in the Indian Ocean. Vector Borne Zoonotic Dis 2006; 6: 115–116

Hochedez P., Jaureguiberry S., Debruyne M. et al. Chikungunya infection in travelers. Emerg Infect Dis, 2006; 12: 1565–1567

Hochedez P., Hausfater P., Jaureguiberry S. et al. Cases of chikungunya fever imported from the islands of the South West Indian Ocean to Paris, France: 80 cases in France. Euro Surveill, 2007; 12: [Epub ahead of print]

Inoue S., Morita K., Matias R.R. et al. Distribution of three arbovirus antibodies among monkeys (*Macaca fascicularis*) in the Philippines. J Med Primatol, 2003; 32: 89–94

Jacups S.P., Whelan P.I. & Currie B.J. Ross River virus and Barmah Forest virus infections: a review of history, ecology, and predictive models, with implications for tropical northern Australia. Vector Borne Zoonotic Dis, 2008; 8: 283-297

Jain M., Rai S. & Chakravarti A. Chikungunya: a review. Trop Doc, 2008; 38: 70-72

Jeandel P., Josse R. & Durand J.P. Exotic viral arthritis: role of alphavirus. Med Trop, 2004; 64: 81-88 (in French)

Josseran L., Paquet C., Zehgnoun A. et al. Chikungunya disease outbreak, Reunion Island. Emerg Infect Dis, 2006; 12: 1994-1995

Jupp P.G., McIntosh B.M., Dos Santos I. et al. Laboratory vector studies on six mosquito and one tick species with chikungunya virus. Trans R Soc Trop Med Hyg, 1981; 75: 15-19

Jupp P.G. & McIntosh B.M. *Aedes furcifer* and other mosquitoes as vectors of chikungunya virus at Mica, northeastern Transvaal, South Africa. J Am Mosq Control Assoc, 1990; 6: 415-420

Kam Y.W., K.S. Ong E., Laurent R et al. Immuno-biology of Chikungunya and implications for disease intervention. Microbes Infect, 2009; 11: 1186-1196

Kennedy A.C., Fleming J. & Solomon L. Chikungunya viral arthropathy: a clinical description. J Rheumatol, 1980; 7: 231-236

Kenney J.L., Volk S.M., Pandya J., et al. Stability of RNA virus attenuation approaches. Vaccine, 2011; 29: 2230-4.

Khan A.H., Morita K., Parquet Md Mdel C. et al. Complete nucleotide sequence of Chikungunya virus and evidence for an internal polyadenylation site. Gen Virol, 2002; 83, 3075-3084

Knudsen A.B. Global distribution and continuing spread of Aedes albopictus. Parassitologia, 1995; 37: 91-97

Labadie K., Larcher T., Joubert C. et al. Chikungunya disease in nonhuman primates involves long-term viral persistence in macrophages. J Clin Invest, 2010; 120: 894-906

Lakshmi V., Neeraja M., Subbalaxmi M.V. et al. Clinical features and molecular diagnosis of Chikungunya fever from South India. Clin Infect Dis, 2008; 46: 1436-1442

Lam S.K., Chua K.B., Hooi P.S. et al. Chikungunya infection—an emerging disease in Malaysia. Southeast Asian J Trop Med Public Health , 2001; 32: 447-451

Lebrun G., Chadda K., Reboux A.H. et al. Guillain-Barré syndrome after chikungunya infection. Emerg Infect Dis, 2009; 15: 495-496

Lemant J., Boisson V., Winer A. et al. Serious acute Chikungunya virus infection requiring intensive care during the Reunion Island outbreak in 2005-2006. Crit Care Med, 2008; 36: 2536-2541

Leo Y.S., Chow A.L.P., Tan L.K. et al. Chikungunya Outbreak, Singapore, 2008. Emerg Infect Dis, 2009 15: 836-837

Levitt N.H., Ramsburg H.H., Hasty S.E. et al. Development of an attenuated strain of chikungunya virus for use in vaccine production. Vaccine, 1986; 4: 157-162

Lidbury B.A., Rulli N.E., Suhrbier A. et al. Macrophage-derived proinflammatory factors contribute to the development of arthritis and myositis after infection with an arthrogenic alphavirus. J Infect Dis, 2008; 197: 1585-1593

Litzba N., Schuffenecker I., Zeller H. et al.Evaluation of the first commercial chikungunya virus indirect immunofluorescence test. J Virol Methods, 2008; 149: 175-179

Mahalingam S., Meanger J., Foster P.S. et al. The viral manipulation of the host cellular and immune environments to enhance propagation and survival: a focus on RNA viruses. J Leukoc Biol, 2002; 72: 429-439

Mahendradas P., Ranganna S.K., Shetty R. et al. Ocular manifestations associated with chikungunya. Ophthalmol, 2008; 115: 287-291

Mallilankaraman K., Shedlock D.J., Bao H. et al. A DNA vaccine against chikungunya virus is protective in mice and induces neutralizing antibodies in mice and nonhuman primates. PLoS Negl Trop Dis, 2011; 5: e928

Mavalankar D., Shastri P. & Raman P. Chikungunya epidemic in India: a major public-health disaster. Lancet Infect Dis, 2007; 7: 306-307

Mavalankar D., Shastri P., Bandyopadhyay T. et al. Increased mortality rate associated with Chikungunya epidemic, Ahmedabad, India. Emerg Infect Dis, 2008; 14: 412-415

Muthumani K., Lankaraman K.M., Laddy D.J. et al. Immunogenicity of novel consensus-based DNA vaccines against Chikungunya virus. Vaccine, 2008; 26: 5128-5134

Ng L.F.P., Chow A., Sun Y.J. et al. IL-1b, IL-6,and RANTES as biomarkers of Chikungunya severity. PLoS One, 2009; 4: e4261

Ozden S., Huerre M., Riviere J.P. et al. Human muscle satellite cells as targets of Chikungunya virus infection. PLoS One, 2007; 2: e527

Panning M., Grywna K., van Esbroeck, M. et al. Chikungunya fever in travelers returning to Europe from the Indian Ocean region, 2006. Emerg Infect Dis, 2008; 14: 416-422

Parola P., de Lamballerie X., Jourdan J. et al. Novel Chikungunya virus variant in travellers returning from Indian Ocean islands. Emerg Infect Dis, 2006; 12: 1493-1499

Pedersen C.E, Robinson D.M., Cole F.E. Isolation of the vaccine strain of Venezuelan equine encephalomyelitis virus from mosquitoes in Louisiana. Am J Epidemiol, 1972; 95:490-496

Pfeffer M., Hanus I., Löscher T. et al. Chikungunya fever in two German tourists returning from the Maldives, September, 2009. Euro Surveill, 2010; 15: pii: 19531

Pialoux G., Gaüzère B.A., Jauréguiberry S. et al. Chikungunya, an epidemic arbovirosis. Lancet Infect Dis, 2007; 7: 319-327

Pile J.C., Henchal E.A., Christopher G.W. et al. Chikungunya in a North American traveler. J Travel Med, 1999; 6: 137-139

Pistone T., Ezzedine K., Schuffenecker I., et al. An imported case of Chikungunya fever from Madagascar: use of the sentinel traveller for detecting emerging arboviral infections in tropical and European countries. Travel Med Infect Dis, 2009;7: 52-4.

Plante K., Wang E., Partidos C.D., et al. Novel Chikungunya Vaccine Candidate with an IRES-Based Attenuation and Host Range Alteration Mechanism. PLoS Pathog, 2011; 7 : e1002142.

Poletti P., Messeri G., Ajelli M. et al. Transmission potential of chikungunya virus and control measures: the case of Italy. PLoS One, 2011; 6: e18860

Powers A.M., Brault A.C., Tesh R.B. et al. Re-emergence of chikungunya and o'nyong-nyong viruses: evidence for distinct geographical lineages and distant evolutionary relationships. J Gen Virol, 2000; 81: 471-479

Precious S.W. Webb H.E. & Bowen E.T.W. Isolation and persistence of Chikungunya virus in cultures of mouse brain cells. J Gen Virol, 1974; 23: 271-279

Quatresous I. E-alert 27 January: chikungunya outbreak in Reunion, a French overseas department. Euro Surveill 2006; 11: E060202.1

Ravi V. Re-emergence of chikungunya virus in India. Indian J Med Microbiol, 2006; 24: 83-84

Ravichandran R. & Manian M. Ribavirin therapy for Chikungunya arthritis. J Infect Dev Ctries, 2008; 2: 140-142.

Receveur M., Ezzedine K., Pistone T. et al. Chikungunya infection in a French traveller returning from the Maldives, October, 2009. Euro Surveill, 2010; 15: 19494

Reiter P., Fontenille D. & Paupy C. Aedes albopictus as an epidemic vector of chikungunya virus: another emerging problem? Lancet Infect Dis, 2006; 6: 463-464

Rezza G., Nicoletti L., Angelini R. et al. CHIKV study group. Infection with Chikungunya virus in Italy: an outbreak in a temperate region. Lancet, 2007; 370: 1840-1846

Robinson M.C. An epidemic of virus disease in Southern Province, Tanganyika Territory, in 1952-1953. I. Clinical features. Trans Royal Society Trop Med Hyg, 1955; 49:28-32

Sam I.C. & AbuBakar S. Chikungunya virus infection. Med J Malaysia 2006; 61: 264–269

Saxena S., Singh M., Mishra N et al. Resurgence of chikungunya virus in India: an emerging threat. Euro Surveill, 2006; 11: E060810.2

Schilte C., Couderc T., Chretien F. et al. Type I IFN controls chikungunya virus via its action on non-hematopoietic cells. J Exp Med, 2010; 207: 429-442

Schuffenecker I., Iteman I., Michault A. et al. Genome microevolution of Chikungunya viruses causing the Indian Ocean outbreak. Plos Medicine, 2006; 3: 1058-1070

Sourisseau M., Schilte C., Casartelli N. et al. Characterization of reemerging chikungunya virus. PLoS Pathogen, 2007; 3: e89

Strauss J.H., Strauss E.M. The alphaviruses: gene expression, replication and evolution. Microbiol Rev, 1994; 58: 491-562

Taubitz W., Cramer J.P., Kapaun A. et al. Chikungunya fever in travelers: clinical presentation and course. Clin Infect Dis, 2007; 45: e1-4

Tsetsarkin K.A., Vanlandingham D.L., McGee C.E. et al. A Single Mutation in Chikungunya Virus Affects Vector Specificity and Epidemic Potential. PLoS Pathog, 2007; 3: 1895-1906

Vazeille M., Moutailler S., Coudrier D. et al. Two Chikungunya Isolates from the Outbreak of La Reunion (Indian Ocean) Exhibit Different Patterns of Infection in the Mosquito, Aedes albopictus. PLoS One, 2007; 2: 1-9

Wang E., Volkova E., Adams A.P. et al. Chimeric alphavirus vaccine candidates for chikungunya. Vaccine, 2008; 26: 5030-5039

Wang D., Suhrbier A., Penn-Nicholson A. et al. A complex adenovirus vaccine against chikungunya virus provides complete protection against viraemia and arthritis. Vaccine, 2011; 29: 2803-2809

Wang E., Kim D.Y., Weaver S.C., et al. Chimeric Chikungunya Viruses are Nonpathogenic in Highly Sensitive Mouse Models, but Efficiently Induce a Protective Immune Response. J Virol, 2011 Jun 22. [Epub ahead of print]

Warter L., Lee C.Y., Thiagarajan R. et al. Chikungunya virus envelope-specific human monoclonal antibodies with broad neutralization potency. J Immunol, 2011; 186: 3258-3264

Wauquier N., Becquart P., Nkoghe D. et al. The acute phase of chikungunya virus infection in humans is associated with strong innate immunity and T CD8 cell activation. J Infect Dis, 2011; 204: 115-123

White A., Berman S. & Lowenthal J.P. Comparative immunogenicities of Chikungunya vaccines propagated in monkey kidney monolayers and chick embryo suspension cultures. Appl Microbiol, 1972; 23: 951-952

Wielanek A.C., Monredon J.D., Amrani M.E. et al. Guillain-Barré syndrome complicating a Chikungunya virus infection. Neurology, 2007; 69: 2105-2107

Wolfe N.D., Kilbourn A.M., Karesh W.B. et al. Sylvatic transmission of arboviruses among Bornean orangutans. Am J Trop Med Hyg, 2001; 64: 310-316

Yergolkar P., Tandale B., Arankalle V. et al. Chikungunya outbreaks caused by African genotype, India. Emerg Infect Dis, 2006; 12: 1580–1583

Zeller H.G. Dengue, arbovirus and migrations in the Indian Ocean. Bull Soc Pathol Exot, 1998; 91: 56-60

Ziegler S.A., Lu L.,. da Rosa A.P. et al. An animal model for studying the pathogenesis of Chikungunya virus infection. Am J Trop Med Hyg, 2008; 79: 133-139

4

Rickettsiosis as Threat for the Traveller

Aránzazu Portillo and José A. Oteo
Hospital San Pedro-Centre of Biomedical Research (CIBIR)
Spain

1. Introduction

Over the past six decades, tourism has experienced continued expansion and diversification becoming one of the largest and fastest growing economic sectors in the world. Many new destinations have emerged alongside the traditional ones of Europe and North America. In the next years an increase of travelling is expected, and the number of related infections will also be higher (http://www.unwto.org/facts/menu.html). Rickettsioses are an important chapter in the field of travel medicine.

Rickettsiae are small gram-negative intracellular bacteria (belonging to the alpha-1 proteobacteria) mainly transmitted by arthropods (lice, fleas, ticks and other acari) with two genera: *Orientia* with a unique specie (*Orientia tsutsugamushi*) and *Rickettsia* with several species. The clinical pictures that they cause are named rickettsioses (Raoult, 2010a).

Rickettsioses have been a threat all along the History and nowadays they are an important cause of morbi-mortality in some areas of the world. To know the distribution of the different diseases caused by these bacteria and how the clinical pictures are recognized may be essential for a quick diagnoses and starting the correct treatment. Some of these infections can be also easily prevented with basic rules. Main rickettsioses with their distribution area are showed in the table 1.

In the 21st Century in most parts of the world hygienic conditions have improved and epidemic typhus is absent. To acquire this condition it is necessary to be in contact with body lice. Furthermore, if people have personal hygiene and change their clothing, body lice are removed. Nevertheless it is possible that if we travel for cooperation to catastrophic areas or other places with poverty, we may take body lice (refugees' camps) and may develop exanthematic typhus.

There are a lot of references of rickettsioses acquired by travellers and considered imported diseases (McDonald et al., 1988; Bottieau et al. 2006; Freedman et al., 2006; Askling et al. 2009; Chen & Wilson, 2009; Jensenius et al., 2009; Stokes & Walters, 2009).

Nowadays ticks cause most travel-associated rickettsioses. Ticks are considered to be one of the most important vectors of infectious diseases in the world, preceded only by mosquitoes. Therefore, tick-borne rickettsioses are endemic all over the world (Hechemy et al., 2006). The majority of travel-associated rickettsioses refer to Sub-Saharan Africa tourists who develop African tick-bite fever (ATBF), mainly transmitted by *Amblyomma hebraeum* (Figure 1). In addition to malaria, ATBF is an important cause of fever in people returning from the tropic (Field et al., 2010). Other reports describe Mediterranean spotted fever (MSF) acquired by tourists bitten by *Rhipicephalus* spp. ticks (Figure 2) when visiting Europe, being more scarce references about other rickettsioses. Flea-borne rickettsioses and chigger-transmitted rickettsioses are less frequent in travellers and tourists, and some of them as murine typhus are associated with poor hygienic conditions. Most travel-acquired rickettsioses are related to outdoors leisure activities, like camping, trekking, hunting, safaris, etc.

It will be impossible to describe all rickettsioses in few pages. Since rickettsioses have very similar clinical pictures and they can be grouped in different syndromes, we will describe these syndromes emphasizing the typical features (i.e.: Presence of eschar or type of rash). Afterwards, distribution can be observed in the table 1. We will also write a specific paragraph for some infections (i.e.: Diseases caused by *Rickettsia akari* and *Orientia tsutsugamushi*).

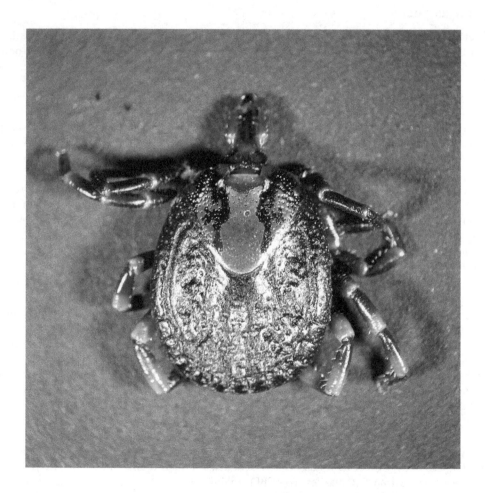

Fig. 1. *Amblyomma hebraeum*, the principal vector of African-tick bite fever (ATBF) in southern Africa.

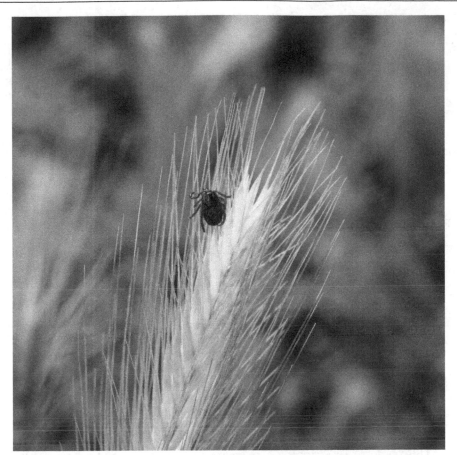

Fig. 2. *Rhipicephalus* spp., the main vector of Mediterranean spotted fever (MSF).

DISEASE	CAUSATIVE AGENT	VECTOR	DISTRIBUTION
Epidemic typhus	*R. prowazekii*	Body lice (*Pediculus humanus corporis*)	Peru, northern Africa, Senegal, Burundi, Rwanda, Russia, sporadic cases in USA associated with flying squirrels. Potentially, all over the world associated to poverty and dirt.
Murine typhus	*R. typhi*	Fleas (*Xenopsylla cheopis* and *Ctenocephalides felis*)	All over the world (more prevalent in tropical and subtropical areas)
Flea-borne spotted fever	*R. felis*	Cat fleas (*Ctenocephalides felis*)	All over the world

DISEASE	CAUSATIVE AGENT	VECTOR	DISTRIBUTION
Scrub typhus	*Orientia tsutsugamushi*	Trombiculid mite larvae (chiggers)	Thailand, Laos, India, Pakistan, Kashmir, Sri-Lanka, Afghanistan, Nepal, China, Japan, Korea, Indonesia. Philippines, Papua-New Guinea, Australia
Rickettsialpox	*R. akari*	Mouse mites (*Liponyssoides sanguineus*)	Eastern Europe, Korea, South Africa, USA
RMSF[1]	*R. rickettsii*	*Dermacentor variabilis* and other American ticks	USA, Mexico, Colombia, Brazil, Argentina, Panama, Costa Rica
RMSF-like	*R. parkeri*	*Amblyomma* spp. ticks	USA, Uruguay, Brazil, Argentina
MSF[2]	*R. conorii conorii, R. conorii israelensis, R. conorii caspia, R. conorii indica*	*Rhipicephalus* spp. ticks	Mediterranean area, Central Europe, Russia, India and Africa
MSF-like	*R. monacensis*	*Ixodes ricinus* ticks	Europe
MSF-like	*R. massiliae*	*Rhipicephalus sanguineus* ticks	Mediterranean area, Argentina, USA?
MSF-like	*R. aeschlimannii*	*Hyalomma marginatum* ticks	Africa, Europe?
DEBONEL / TIBOLA[2]	*R. slovaca R. rioja R. raoultii*	*Dermacentor marginatus* ticks	Europe
LAR[4]	*R. sibirica mongolitimonae*	*Hyalomma* spp. and *Rhipicephalus pusillus* ticks	Europe, Africa.
ATBF[5]	*R. africae*	*Amblyomma* spp. ticks	Sub-Saharan Africa and West Indies
Siberian tick typhus	*R. sibirica sibirica*	*Dermacentor* spp. ticks	Russia, Pakistan, China
R. helvetica infection	*R. helvetica*	*Ixodes ricinus* ticks	Central and northern Europe, Asia
Japanese spotted fever	*R. japonica*	Ticks	Japan
Queensland tick typhus	*R. australis*	*Ixodes* spp. ticks	Eastern Australia
Flinder's Island spotted fever	*R. honei*	Ticks	Australia, Southeast Asia
Far Eastern spotted fever	*R. heilonjgiangensis*	*Dermacentor* spp. ticks	Eastern Asia

[1]RMSF: Rocky Mountain spotted fever; [2]MSF: Mediterranean spotted fever; [3]DEBONEL/TIBOLA: *Dermacentor*-borne, necrosis, erythema, lymphadenopathy/Tick-borne lymphadenopathy; [4]LAR: Lymphangitis-associated rickettsiosis; [5]ATBF: African tick-bite fever.

Table 1. *Rickettsia* spp. causing medical diseases, vectors and distribution

2. Typhus syndrome

Typhus syndrome refers to a febrile syndrome with mental status impairment and rash. It is caused by *Rickettsia prowazekii* (epidemic typhus) and *Rickettsia typhi* (formerly, *R. mooseri*). *Rickettsia felis* may also produce a typhus syndrome named flea-borne spotted fever, which is similar to *R. typhi* infection (perhaps less severe) (Walker & Raoult, 2010; Dumler & Walker 2010; Oteo et al., 2006).

Nowadays epidemic typhus is only present in some regions of Africa, Russia and in Peru. It is associated with bad hygienic conditions that are necessary for body lice parasitization. Sporadic cases associated with contact with flying squirrels and their parasite arthropods, which have been involved as new reservoirs of the infection, have also been reported in USA. A possible source of *R. prowazekii* infection may be a recrudescent case (Brill-Zinsser disease) of *R. prowazekii* infection. If hygienic conditions are altered and an epidemic of body lice appears may be an epidemic of typhus, as occurred in Burundi with hundreds of affected people (Raoult et al., 1998). Some cases of louse-borne typhus in travellers have been published (Zanetti et al., 1998; Kelly et al., 2002).

Endemic typhus or murine typhus is associated with the presence of fleas. The main vector is the rat flea (*Xenopsylla cheopis*) associated with dirt and poor hygienic conditions. Flea-borne spotted fever is associated with the cat flea, and in this case bad hygienic conditions are not necessary. Murine typhus and flea-borne spotted fever are distributed all over the world. Although they are more frequent in tropical and subtropical areas, cases have also been reported in the Mediterranean area (Greece, Italy, Spain, France and Portugal) (Bernabeu-Wittel et al., 1999; Angel-Moreno et al., 2006; Gikas et al,. 2009; Pérez-Arellano et al., 2005; Oteo et al., 2006).

The clinical pictures of murine typhus and flea-borne spotted fever are less severe than the one of epidemic typhus. Thus, 1-2 weeks after the flea exposure, patients begin with fever, headache, myalgia, nausea and vomiting. Rash can be difficult to see in some cases, but is present until 80%. For *R. typhi* infection, rash is macular or maculo-papular and typically affects trunk and less frequently extremities. In epidemic typhus, petechial rash is more frequent than in endemic typhus, and cough, nausea and vomiting are frequent features. On the contrary of tick-borne rickettsioses or scrub typhus, an inoculation eschar (*tache noire*) is not observed. In most cases, fever and rash disappear in a few weeks but complications can be developed (central nervous, kidney involvement with renal insufficiency, respiratory failure, etc.). These complications are more frequent for epidemic typhus and in older people or patients suffering chronic diseases (Walker & Raoult, 2010; Dumler & Walker 2010). In all these conditions a raise in hepatic enzymes, C reactive protein as well as in leucocytes and platelets counts can be observed. We can also observe hepatosplenomegaly. In severe cases mainly associated with epidemic typhus, evolution to a multiple-organ dysfunction syndrome and coagulation disorders may appear.

Some references related to travellers are: Zanetti et al., 1998; Niang et al., 1999; Kelly et al., 2002; Jensenius et al., 2004; Azuma et al., 2006; Angelakis et al., 2010; Walter et al., 2011.

3. Tick-borne spotted fever

Tick-borne spotted fever are worldwide distributed and the clinical picture is very similar, although the severity is different related with the *Rickettsia* species involved.

ATBF and MSF are the most frequent tick-borne spotted fever rickettsioses in travellers (Smoak et al., 1996; Fournier et al., 1998; Oteo et al., 2004a; Raoult et al., 2001; Caruso et al., 2002; Jensenius et al., 2003; Roch et al., 2008; Tsai et al., 2008; Consigny et al., 2009; Stephany et al., 2009; Althaus et al., 2010; Jensenius et al., 2004; Boillat et al., 2008; Laurent et al., 2009). For this reason, we will refer to these conditions taking into account that few differences in the incubation period and severity may exist. For Rocky Mountain spotted fever (RMSF) and MSF caused by *R. conorii israelensis*, higher mortality than with the rest of spotted fever rickettsioses has been communicated (de Sousa et al., 2003). Some features of the main spotted fever rickettsioses are shown in table 2.

From 4 to 21 days after the tick bite, fever suddenly starts in 100% cases (less severe in ATBF). A characteristic inoculation lesion (eschar) (figure 3) is typically found until 72% of MSF cases and until 95% for ATBF. Multiple eschars are observed in some cases. This is more frequent in ATBF. Fever is accompanied of chills, headache, etc. (table 2). From 3 to 5 days after the onset of fever, the rash appears. This is a maculo-papular rash with purpuric elements in some cases (figure 4). It is more frequent in extremities and typically affects palms and soles. In ATBF the rash can be vesicular (figure 5), as occurs in *R. akari* and *R. australis* infections. For *R. sibirica mongolitimonae* infection, known as lymphangitis-associated rickettsiosis (LAR), lymphangitis from the eschar may appear in approximately

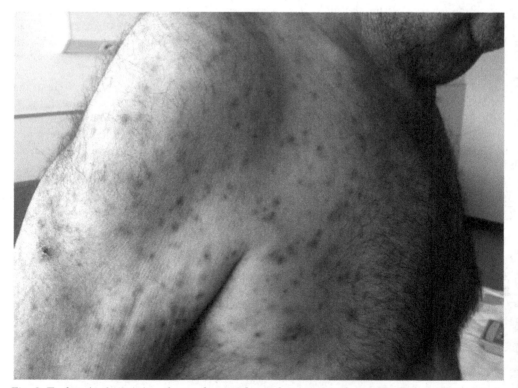

Fig. 3. Eschar (*tache noire*) and maculo-papular rash in a patient with Mediterranean spotted fever.

50% cases. It also can be observed in ATBF (Figure 6). There are few reported cases of tick-borne spotted fever caused by other of *Rickettsia* species (*R. monacensis, R. aeschlimannii, R. massiliae, R. helvetica, R. sibirica mongolitimonae, R. parkeri, R. japonica* and *R. honei*, among others) but it seems that the clinical pictures are very similar to the one of MSF cases. Data about the incidence of these infections among travellers to endemic areas are very scarce (Jensenius et al., 2004; Socolovschi et al., 2010).

For *R. helvetica* infections rash can be absent and fever is often the unique clinical manifestation. All these diseases are more frequent in spring and summer, when the vectors are more active. In all these conditions a raise in hepatic enzymes, C reactive protein and in leucocytes and platelets counts can be observed. We can also observe hepatosplenomegaly. In severe cases mainly associated to RMSF or MSF, evolution to a multiple-organ dysfunction syndrome and coagulation disorders may appear.

Distribution of human cases of tick-borne rickettsioses in Europe, Africa and Americas are showed in figures 7-10. Human cases of tick-borne rickettsioses and scrub typhus in Asia and Oceania are showed in figure 11.

DISEASE	RASH	SPECIFITIES	ESCHAR	FEVER
MSF[1]	>95%	10% purpuric rash	72%. Multiple in 32% (children)	100%
RMSF[2]	90%	45% purpuric rash	<1%	100%
ATBF[3]	30%	Vesicular rash	100%. Frequently multiple	100%
DEBONEL/TIBOLA[4]	Possible	Lymph nodes	100%. Larger than in other rickettsioses	30%
LAR[5]	>90%	50% lymphangitis	Frequent	100%
R. aeschlimannii infection	Possible	-	Possible	100%
R. helvetica infection	Possible	-	Absent	Not always
R. massilliae infection	Possible	Rash can be purpuric	Possible	100%
R. monacensis infection	Possible	-	?	100%
Queensland tick typhus	100%	Vesicular rash	65%	100%
Flinder's Island spotted fever	85%	8% purpuric rash	28%	100%
Siberian tick typhus	100%	-	77%	100%
Japanese spotted fever	100%	-	90%	100%
Far eastern spotted fever	Possible	-	Possible	100%

[1]MSF: Mediterranean spotted fever; [2]RMSF: Rocky Mountain spotted fever; [3]ATBF: African tick-bite fever; [4]DEBONEL/TIBOLA: *Dermacentor*-borne, necrosis, erythema, lymphadenopathy/Tick-borne lymphadenopathy; [5]LAR: Lymphangitis-associated rickettsiosis.

Table 2. Main clinical characteristics of tick-borne rickettsioses

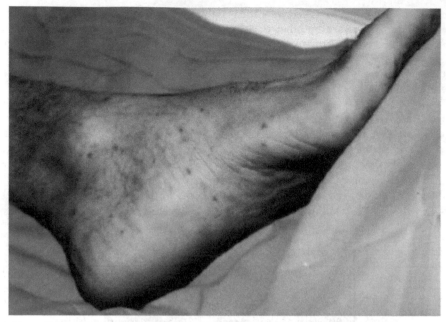

Fig. 4. Vasculitic rash affecting soles in a patient with Mediterranean spotted fever.

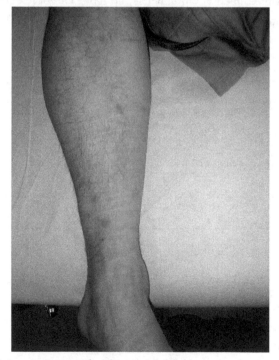

Fig. 5. Vesicular rash in a patient with African-tick bite fever.

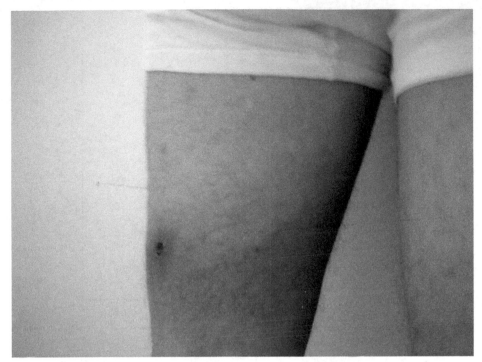

Fig. 6. Eschar and lymphangitis in a patient with African tick-bite fever.

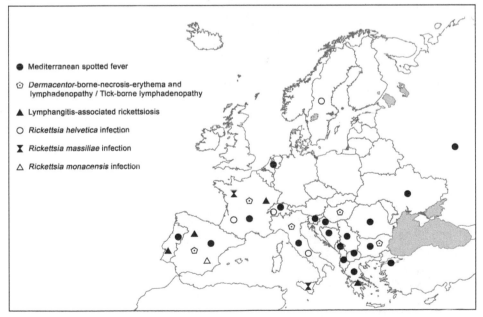

Fig. 7. Map showing distribution of human cases of tick-borne rickettsioses in Europe.

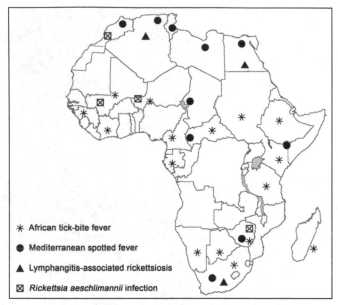

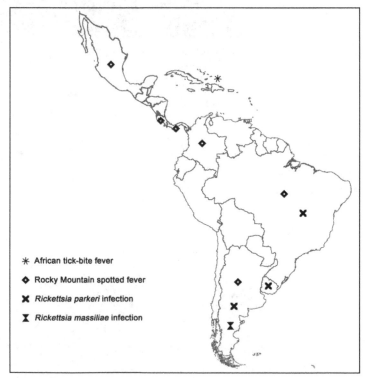

Fig. 8. Map showing distribution of human cases of tick-borne rickettsioses in Africa.

Fig. 9. Map showing distribution of human cases of tick-borne rickettsioses in Latin America.

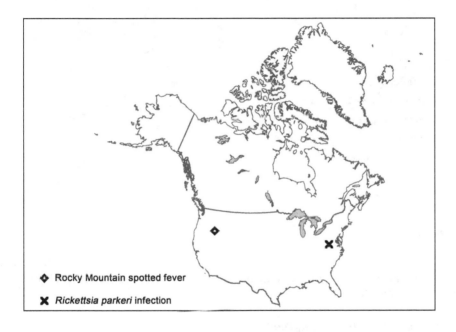

Fig. 10. Map showing distribution of human cases of tick-borne rickettsioses in North America.

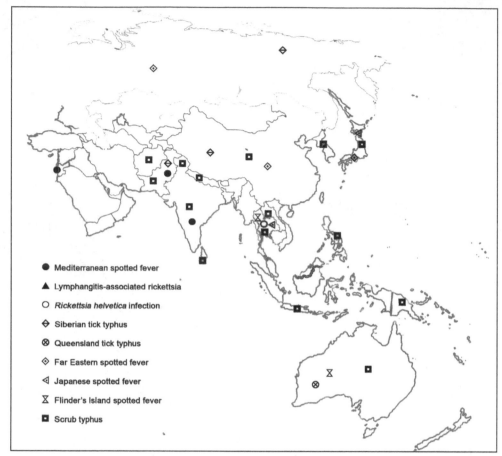

Fig. 11. Map showing distribution of human cases of tick-borne rickettsioses and srub typhus in Asia and Oceania.

4. Eschar and lymphadenopathy

This clinical syndrome has been recently reported in Europe, where it is named TIBOLA (TIck-BOrne LimphAdenopaty) or DEBONEL (*DErmacentor*-BOrne Necrosis-Erythema-Lymphadenopathy). *R. slovaca*, *R. rioja* and *R. raoultii* are the etiological agents, and *Dermacentor marginatus* is the main vector. This tick species is distributed all over Europe as well as in the North of Africa. Since this rickettsiosis appears in the coldest months of the year, the risk of acquisition for the travellers is lower than for the rickettsioses that are prevalent in spring and summer. In most cases (>90%) the tick-bite is located on the scalp (head) and always in the upper site of the body. After 1-15 days (mean: 4.8 days) of incubation period, the characteristic skin lesion starts as a crusted lesion at the site of the tick-bite (frequently on the scalp). A honey-like discharge from the lesion is observed in some cases. Few days later, a necrotic eschar appears (figure 12). This eschar is usually bigger than the one observed in MSF cases, and it is surrounded by an erythema. When the tick-bite is out of the head, the skin lesion resembles the erythema migrans of Lyme disease. Other typical manifestation, which is always present when the bite is on the head, is the presence of regional and very painful lymphadenopathies.

On the contrary of other rickettsioses, in DEBONEL/TIBOLA there are not systemic clinical signs (or they are rare), such as fever or maculo-papular rash (Oteo et al., 2004b). The clinical course is sub-acute and no severe complications have been described.

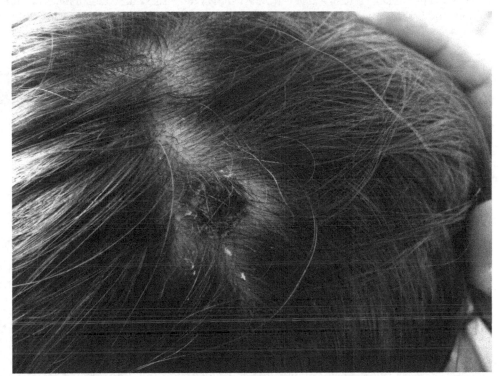

Fig. 12. DEBONEL/TIBOLA patient with the typical crusted lesion on the scalp.

5. Scrub typhus

The etiological agent of scrub typhus is *Orientia tsutsugamushi*, which is transmitted by chigger bites (trombiculid mite larvae). It is mainly distributed in Afghanistan, India, Pakistan, Sri-Lanka, Kashmir, China, Nepal, Japan, Korea, Vietnam, Indonesia, Laos, Philippines, Papua New Guinea and Australia (Figure 11). Cases are mainly observed in autumn and spring, in temperate zones where the bite of this arthropod, which is on vegetation, is frequent. The incubation period is about 10 or more days and the clinical signs and symptoms are similar to typhus syndrome, including the rash which is transient and easily missed. A difference with typhus syndrome is the presence of eschar that is frequently multiple. The presence of regional lymphadenopathy is also more frequent. The mortality can be high despite the correct antimicrobial treatment. Outbreaks related to military operations have been reported (Pages et al., 2010). Most travel acquired cases of scrub typhus occur in patients returning from Southeast Asia (Jensenius et al., 2004, 2006).

6. Rickettsialpox

Rickettsialpox is a worldwide (North America, Eastern Europe, Korea and southern Africa) rickettsiosis caused by *Rickettsia akari* and transmitted by the bite of the mouse mite *Lyponyssoides sanguineus*. We can consider it a remerging infection since several cases have been detected in New York City after September 11 attacks (Paddock et al., 2003). Patients have fever, a prominent eschar -which is the best sign of the disease- and rash that, as occurs in ATBF and Queensland tick typhus, may be vesicular. Palms and soles are not involved. The presence of regional lymphadenopathy is common. Patients recover without treatment in most cases (Raoult, 2010b).

7. Laboratory diagnostic tools

As occurs for all infectious diseases, the most definitive diagnostic method is the rickettsial isolation in culture. The main problem is that *Rickettsia* spp. are strictly intracellular bacteria, conventional growth media cannot be used, and a laboratory with P3 safety level (not generally available in clinical microbiology labs) is necessary. Furthermore, culture is not very sensitive and the yield decreases when clinical samples are taken after antibiotic treatment or when samples are not processed within 24 hours. It is a slow technique that is used for research purposes but not for the routine clinical practice. Centrifugation shell-vial technique is a commercially available adaptation of cell cultures that is easier to handle, faster and less hazardous. Isolation attempts on cell cultures may be performed using buffy coat or tissue samples (eschar biopsies when possible). If not processed within 24 h, samples must be frozen at -70°C or in liquid nitrogen.

Detection of rickettsiae by Giménez or Giemsa staining from blood and tissue samples would allow the confirmation of the diagnosis, but these techniques are non-specific and their sensitivity is very low.

In some laboratories molecular biology tools, such as polymerase chain reaction (PCR) and sequencing, are also available. PCR-based assays from anticoagulated blood, biopsies and arthropod tissue samples targeting *Rickettsia* spp. genes are quite sensitive and useful for a quick diagnosis of these infections. The evaluation of several primer sets for the molecular diagnosis of rickettsioses demonstrated that the performance of three sequential PCRs (nested or semi-nested ones) allowed the detection and identification of *Rickettsia* species in a high percentage of the samples with previous clinical diagnosis or microbiological confirmation (serological analysis) of rickettsiosis (Santibáñez et al., 2011). Blood and tissue samples should be stored at -20°C or lower if PCR-based diagnosis is delayed for more than 24 hours. The European guidelines for the diagnosis of tick-borne bacterial diseases contain useful information for clinicians and microbiologists (Brouqui et al., 2004).

Indirect diagnostic tests and specifically, immunofluorescence assays (IFA) are considered the standard tests. Besides, since most traveller patients are investigated after returning, IFA are the most available tools for diagnosis. Acute and convalescent sera (collected 4-6 weeks after the onset of the illness) should be taken. In many cases we cannot observe seroconvertion but a high titre of antibodies. Cross-reactions among *Rickettsia* spp. make very difficult to definitively identify the causative agent by means of IFA. This can only be achieved in reference centres in which different antigens and other serological assays, such as western-blot, are available. Serum samples can be preserved at -20°C or lower for several months without significant degradation of antibodies.

Ticks removed from patients can be used as tools for the diagnosis of tick-borne rickettsioses. The strategy includes the identification of the tick to the species level, and the detection or isolation of rickettsias (Table 3).

1. Identification of the ticks to the species level

2. Detection of bacteria in ticks with the use of staining tests (haemolymph for viable ticks; salivary glands if ticks were frozen), or PCR-based methods (using one-half of the tick, the other half being kept frozen). PCR may also be done using only ticks that stain positive.

3. Sequencing of the amplified PCR fragment and comparison with available sequences in sequence databases.

4. If there is 100% similarity between the tested sequence and the corresponding sequence of a known organism, the presumptive identification is confirmed

5. If the tested sequence appears to be different from all corresponding sequences available, the organism is probably a new strain and should be isolated and characterized from the stored frozen part of the tick

Table 3. Strategy for detecting and/or isolating rickettsias from ticks

Diagnostic scores with epidemiological, clinical and laboratory tests for some tick-borne rickettsioses (ATBF and MSF) have been proposed (Tables 4 and 5).

a. Direct evidence of *R. africae* infection by culture and/or PCR
   or

b. Clinical and epidemiological features highly suggestive of ATBF, such as multiple inoculation eschars and/or regional lymphadenitis and/or a vesicular rash and/or similar symptoms among other members of the same group of travellers coming back from an endemic area (sub-Saharan Africa or French West Indies)
   and

   Positive serology against spotted fever group rickettsiae
   or

c. Clinical and epidemiological features consistent with a spotted fever group rickettsiosis such as fever and/or any cutaneous rash and/or single inoculation eschar after travel to sub-Saharan Africa or French West Indies
   and

   Serology specific for a recent *R. africae* infection (seroconversion or presence of IgM ‡ 1:32), with antibodies to *R. africae* greater than those to *R. conorii* by at least two dilutions, and/or a Western blot or cross-absorption showing antibodies specific for *R. africae*

Table 4. Diagnostic criteria for African-tick bite fever (ATBF). A patient is considered to have ATBF when criteria A, B or C are met

CRITERIA	SCORE[a]
Epidemiological criteria	
Stay in endemic area	2
Occurrence in May–October	2
Contact (certain or possible) with dog ticks	2
Clinical criteria	
Fever > 39°C	5
Eschar	5
Maculopapular or purpuric rash	5
Two of the above criteria	3
All three of the above criteria	5
Non-specific laboratory findings	
Platelets < 150 G/L	1
SGOT or SGPT > 50 U/L	1
Bacteriological criteria	
Blood culture positive for *Rickettsia conorii*	25
Detection of *Rickettsia conorii* in a skin biopsy	25
Serological criteria	
Single serum and IgG > 1/128	5
Single serum and IgG > 1/128 and IgM > 1/64	10
Four-fold increase in two sera obtained within a 2-week interval	10

SGOT, serum glutamate–oxaloacetate transaminase; SGPT, serum glutamate–pyruvate transaminase.
[a]A positive diagnosis is made when the overall score is ≥ 25.

Table 5. Diagnostic criteria for Mediterranean spotted fever caused by *Rickettsia conorii*

8. Prophylaxis

An important chapter in the field of rickettsioses is related to prophylaxis. Since the majority of rickettsioses associated to travels are transmitted by ticks, the main preventive measure is to avoid tick-bites. Measures to avoid chiggers' attacks are the same as the ones used against ticks. Only fleas can be more difficult to avoid when cats and other pets are abundant. If there is risk of getting lice, hygiene measures such as changing clothing (they live in the seams of clothing) may be sufficient.

How can we avoid tick-bites? There are some rules that can be useful to avoid arthropod-bites:

1. You must not wear dark clothes to see the ticks and remove them before attaching. Curiously, dark clothes attract less arthropods than clear ones. But, in our opinion, to look for the arthropods and remove them as soon as possible is more effective.
2. For outdoor activities (grass areas or mountains) you do not have to exposure your body to ticks. Thus, it is very useful to wear clothing that covers the majority of your body. The trousers must be tucked in your shocks with boots. Long sleeves shirt must be tucked into trousers. You must also wear a cap (especially children).
3. Permethrin-based repellents can be used on clothing, although their effect is short in time and the application should be repeated every few hours.
4. A careful inspection of clothing and body looking for ticks after returning from outdoors activities in endemic areas as well as removing them correctly has been

effective for the prevention of Lyme disease. The tick needs at least 24-48 hours for the transmission of *Borrelia burgdorferi*. This measure can be less efficient for *Rickettsia* spp. because these microorganisms can be transmitted since the first hours. But, anyway, the removal of the tick has to be done.

5. The contact with parasitized pets and wild animals must be avoided.

There are two questions that physicians have linked up with tick-bites: How must I remove the tick? Must I take prophylactic drugs after a tick-bite?

The first question is easy to answer. The most useful method to remove an attached tick is using forceps. Smooth forceps (without teeth) must be introduced between the tick's head and the skin in a 90° angle and then pull (Oteo et al., 1996). Other traditional methods as using oil, burning or freezing must be forgotten.

The other question is the use of prophylactic drugs after arthropod bites. There are no studies to answer this question. The transmission of rickettsias may be very quick, so we cannot extrapolate the recommendations for Lyme disease. Anyway, when people have been bitten by several ticks in an endemic area for a determinate disease (i.e.: Kruger National Park in South Africa and ATBF) and if the patient is anxious, we can offer doxycycline. It has been demonstrated that 3 doses of 100 mg. every 12 hours is safety and sufficient as treatment for the majority of rickettsioses. We must be cautious with the sun to avoid photo-sensibility. Children can take doxycycline for a short period of time. It is only contraindicated for pregnant women and in this case we can use macrolides (i.e. azythromycin).

Vaccine approaches for prevention of rickettsial diseases have been developed since the past century, but currently no vaccine is available. Major surface protein antigens (OmpA and OmpB) of *R. rickettsii* and *R. conorii* are candidate vaccine antigens. Molecular biology techniques such as selection, cloning and expression of genes encoding *R. prowazekii* virulence-associated proteins, offer the opportunity to develop new rickettsial vaccines against typhus group rickettsiae. Further research is needed to develop effective vaccines without undesirable toxic reactions (Azad & Radulovic, 2003; Walker, 2009).

9. Treatment

The treatment of rickettsiosis should be initiated as soon as possible. Antibiotics are very effective and may avoid severe complications and death. In all cases if rickettsiosis is suspected, samples should be sent for laboratory confirmation. In DEBONEL/TIBOLA, in which the clinical signs and symptoms are less severe, recovery without antimicrobials occurs but the use of antibiotics shortens the clinical course and improves the clinical picture (Ibarra et al., 2005).

Doxycycline is the most useful drug in children and adults. Doxycycline can be administered in short course (100 mg. every 12 hours for one day) for the treatment of typhus and scrub typhus. In the case of MSF, 2 doses of 200 mg./12 hous are also very effective (in children, 5 mg./kg./12hours); although most physicians use 100 mg. every 12 hours for 3-7 days after fever disappears. The same can be recommended for ATBF. This antibiotic regimen could probably be followed in other tick-borne rickettsioses but there are not good evidences (clinical assays) to support a recommendation. In RMSF the administration of doxycycline for 7 days is recommended. Other drugs that can be prescribed when not using doxycycline (allergy or pregnancy) are chloramphenicol (50-75 mg./kg./day given in 4 doses for 7-10 days) and azythromycin (500 mg./day for 5 days). Doxycycline for 7 days is the treatment of choice for rickettsialpox. Although there is *in vitro* susceptibility to quinolones, the use of these drugs has been associated with worse clinical course (Botelho-Nevers et al., 2011).

10. Conclusion

In conclusion, rickettsioses are a worldwide threat that must be suspected in travellers returning from endemic areas. Most cases are caused by tick-bites, although in some areas of the world old diseases as typhus are present, and the risk exists. Rickettsiosis must be suspected in all patients with fever, exanthema with or without rash. Starting treatment with doxycycline when possible may be essential to rapidly recover and avoid complications. ATBF along with malaria is the leading cause of fever after returning from Sub-Saharan Africa.

11. Acknowledgment

We are grateful to all members from the Centre of Rickettsiosis and Arthropod-Borne Diseases, Hospital San Pedro-Centre of Biomedical Research (CIBIR), Logroño (La Rioja), Spain.
Financial support was provided in part by a grant from 'Instituto de Salud Carlos III' (EMER 07/033), Ministerio de Ciencia e Innovación (Spain).

12. References

Althaus, F., Greub, G., Raoult, D. & Genton, B. (2010). African tick-bite fever: a new entity in the differential diagnosis of multiple eschars in travelers. Description of five cases imported from South Africa to Switzerland. *International Journal of Infectious Diseases*, Vol.14, Suppl.3 (September 2010), pp. e274-276, ISSN 1201-9712

Angelakis, E., Botelho, E., Socolovschi, C., Sobas, C.R., Piketty, C., Parola, P. & Raoult, D. (2010). Murine typhus as a cause of fever in travelers from Tunisia and Mediterranean areas. *Journal of Travel Medicine*, Vol.17, No.5, (September 2010), pp. 310-315, ISSN 1195-1982

Angel-Moreno, A., Bolaños, M., Santana, E., Pérez-Arellano, J.L. (2006). Murine typhus imported from Senegal in a travelling immigrant. *Enfermedades Infecciosas y Microbiología Clínica*, Vol.24, No.6, (June-July 2006), pp. 406-407, ISSN 0213-005X

Askling, H.H., Lesko, B., Vene, S., Berndtson, A., Björkman, P., Bläckberg, J., Bronner, U., Follin, P., Hellgren, U., Palmerus, M., Ekdahl, K., Tegnell, A. & Struwe J. (2009). Serologic analysis of returned travelers with fever, Sweden. *Emerging Infectious Diseases*, Vol.15, No.11, (November 2009), pp. 1805-1808, ISSN 1080-6059

Azad, A.F. & Radulovic, S. (2003). Pathogenic rickettsiae as bioterrorism agents. *Annals of the New York Academy of Sciences*, Vol.990 (June 2003), pp. 734-8, ISSN 0077-8923

Azuma, M., Nishioka, Y., Ogawa, M., Takasaki, T., Sone, S. & Uchiyama, T. (2006). Murine typhus from Vietnam, imported into Japan. *Emerging Infectious Diseases*, Vol.12, No.9, (September 2006), pp. 1466-1468, ISSN 1080-6059

Bernabeu-Wittel, M., Pachón, J., Alarcón, A., López-Cortés, L.F., Viciana, P., Jiménez-Mejías, M.E., Villanueva, J.L., Torronteras, R. & Caballero-Granado, F.J. (1999). Murine typhus as a common cause of fever of intermediate duration: a 17-year study in the south of Spain. *Archives of Internal Medicine*, Vol.159, No.8, (April 1999), pp. 872-876, ISSN 0003-9926

Boillat, N., Genton, B., D'Acremont, V., Raoult, D. & Greub, G. (2008). Fatal case of Israeli spotted fever after Mediterranean cruise. *Emerging Infectious Diseases*, Vol.14, No.12, (December 2008), pp. 1944-1946, ISSN 1080-6059

Botelho-Nevers, E., Rovery, C., Richet, H. & Raoult, D. (2011). Analysis of risk factors for malignant Mediterranean spotted fever indicates that fluoroquinolone treatment has a deleterious effect. *Journal of Antimicrobial Chemotherapy*, Vol.66, (June 2011), pp. 1821-1830, ISSN 0305-7453

Bottieau, E., Clerinx, J., Schrooten, W., Van den Enden, E., Wouters, R., Van Esbroeck, M., Vervoort, T., Demey, H., Colebunders, R., Van Gompel, A. & Van Den Ende, J. (2006). Etiology and outcome of fever after a stay in the tropics. *Archives of Internal Medicine*, Vol.166, No.15, (August 2006), pp. 1642-1648, ISSN 0003-9926

Brouqui, P., Bacellar, F., Baranton, G., Birtles, R.J., Bjoërsdorff, A., Blanco, J.R., Caruso, G., Cinco, M., Fournier, P.E., Francavilla, E., Jensenius, M., Kazar, J., Laferl, H., Lakos, A., Lotric-Furlan, S., Maurin, M., Oteo, J.A., Parola, P., Perez-Eid, C., Peter, O., Postic, D., Raoult, D., Tellez, A., Tselentis, Y. & Wilske, B.; ESCMID Study Group on *Coxiella, Anaplasma, Rickettsia* and *Bartonella*; European Network for Surveillance of Tick-Borne Diseases. (2004). Guidelines for the diagnosis of tick-borne bacterial diseases in Europe. *Clinical Microbiology and Infection*, Vol.10, (December 2004), pp. 1108-1132, ISSN 1198-743X

Caruso, G., Zasio, C., Guzzo, F., Granata, C., Mondardini, V., Guerra, E., Macrì, E. & Benedetti, P. (2002). Outbreak of African tick-bite fever in six Italian tourists returning from South Africa. *European Journal of Clinical Microbiology & Infectious Diseases*, Vol.21, No.2, (February 2002), pp. 133-136, ISSN 0934-9723

Chen LH, Wilson ME. (2009). Tick-borne rickettsiosis in traveler returning from Honduras. *Emerging Infectious Diseases*, Vol.15, No.8, (August 2009), pp. 1321-3, ISSN 1080-6059

Consigny, P.H., Schuett, I., Fraitag, S., Rolain, J.M., Buffet, P. (2009). Unusual location of an inoculation lesion in a traveler with African tick-bite fever returning from South Africa. *Journal of Travel Medicine*, Vol.16, No.6, (November-December 2009), pp. 439-440, ISSN 1195-1982

de Sousa, R., Nóbrega, S.D., Bacellar, F., Torgal, J. (2003). Mediterranean spotted fever in Portugal: risk factors for fatal outcome in 105 hospitalized patients. *Annals of the New York Academy of Sciences*, Vol.990 (June 2003), pp. 285-294, ISSN 1749-6632

Dumler J.S. & Walker, D.H. (2010). *Rickettsia tyhi* (Murine typhus), In: *Mandell, Douglas, and Bennett´s Principles and Practice of Infectious Diseases*, Mandell G.L., Bennett J.E., Dolin R. (Eds.), pp. 2525-2528, Churchill Livingstone Elsevier, ISBN 978-0-4430-6839-3, Philadelphia-USA.

Field, V., Gautret, P., Schlagenhauf, P., Burchard, G.D., Caumes, E., Jensenius, M., Castelli, F., Gkrania-Klotsas, E., Weld, L., Lopez-Velez, R., de Vries, P., von Sonnenburg, F., Loutan, L. & Parola, P.; EuroTravNet network. (2010). Travel and migration associated infectious diseases morbidity in Europe, 2008. *BMC Infectious Diseases*, Vol.10, (November 2010), 330, ISSN 1471-2334

Fournier, P.E., Roux, V., Caumes, E., Donzel, M. & Raoult, D. (1998). Outbreak of *Rickettsia africae* infections in participants of an adventure race in South Africa. *Clinical Infectious Diseases*, Vol.27, No.2, (August 1998), pp. 316-323, ISSN 1058-4838

Freedman, D.O., Weld, L.H., Kozarsky, P.E., Fisk, T., Robins, R., von Sonnenburg, F., Keystone, J.S., Pandey, P. & Cetron, M.S.; GeoSentinel Surveillance Network.

(2006). Spectrum of disease and relation to place of exposure among ill returned travelers. *The New England Journal of Medicine*, Vol.354, No.2, (January 2006), pp. 119-130, ISSN 0028-4793

Gikas, A., Kokkini, S., Tsioutis, C., Athenessopoulos, D., Balomenaki, E., Blasak, S., Matheou, C., Tselentis, Y. & Psaroulaki, A. (2009). Murine typhus in children: clinical and laboratory features from 41 cases in Crete, Greece. *Clinical Microbiology and Infection*, Vol.15, Suppl. 2 (December 2009), pp. 211-212, ISSN 1198-743X

Hechemy, K.E., Oteo, J.A., Raoult, D., Silverman, D.J. & Blanco, J.R. (2006). A century of rickettsiology: emerging, reemerging rickettsioses, clinical, epidemiologic, and molecular diagnostic aspects and emerging veterinary rickettsioses: an overview. *Annals of the New York Academy of Sciences*, Vol.1078 (October 2006), pp. 1-14, ISSN 0077-8923

Ibarra, V., Blanco, J.R., Portillo, A., Santibáñez, S., Metola, L., Oteo, J.A. (2005). Effect of antibiotic treatment in patients with DEBONEL/TIBOLA. *Annals of the New York Academy of Sciences*, Vol.1063 (December 2005), pp. 257-258, ISSN 0077-8923

Jensenius, M., Davis, X., von Sonnenburg, F., Schwartz, E., Keystone, J.S., Leder, K., Lopéz-Véléz, R., Caumes, E., Cramer, J.P., Chen, L. & Parola, P.; GeoSentinel Surveillance Network. (2009). Multicenter GeoSentinel analysis of rickettsial diseases in international travelers, 1996-2008. *Emerging Infectious Diseases*, Vol.15, No.11, (November 2009), pp. 1791-1798, ISSN 1080-6059

Jensenius, M., Fournier, P.E. & Raoult, D. (2004). Rickettsioses and the international traveler. *Clinical Infectious Diseases*, Vol.39, No.10, (November 2004), pp. 1493-1499, ISSN 1058-4838

Jensenius, M., Fournier, P.E., Vene, S., Hoel, T., Hasle, G., Henriksen, A.Z., Hellum, K.B., Raoult, D. & Myrvang, B.; Norwegian African Tick Bite Fever Study Group. (2003). African tick bite fever in travelers to rural sub-Equatorial Africa. *Clinical Infectious Diseases*, Vol.36, No.11, (June 2003), pp. 1411-1417, ISSN 1058-4838

Jensenius, M., Montelius, R., Berild, D. & Vene, S. (2006). Scrub typhus imported to Scandinavia. *Scandinavian Journal of Infectious Diseases*, Vol.38, No.3, pp. 200-202, ISSN 0036-5548

Kelly, D.J., Richards, A.L., Temenak, J., Strickman, D., Dasch, G.A. (2002). The past and present threat of rickettsial diseases to military medicine and international public health. *Clinical Infectious Diseases*, Vol.34, Suppl.4, (June 2002), pp. S145-169, ISSN 1058-4838

Laurent, M., Voet, A., Libeer, C., Lambrechts, M., Van Wijngaerden, E. (2009). Mediterranean spotted fever, a diagnostic challenge in travellers. *Acta Clinica Belgica*, Vol.64, No.6, (November-December 2009), pp. 513-516, ISSN 0001-5512

McDonald, J.C., MacLean, J.D. & McDade, J.E. (1988). Imported rickettsial disease: clinical and epidemiologic features. *American Journal of Medicine*, Vol.85, No.6, (December 1988), pp. 799-805, ISSN 0002-9343

Niang, M., Brouqui, P., Raoult, D. (1999). Epidemic typhus imported from Algeria. *Emerging Infectious Diseases*, Vol.5, No.5, (September-October 1999), pp. 716-718, ISSN 1080-6059

Oteo, J.A., Ibarra, V., Blanco, J.R., Martínez de Artola, V., Márquez, F.J., Portillo, A., Raoult, D., Anda, P (2004b). *Dermacentor*-borne Necrosis Erythema and Lymphadenopathy:

Clinical and epidemiological features of a new tick-borne disease. *Clinical Microbiology and Infection*, Vol.10, pp. 327-331, ISSN 1198-743X

Oteo, J.A., Martínez de Artola, V., Gómez-Cadiñanos, R., Casas, J.M., Blanco, J.R. & Rosel, L. (1996). Evaluation of methods of tick removal in human ixodidiasis. *Revista Clínica Española* Vol.196, No.9, (September 1996), pp. 584-587, ISSN 0014-2565

Oteo, J.A., Portillo, A., Blanco, J.R., Ibarra, V. & Santibáñez, S. (2004a). Medicina Clínica, Vol.122, No.20, (May 2004), pp. 786-788, ISSN 0025-7753

Oteo, J.A., Portillo, A., Santibáñez, S., Blanco, J.R., Pérez-Martínez, L. & Ibarra, V. (2006). Cluster of cases of human *Rickettsia felis* infection from southern Europe (Spain) diagnosed by PCR. *Journal of Clinical Microbiology*, Vol.44, No.7, (July 2006), pp. 2669-2671, ISSN 0095- 1137

Paddock, C.D., Zaki, S.R., Koss, T., Singleton, J. Jr., Sumner, J.W., Comer, J.A., Eremeeva, M.E., Dasch, G.A., Cherry, B. & Childs, J.E. Rickettsialpox in New York City: a persistent urban zoonosis. *Annals of the New York Academy of Sciences*, Vol.990, (June 2003), pp. 36-44, ISSN 1749-6632

Pages F., Faulde M., Orlandi-Pradines E. & Parola P. (2010). The past and present threat of vector-borne diseases in deployed troops. *Clinical Microbiology and Infection*, Vol.16, No.3, (March 2010), pp. 209-224, ISSN 1198-743X

Pérez-Arellano, J.L., Fenollar, F., Angel-Moreno, A., Bolaños, M., Hernández, M., Santana, E., Hemmersbach-Miller, M., Martín, A.M. & Raoult, D. (2005). Human *Rickettsia felis* infection, Canary Islands, Spain. *Emerging Infectious Diseases*, Vol.11, No.12, (December 2005), pp. 1961-1964, ISSN 1080-6059

Raoult D. (2010b). *Rickettsia akari* (Rickettsialpox), In: *Mandell, Douglas, and Bennett´s Principles and Practice of Infectious Diseases*, Mandell G.L., Bennett J.E., Dolin R. (Eds.), pp. 2509-2510, Churchill Livingstone Elsevier, ISBN 978-0-4430-6839-3, Philadelphia-USA.

Raoult, D. (2010a). Introduction to Rickettsioses, Ehrlichioses, and Anaplasmosis, In: *Mandell, Douglas, and Bennett´s Principles and Practice of Infectious Diseases*, Mandell G.L., Bennett J.E., Dolin R. (Eds.), pp. 2495-2498, Churchill Livingstone Elsevier, ISBN 978-0-4430-6839-3, Philadelphia-USA.

Raoult, D., Fournier, P.E., Fenollar, F., Jensenius, M., Prioe, T., de Pina, J.J., Caruso, G., Jones, N., Laferl, H., Rosenblatt, J.E. & Marrie, T.J. (2001). *Rickettsia africae*, a tick-borne pathogen in travelers to sub-Saharan Africa. *The New England Journal of Medicine*, Vol.344, No.20, (May 2001), pp. 1504-1510, ISSN 0028-4793

Raoult, D., Ndihokubwayo, J.B., Tissot-Dupont, H., Roux, V., Faugere, B., Abegbinni, R. & Birtles, R.J. (1998). Outbreak of epidemic typhus associated with trench fever in Burundi. *Lancet*, Vol.352, No.9125, (August 1998), pp. 353-358, ISSN 0140-6736

Roch, N., Epaulard, O., Pelloux, I., Pavese, P., Brion, J.P., Raoult, D. & Maurin M. (2008). African tick bite fever in elderly patients: 8 cases in French tourists returning from South Africa. *Clinical Infectious Diseases*, Vol.47, No.3, (August 2008), pp. e28-35, ISSN 1058-4838

Santibáñez, S., Portillo, A., Santibáñez, P., Ibarra, V., Palomar, A., Oteo, J.A. (2011). Utility of five PCR targets for molecular diagnosis of human rickettsioses, *Proceedings of the 6th International Meeting on Rickettsiae and Rickettsial Diseases*, Heraklion, Crete, Greece, June 2011.

Smoak, B.L., McClain, J.B., Brundage, J.F., Broadhurst, L., Kelly, D.J., Dasch, G.A. & Miller, R.N. (1996). An outbreak of spotted fever rickettsiosis in U.S. Army troops deployed to Botswana. *Emerging Infectious Diseases*, Vol.2, No.3, (July-September 1996), pp. 217-221, ISSN 1080-6059

Socolovschi, C., Barbarot, S., Lefebvre, M., Parola, P. & Raoult, D. (2010). *Rickettsia sibirica mongolitimonae* in traveler from Egypt. *Emerging Infectious Diseases*, Vol.16, No.9, (September 2010), pp.1495-1496, ISSN 1080-6059

Stephany, D., Buffet, P., Rolain, J.M., Raoult, D. & Consigny, P.H. (2009). *Rickettsia africae* infection in man after travel to Ethiopia. *Emerging Infectious Diseases*, Vol.15, No.11, (November 2009), pp. 1867-1870, ISSN 1080-6059

Stokes, P.H. & Walters, B.J. (2009). Spotted fever rickettsiosis infection in a traveler from Sri Lanka. *Journal of Travel Medicine*, Vol.16, No.6, (November-December 2009), pp. 436-438, ISSN 1195-1982

Tsai, Y.S., Wu, Y.H., Kao, P.T., Lin, Y.C. (2008). African tick bite fever. *Journal Formosan Medical Association*, Vol.107, No.1, (January 2008), pp. 73-76, ISSN 0929-6646

Walker, D.H. & Raoult, D. (2010). *Rickettsia prowazekii* (Epidemic or louse-borne typhus), In: *Mandell, Douglas, and Bennett´s Principles and Practice of Infectious Diseases*, Mandell G.L., Bennett J.E., Dolin R. (Eds.), pp. 2521-2524, Churchill Livingstone Elsevier, ISBN 978-0-4430-6839-3, Philadelphia-USA.

Walker, D.H. (2009). The realities of biodefense vaccines against Rickettsia. *Vaccine*, Vol. 27, Suppl. 4 (November 2009), pp. D52-5, ISSN 0264-410X

Walter, G., Botelho-Nevers, E., Socolovschi, C., Raoult, D. & Parola, P. (2011). Murine typhus in returned travelers: a report of thirty-two cases, *Proceedings of the 6th International Meeting on Rickettsiae and Rickettsial Diseases*, Heraklion, Crete, Greece, June 2011.

Zanetti, G., Francioli, P., Tagan, D., Paddock, C.D. & Zaki, S.R. (1998). Imported epidemic typhus. *Lancet*, Vol.352, No.9141, (November 1998), pp. 1709, ISSN 0140-6736

5

Human Ehrlichioses and Rickettsioses in Cameroon

Lucy Ndip[1], Roland Ndip[1], David Walker[2] and Jere McBride[2]
[1]University of Buea
[2]University of Texas Medical Branch, Galveston
[1]Cameroon
[2]USA

1. Introduction

Human ehrlichioses and rickettsioses are important arthropod borne infectious diseases which are transmitted by ticks, mites, lice and fleas. Infections result in mild to fatal outcomes, with clinical presentations that resemble other tropical infectious diseases such as malaria making clinical diagnosis difficult. Despite recognition as important causes of life-threatening diseases in the United States, the geographic distribution of these diseases worldwide remains undefined due to their recent emergence, challenges in diagnosis and lack of comprehensive epidemiological studies needed to determine incidence in developing countries. Recently, the transfer of technological developments to other parts of the world especially developing countries has encouraged basic epidemiological inquiry and generated scientific interest in understanding the epidemiology of these tick borne diseases and their role as causes of undifferentiated febrile illnesses. In this chapter, we review the current knowledge of human monocytotropic ehrlichiosis (HME) and spotted fever rickettsiosis (African tick bite fever) in Cameroon.

2. Ehrlichiosis

2.1 Etiologic agents

Ehrlichioses are diseases caused by small (approximately 0.4–1.5 μm diameter) Gram negative, obligately intracellular bacteria belonging to the genus *Ehrlichia* of the family Anaplasmataceae, Order Rickettsiales and the alpha sub-division Proteobacteria (Dumler et al., 2001). Although they have a characteristic Gram negative cell wall structure, they lack the necessary enzymes to synthesize cell membrane components such as lipopolysaccharide and peptidoglycan (Lin & Rikihisa, 2003). As intracellular pathogens, *Ehrlichia* reside in cytoplasmic membrane-bound vacuoles inside host cells (granulocytes or monocytes) forming microcolonies called morulae, derived from the Latin word "morus" for mulberry (Popov et al., 1995; Paddock et al., 1997; Ismail et al., 2010). These morulae (ranging in size from 1.0 to 6.0 μm in diameter) may contain 1 to >40 organisms of uniform or mixed cell types (Popov et al., 1995; Rikihisa, 1999).

Organisms in the family *Anaplasmataceae* were first described in 1910 when Theiler described *Anaplasma marginale*, the etiologic agent of an economically important and severe disease of cattle (Mahan, 1995). This discovery was followed shortly thereafter by the description of *E. ruminantium* (formerly *Cowdria ruminantium*) by Cowdry in 1925; *E. canis* by Donatien and Lestoquard in 1935; and *A. phagocytophilum* (formerly *E. phagocytophila*) by Gordon in 1940. Hence, the genus *Ehrlichia* was established in 1945 in honour of the German microbiologist Paul Ehrlich (Uilenberg, 1983).

Ehrlichia species cause significant diseases in their natural hosts (livestock and companion animals) and emerging zoonoses in humans (McBride & Walker, 2010). The first human ehrlichial infection (sennetsu fever) was reported in 1953 (Rapmund, 1984; Dumler et al., 2007). Sennetsu fever, caused by *Neorickettsia sennetsu*, was identified in Japan and Malaysia (Dumler et al., 2001; Dumler et al., 2007). However, recent phylogenetic reclassifications based on molecular analysis revealed that *E. sennetsu* is not a member of the *Ehrlichia* genus (Dumler et al., 2001). Presently, the genus *Ehrlichia* consists of five recognized species including *E. canis, E. chaffeensis, E. ewingii, E. muris,* and *E. ruminantium,* all of which are at least 97.7% similar in 16S rRNA gene sequence (Perez et al., 1996; Paddock et al., 1997; Dumler et al., 2001; Perez et al., 2006).

Ehrlichiae have relatively small genomes (0.8–1.5 Mb) with low G+C content and a high proportion of non-coding sequences but can synthesize all nucleotides, vitamins and cofactors (Dunning et al., 2006). They also have small subsets of genes associated with host-pathogen interactions (Ismail et al., 2010). *E. chaffeensis* have immunodominant outer membrane proteins (OMP-1/MSP2/P28) (Ohashi et al., 1998; Yu et al., 2000; Huang et al., 2008), and in infected macrophages ehrlichiae express the p28-Omp 19 and 20 genes as dominant protein products (Ganta et al., 2009; Peddireddi et al., 2009). Ehrlichiae also express several targets of the humoral immune response including tandem repeat and ankyrin repeat containing proteins (Yu et al., 1997; Sumner et al., 1999; McBride et al., 2003; McBride et al., 2007). *E. chaffeensis*, a human pathogen that was first recognised in the United States in 1986 and isolated in 1991 (Maeda et al., 1987; Dawson et al., 1991) is the cause of human monocytotropic ehrlichiosis (HME) (Anderson et al., 1992), a moderate to severe disease with a case fatality rate of 3% (Fishbein et al., 1994; McBride & Walker, 2010). *E. chaffeensis* is an obligately intracellular bacterium that primarily infects mononuclear leukocytes and replicates by binary fission. *E. chaffeensis* morulae can be detected in peripheral blood smears obtained from infected patients when observed with a light microscope (Rikihisa, 1991). When tissues (including clinical samples), mononuclear leucocytes or cell lines of mammalian origin infected with *E. chaffeensis* are viewed by electron microscopy, two distinct morphologic cell types are identified: a predominantly coccoid form which has a centrally condensed nucleoid DNA and ribosomes (dense-cored cells) measuring between 0.4 and 0.6 μm in diameter and reticulate or the coccobacillary form, which measures about 0.4 to 0.6 μm by 0.7 to 1.9 μm (Paddock et al., 1995; Popov et al., 1997).

2.2 Vectors and reservoirs

Investigative studies following the discovery of *E. chaffeensis* in the late 1980s revealed that the agent is transmitted to humans by the tick *Amblyomma americanum*, commonly referred to as the lone star tick which has a limited geographic distribution to the United States (Anderson et al., 1993). Molecular analysis (PCR) has demonstrated *E. chaffeensis* DNA in adult *A. americanum* ticks collected from different states. The increased recognition of *E. chaffeensis* as an emerging problem has evoked renewed interest in this and other tick borne diseases, and this has stimulated epidemiologic investigations of this pathogen and its vector in other regions where the tick *A. americanum* is not found. Results not only indicate that *E. chaffeensis* has a wider distribution than the United States (Ndip et al., 2010), but also indicates that the pathogen exists outside of the known range of *A. americanum* and is harbored by other tick species. These tick species include *Ixodes pacificus* in California (Kramer et al., 1999), *Dermacentor variabilis* in Missouri (Roland et al., 1998), *Ixodes ricinus* in Russia (Alekseev et al., 2001), *Amblyomma testudinarium* in China, (Cao et al., 2000), *Haemaphysalis longicornis* (Lee et al., 2003), and *Ixodes persulcatus* (Kim et al., 2003) in Korea.

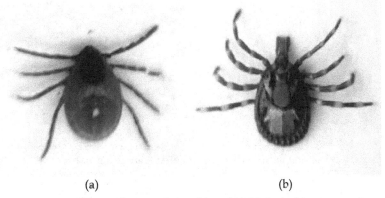

(a) (b)

Fig. 1. a) *Rhipicephalus sanguineus* (brown dog tick) and b) Male *Amblyomma variegatum* tick (courtesy Laboratory for Emerging Infectious Diseases, University of Buea)

Studies carried out by Ndip and colleagues in Cameroon identified *Ehrlichia chaffeensis* in *Rhipicephalus sanguineus* ticks. *R. sanguineus*, commonly known as the brown dog tick (Figure 1a) is a species that infests canids worldwide. In one study in Limbe, Cameroon, a very high prevalence of *E. chaffeensis* was detected in *R. sanguineus* ticks infesting dogs inhabiting one kennel (Ndip et al., 2010). *E. chaffeensis* DNA was detected in 33 (56%) of 63 *R. sanguineus* ticks collected from five dogs as opposed to 4 (6%) ticks infected with *E. canis*. Furthermore, co-infection with more than one pathogen was not uncommon. The *E. chaffeensis* strain circulating in Cameroon is similar to the North American strain AF403710 based on the analysis of the 378 bp fragment of the disulphide bond formation (Dsb) protein gene (Ndip et al., 2010). Earlier reports revealed *E. canis*, *E. chaffeensis*, and *E. ewingii* in *R. sanguineus* ticks collected from 51 dogs from different localities in Cameroon (Figure 2), suggesting that dogs could be a reservoir for *E. chaffeensis* and that *R. sanguineus* is the probable vector (Ndip et al., 2007).

In the United States, the white-tailed deer (*Odocoileus virginianus*) has been recognised as the primary natural reservoir of *E. chaffeensis* (Dugan et al., 2000). However, animals such as goats, dogs, and coyotes have also been identified as reservoirs which could play a limited role in the transmission of the pathogen to humans (Breitschwerdt et al., 1998; Dugan et al., 2000; Kocan et al., 2000). Unlike rickettsial species, ehrlichial species are not transmitted trans-ovarially (ie., larvae are uninfected) suggesting that the pathogen is maintained transstadially after the infection is acquired (Ismail et al., 2010). Although the reservoirs for *E. chaffeensis* in Cameroon have not yet been conclusively identified, preliminary studies detected antibodies reactive to *E. chaffeensis* in 56% of goats analysed suggesting a probable role of goats in maintaining the pathogen in nature. Moreover, *E. chaffeensis* DNA was detected in 17% of ticks collected from these animals (Ndip, unpublished data).

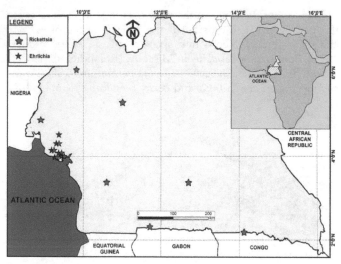

Fig. 2. Known distribution of ehrlichiae and rickettsiae in Cameroon

2.3 Clinical manifestations

The comprehensive data available in literature today on symptoms observed in HME infection is based on cases reported to the United States' Centers for Disease Control and Prevention in addition to a series of patients studied since the disease was described. After exposure to an infecting tick, an incubation period of 1 to 2 weeks (median, 9 days) ensues after which patients develop a febrile illness (often >39°C) characterized by general malaise, low-back pain, or gastrointestinal symptoms (Paddock & Childs, 2003). These signs and symptoms most often resemble manifestations caused by other infectious and non-infectious causes. After 3 to 4 days, symptoms progress and patients may seek medical attention presenting with fever (>95%), headache (60 to 75%), myalgias (40 to 60%), nausea (40 to 50%), arthralgias (30 to 35%), and malaise (30 to 80%) (Fishbein et al., 1994).

Some patients (10-40%) may present with cough, pharyngitis, diarrhea, or abdominal pain and may even progress to changes in mental status (Fishbein et al., 1994; Olano et al., 2003). Some populations especially HIV-infected patients (Paddock et al., 2001) and children (Jacobs & Schutze, 1997) may develop a rash on the extremities, trunk and face (Edwards, 1991). Hematological changes include leukopenia in approximately 60 to 70% of patients and thrombocytopenia (Fishbein et al., 1994; Olano & Walker, 2002). Liver enzymes (hepatic transaminases) may become slightly elevated (Nutt & Raufman, 1999). About 60 to 70% of patients require hospitalization and untreated cases last for 2-3 weeks or progress to a fatal outcome during the second week (Fishbein et al., 1994; Standaert et al., 2000). About 20% of patients develop neurologic signs, cough or other respiratory symptoms (Fishbein et al., 1994; Olano et al., 2003). Case-fatality ratio is approximately 3% (McQuiston et al., 2003) with risk factors for severe or fatal disease including older age (Paddock et al., 2001), underlying debilitating diseases such as HIV infection, immunosuppressive therapies (Olano & Walker, 2002) and sickle cell disease (Paddock & Childs, 2003).

These reported symptoms are quite similar to those manifested by Cameroonian HME patients. In one series of 206 acutely ill patients studied, 30 (14.6%) demonstrated anti-ehrlichial IgM antibodies, and these probable HME patients presented with headache (83%), fatigue (37%), abdominal pain (47%), joint pain (60%), anorexia (37%) and diarrhoea (13%) in addition to fever (>38°C). Their mean hematocrit, AST and ALT values were 48±21%, 46±23% and 36± 21%, respectively. Five (17%) of the patients were anaemic while 10 (33%) and 5 (17%) had abnormal AST and ALT values, respectively (Ndip, unpublished data). In another series of 118 acutely ill febrile patients studied with HME diagnosed by detection of E. chaffeensis DNA in patient's blood (n=12), these patients presented with fever (100%), headache (seen in 72% of the patients), arthralgia (58%), myalgia (42%), cough (17%) and a diffuse maculopapular rash (17%). The rash was present on the trunk of one patient and the arms of another. One patient of the 12 with detectable E. chaffeensis DNA required hospitalization (see Table 1) (Ndip et al., 2009).

2.4 Epidemiology
The epidemiology and ecology of HME worldwide is not well documented. Since its description in 1986 more than 1000 cases of HME from at least 30 U.S. states have been reported to the Centers for Disease Control and Prevention in Atlanta, Georgia with nearly all occurring in the southeastern and south-central United States where the vector, A. americanum is common (Paddock & Childs, 2003; Dumler et al., 2007). However, the evidence of the disease and/or the pathogen is increasingly being reported in other parts of the world. This includes Africa (Uhaa et al., 1992; Brouqui et al., 1994; Ndip et al., 2009; Ndip et al., 2010), Israel (Dawson et al., 1991; Keysary et al., 1999; Brouqui & Dumler, 2000), Latin America (Gongora-Biachi et al., 1999; Calic et al., 2004;) and Asia (Heppner et al., 1997; Cao et al., 2000; Heo et al., 2002; Kim et al., 2003; Park et al., 2003, Lee & Chae, 2010).

In Cameroon, HME has been identified in patients along the coast of Cameroon, in Buea (4°10'0''N9°14'0''E), Limbe (4°01'N 9°13'13''E), Muyuka (4°43'18''N 9°38'27''E), Tiko (4°4'0''N 9°22'60''E), and Kumba (4°38'38'' N9°26'19''E) and the agent, E. chaffeensis, in ticks collected from Limbe (Figure 2). HME was observed in both males and females as well as in children and adults although results suggested that older age was a risk factor for the disease (Ndip et al., 2009). The majority of the patients were adults which suggests that exposure to infected ticks may have occurred during outdoor activities such as farming. Another risk factor is that of owning a companion or domestic animal since most Cameroonian HME patients indicated they had tick-infested pets and domestic animals.

2.5 Microbiological diagnosis
The diagnosis of HME requires specialized microscopy equipment and skills which are not readily available in many diagnostic laboratories. Several methods have been proposed for the diagnosis of HME (Paddock & Childs, 2003; Ismail et al., 2010), including serologic tests such as immunofluorescent assay (IFA), western immunoblot employing specific proteins or ehrlichial whole cell antigens or the recently developed Ehrlichia recombinant protein or peptide ELISA for detection of the antibody (Cardenas et al., 2007; Luo et al., 2010; O'Connor et al., 2010). Though these tests can be used to confirm diagnosis retrospectively, some patients may not sero-convert during the early days of the disease and cannot be diagnosed with serologic tests. However, collecting paired sera (at acute and convalescent phases of illness) is confirmatory as a four-fold rise in titer indicates current infection. However, this

always presents a problem because patients who recover may not return to the hospital for follow up. Moreover, another issue with the interpretation of serological tests such as IFA is cross-reactive antibodies against other organisms, including *Anaplasma* species. PCR has also been employed to identify ehrlichial DNA in acutely ill patients when antibodies have not reached detectable levels. Several genes have been proposed and used including the VLPT gene (TRP32), TRP36, 16S rRNA, the TRP120, the Dsb, 28-kDa outer membrane protein gene have been used as genus or species specific targets (Yu et al., 1999; Doyle et al., 2005). IFA, western blot and PCR have been used to study the prevalence of ehrlichiae in blood of acutely ill patients, reservoirs, or in suspected tick vectors and anti-ehrlichial antibody in sera (Ndip et al., 2005; Ndip et al., 2007; Ndip et al., 2009; Ndip et al., 2010). Figure 3 shows IFA photomicrographs of whole cell of *E. chaffeensis* reacting with antibodies in an HME patient serum. A rapid method to detect *E. chaffeensis* is the observation of morulae in smears of peripheral blood buffy coat using the Diff Quik or Giemsa stain. However, this technique is very insensitive, and morulae are detected in leukocytes in only 10% of HME patients.

Patients	1	2	3	4	5	6	7	8	9	10	11	12
Gender	F	F	M	F	M	M	F	M	F	F	M	M
Age (yr)	63	40	5	23	22	20	21	1	16	26	35	25
Location	A	B	C	D	C	D	A	C	A	A	B	A
Clinical Manifestations												
Fever >38°C	Yes	Yes	Yes	Yes	Yes	Yes	Yes	Yes	Yes	Yes	Yes	Yes
*Day(s)	6	8	4	7	4	3	1	1	2	7	2	2
Headache	Yes	Yes	Yes	No	No	Yes	Yes	No	Yes	Yes	Yes	No
Myalgia	Yes	Yes	No	No	No	Yes	No	No	Yes	No	Yes	No
Arthralgia	Yes	Yes	No	No	No	Yes	Yes	No	Yes	Yes	Yes	No
Rash	No	No	No	Yes	No	No	No	Yes	No	No	No	No

*Days after onset (i.e., before collection of sample).
Locations: A - Buea , B – Limbe, C – Tiko, D - Muyuka

Table 1. Epidemiologic and clinical characteristics of twelve Cameroonian patients with HME

2.6 Treatment

The drug of choice for the treatment of *E. chaffeensis* infection is the tetracyclines (particularly doxycycline) and their derivatives. Generally, between 1 and 3 days after a patient with HME commences treatment with doxycycline, the patient becomes afebrile (Olano & Walker, 2002). However, treatment may continue for up to 10 days or at least 3 days after the patient becomes afebrile (Chapman et al., 2006). Clinical experience and *in-vitro* susceptibility testing of *E. chaffeensis* to some classes of antibiotics have revealed that fluoroquinolones, penicillins, aminoglycosides, macrolides and cotrimoxazole are not effective therapeutics (Dumler et al., 1993; Brouqui et al., 1994; Brouqui & Raoult, 1994; McBride & Walker, 2010).

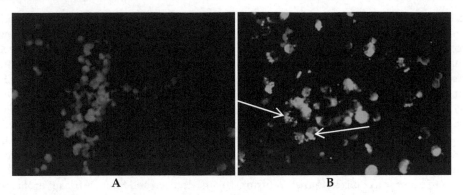

Fig. 3. Reactions of patient serum with *Ehrlichia chaffeensis* antigen and staining with Fluorescein isothiocynate (FITC)-labelled goat, IgG anti-human antibody (X40 magnification). **A**: Negative IFA slide, no inclusion bodies in cells. **B**: Positive IFA slide with morulae in monocytes (arrows) (Courtesy Laboratory for Emerging Infectious Diseases, University of Buea).

3. Rickettsiosis

3.1 The Genus *Rickettsia*

Rickettsial organisms are Gram-negative bacteria belonging to the order Rickettsiales, Family Rickettsiaceae and the Genus *Rickettsia*. They are strict intracellular parasites that are transmitted by arthropods including fleas, lice, mites and ticks (Kelly et al., 1992). These organisms are typically short rods (coccobacilli) measuring about 0.8-2.0µm in length and 0.3-0.5µm in diameter. They exhibit most of the biochemical and morphological characteristics of the Gram-negative cell (Gimenez, 1964; La Scola & Raoult, 1997). Based on antigenic characteristics, species of the genus *Rickettsia* have been divided into three groups; namely the typhus group (TG), the spotted fever group (SFG) and the transitional group (TRG). The TG has two members (*R. prowazekii* and *R. typhi*), which are mainly transmitted by lice and fleas, respectively (Raoult & Roux, 1997). The largest of the antigenic groups is the SFG that is made up of the tick-transmitted pathogens (except *R. bellii* and *R. canadensis*) (Parola et al., 2005). It has been grouped into several genogroups based on the *16S rRNA*, the *gltA*, *ompA*, *ompB* and *sca2* sequences. These groups include the *R. rickettsii* group, the *R. massiliae* group and *R. helvetica* group. The transitional group includes *R. akari*, *R. australis*, and *R. felis*. There are many ancestral organisms including *R. canadensis* and *R. bellii* (Parola et al., 2005), as well as numerous rickettsiae in herbivorous insects, and other hosts (leaches and amoeba). Also in the family Rickettsiaceae is *Orientia tsutsugamushi*, which is transmitted by *Leptotrombidium deliense* (Tamura et al., 1995).

Rickettsial organisms are of worldwide occurrence, although species/vector differences may exist along various geographical lines. In Africa, several species have been reported. These include *R. conorii* Malish strain, the cause of Mediterranean spotted fever or "boutonneuse fever". It was first documented in Tunis (Conor & Bruch, 1910), and today the disease continues to be reported in Tunisia (Romdhane et al., 2009; Sfar et al., 2009) and South Africa. The infection has the characteristic of a papular rash, in addition to an eschar at the site of the tick bite (Anton et al., 2003). The pathogen is transmitted by *R. sanguineus* ticks, and is considered an urban disease (Font & Segura, 1983). Human infections with another strain of *R. conorii* (Israeli spotted fever strain) have been recently documented in Tunisia (Znazen et al., 2011). *R. conorii* Astrakhan strain is the cause of Astrakhan fever first detected in Astrakhan, Russia in the 1970s and transmitted by *R. sanguineus* and *R. pumilio* ticks (Parola et al., 2005). The Astrakhan strain has also been isolated from a patient in Chad (Fournier et al., 2003). *R. sibirica* mongolitimonae strain was identified in *Hyalomma truncatum* ticks in Niger in 2001 (Parola et al., 2001) and the first human case in Africa was documented in South Africa (Pretorius & Birtles, 2004). Other cases have been reported to have been acquired in Algeria (Fournier et al., 2005) and Egypt (Socolovschi et al., 2010). Another species, *R. aeschlimannii*, which was first isolated in *H. marginatum* ticks in Morocco (Beati et al., 1997) and later detected in *H. marginatum rufipes* in Mali and Niger, have been known to cause infections in tourists returning from Morocco and South Africa (Parola et al., 2001). *R. massiliae*, first isolated from *R. sanguineus* ticks in Marseille, France (Parola et al., 2005) was detected in *R. muhsame*, *R. lunalatus* and *R. sulcatus* from Central African Republic (Dupont et al., 1994) and in *R. muhsame* ticks collected from cattle in Mali 2001) and Ivory Coast (Berrelha et al., 2009). *Rickettsia felis* is a recently identified pathogen which was first detected in *Ctenocephalides felis* fleas (Bouyer et al., 2001). In Africa, the agent has been reported in Ivory Coast (Berrelha et al., 2009) and Senegal (Socolovsch et al., 2010), and human infections have been reported in Kenya (Richards et al., 2010). *Rickettsia africae*, the etiologic agent of African tick bite fever appears to be the most prevalent rickettsiosis in Africa. The disease was first reported in Mozambique and South Africa (McQuiston et al., 2004). The first isolate (*R. africae* strain ESF-5), was recovered from *A. variegatum* ticks in Ethiopia although it was only characterized as *R. africae* later (Roux et al., 1996). The agent was later isolated in *A. hebraeum* ticks in Zimbabwe in 1990, and in 1992, the first isolate from a patient was obtained (Kelly et al., 1991; Kelly et al., 1994). The pathogen has been detected in many other African countries including Senegal (Mediannikov et al., 2010), Ethiopia (Stephany et al., 2009) and Cameroon (Ndip et al., 2004a; Ndip et al., 2004b). In the following, we give a synopsis of our current knowledge of African tick bite fever in Cameroon.

3.2 Causative organism
R. africae, a member of the SFG is the only species that has been detected in Cameroon. The organism which measures about 0.4 μm by 1.0 μm, has an outer slime layer and a trilaminar cell wall which contains immunogenic lipopolysaccharide antigens responsible for cross-reactivity with the other SFG rickettsiae (Hechemy et al., 1989; Kelly et al., 1996). Like other Gram-negative organisms, rickettsiae have outer membrane proteins (dubbed OmpA and OmpB) present as species-specific antigens (Fournier et al., 1998; Roux & Raoult, 2000). The organism lives freely in the cytoplasm and usually infects endothelial cells. According to phylogenetic studies, this rickettsial species, which belongs to the *R. rickettsii* group is closely related to *R. parkeri* in North America and *R. sibirica* in northeast Asia (Parola et al., 2005).

3.3 Tick vectors and reservoirs
R. africae is a tick-borne pathogen, and ticks serve both as vectors and reservoirs. The pathogen is maintained in the tick through trans-stadial and trans-ovarial transmission, and this situation indicates the potential for transmission to humans by all stages (larvae, nymphs, and adults) of the feeding ticks. Ixodid ticks (hard ticks) of the genus *Amblyomma* have been recognized as the vectors (Kelly, 2001). In Cameroon, *A. variegatum* (Figure 1b)

has been identified as the potential vector with about 75% of ticks (male and female) collected from cattle found to be infected with *R. africae* (Ndip et al., 2004b). Reports from other studies have indicated that *R. africae* infection in *Amblyomma* ticks frequently has a high prevalence (up to 100%) reported in ticks collected in some disease-endemic countries (Dupont et al., 1994; Parola et al., 2001). Like any other tick borne disease, the ecological characteristics of the vector influence the epidemiology of the disease. The ticks are usually found all year round, but they peak during and after the rainy season when humidity is very high (Walker et al., 2003). *Ambylomma* are predominantly cattle ticks, and infestation of cattle can be very high (Kelly & Mason, 1991). *A. variegatum*, commonly found in central and west Africa typically enjoys a wide variety of different habitats although they have a preference for semi-arid and humid areas with tall grass, trees, and/or bush cover. These ticks usually quest on vegetation and would usually attack legs although they may crawl to other areas such as groin and perineum where they attach (Jensenius et al., 2003).

3.4 Clinical presentation
Since the description of ATBF in 1992, most of the knowledge available regarding the disease has been documented in travelers who become infected with *R. africae* during travel in Africa. After inoculation from a tick bite, the bacteria invade the vascular endothelial system causing a focal or disseminated vasculitis. Endothelial cells of small blood vessels become infected leading to the destruction of the endothelial cells (Toutous-Trellu et al., 2003) of the host where they have multiplied and eventually injured the host cells, leading to the disease symptoms. Multiple eschars typical of ATBF develop at the sites of tick bite, and following an incubation period between 5 and 7 days (up to two weeks in some cases), after the tick bite a febrile illness develops (Raoult et al., 2001). In most cases, symptoms of ATBF are usually mild and include headaches, nausea, chills, myalgia, lymphadenopathy and prominent neck ache (Jensenius et al., 2003; Raoult et al., 2001). Although there have been some controversies over the differences in the clinical presentations of African tick bite fever, our study of acutely ill patients in Cameroon revealed that the some individuals may manifest severe symptoms while in others the symptoms are mild. However, symptoms reported include fever >38°C (100%), headache (71%), myalgia (71%), arthralgia (57%), rash (15%) and pulmonary signs (28%).

3.5 Epidemiology
ATBF has been recognized as an emerging problem in sub-Saharan Africa, especially for international travelers to rural areas (Jensenius et al., 2003). Most of the victims reported are tourists who visit game reserves or participate in outdoor activities such as running, trekking and hiking in forested areas, usually inhabited by *Amblyomma* ticks. The patients acquire the disease in rural Africa, but most often symptoms manifest only after they have returned to their various countries in Europe and America. The first report suggesting that rickettsiosis could be prevalent in Cameroon was published in 1968 (Maurice et al., 1968). The report based on a serologic survey that used an unreliable technique demonstrated rickettsial antibodies in cattle and humans in the northern region of Cameroon and in other animals in the south of the country (Maurice et al., 1968; Le et al., 1977). Efforts to determine the epidemiology and ecology later re-emerged in 2004 when anti-rickettsial IgM antibodies were detected in some Cameroonian patients along the coastal region of Cameroon (Ndip et

al., 2004a). These results were further confirmed by detection of *R. africae* DNA in about 6% of acutely ill febrile patients (Ndip et al., 2004b). Human infections or the agent has been detected in all regions of southern Cameroon where epidemiologic investigations have been made (Figure 3). According to these studies, age appeared to be a risk factor of acquiring the disease, and it is suggested that activities such as game hunting usually constitutes a risk factor (Ndip et al., 2011). Other activities which could predispose to infection include cattle rearing and exposure to tick habitats.

Cameroon is a sub-saharan tropical country with a vast equatorial forest providing a good habitat for ticks (especially *A. variegatum* ticks). Individuals residing in lowland rainforest habitats have a higher risk of acquiring ATBF probably because these habitats are ideal for *A. variegatum* ticks because of their moderate canopy cover, providing microclimates favoring tick survival (Ndip et al., 2011). Although ATBF has been shown to be prevalent in the southern part of Cameroon (Figure 2), the actual epidemiology of the disease through wider disease surveillance needs to be documented.

3.6 Diagnosis

Diagnosis of ATBF can be achieved by either serological analysis of acute and convalescent serum samples or molecular detection of the DNA of the bacterium by real-time or conventional PCR. Target genes that have been utilized include the rickettsial *gltA* and *ompA* genes. For serological diagnosis, the indirect immunofluorescent test has been used in conjunction with western blot assay to detect antibodies reactive with whole cells or specific proteins of cell lysates of *R. africae*. However, these tests are not very reliable in distinguishing species because cross-reactivity may be observed among the SFG rickettsiae. However, some authors have proposed that a fourfold or greater titer for *R. africae* compared to other species is confirmatory (Raoult et al., 2001; Ndip et al., 2004a). The western immunoblot assay can also be used to detect antibodies against species-specific OmpA and OmpB proteins.

3.7 Treatment

The drug of choice for the treatment of ATBF is doxycycline (100 mg twice daily) for 3-7 days. *In-vitro* studies also indicate that *R. africae* is susceptible to tetracyclines, fluoroquinolones, some macrolides and chloramphenicol (Rolain et al., 1998). Mild cases of ATBF have also been shown to recover naturally (Jensenius et al., 1999).

4. Prevention of ehrlichiosis and rickettsiosis

Studies in Cameroon indicate that one risk factor for contracting *E. chaffeensis* infection and ATBF appears to be exposure to potential tick vectors. Many reports involving acquisition of rickettsial diseases have also indicated that exposure to ticks during safari tours and visit to parks constitute an important risk factor. Therefore, an important method of preventing ehrlichiosis and rickettsiosis is by reducing contact with infected ticks. Personal protective measures are quite important, including wearing light colored clothes when walking in tick infested areas, using insect repellents and examination of clothing after a visit to a tick infested area, and prompt removal of attached tick can all reduce the risk of infection. Companion animals and other domesticated animals should be taken care of and tick infestation controlled.

4.1 Conclusions

These data emphasize the importance of ehrlichiosis and ATBF as prevalent diseases in an indigenous Cameroonian population. Although these diseases present as febrile illnesses, they are rarely considered when evaluating patients with acute, undifferentiated febrile illnesses. This situation can be attributed in part to lack of adequate knowledge of the epidemiology and ecology of the disease to prompt diagnosis; unavailability of specific laboratory tests, equipment, and expertise and also the limited economic resources. Sharing new knowledge on these diseases and techniques to facilitate diagnosis are important factors that can change the types and frequencies of diseases diagnosed in febrile patients and necessitate surveillance for these diseases. Future efforts will attempt to address other issues requiring investigations such as the full description of the clinical spectrum of these diseases in African patients and risk factors for severe illness.

5. References

Alekseev, A.N., Dubinina, H.V., Semenov, A.V. & Bolshakov, C.V. (2001). Evidence of ehrlichiosis agents found in ticks (Acari: Ixodidae) collected from migratory birds. *Journal of Medical Entomolology*. 38 : 471-474.

Anderson, B.E., Sims, K.G., Olson, J.G., Childs, J.E., Piesman, J.F., Happ, C.M., Maupin, G.O. & Johnson, B.J. (1993). *Amblyomma americanum*: a potential vector of human ehrlichiosis. *American Journal of Tropical Medicine & Hygiene*. 49:239-244.

Anderson, B.E., Sumner, J.W., Dawson, J.E., Tzianabos, T., Greene, C.R., Olson, J.G., Fishbein, D.B., Olsen-Rasmussen, M., Holloway, B.P., George, E.H., et al. (1992). Detection of the etiologic agent of human ehrlichiosis by polymerase chain reaction. *Journal of Clinical Microbiology*. 30: 775-780.

Anton, E., Font, B., Munoz, T., Sanfeliu, I. & Segura, F. (2003). Clinical and laboratory characteristics of 144 patients with Mediterranean spotted fever. *European Journal of Clinical Microbiology & Infectious Diseases*. 22:126-128.

Beati, L., Meskini, M., Thiers, B. & Raoult, D. (1997). *Rickettsia aeschlimannii* sp. nov., a new spotted fever group rickettsia associated with *Hyalomma marginatum* ticks. *International Journal of Systematic Bacteriology*. 47:548-554.

Berrelha, J., Briolant, S., Muller, F., Rolain, J.M., Marie, J.L., Pages, F., Raoult, D. & Parola, P. (2009). *Rickettsia felis* and *Rickettsia massiliae* in Ivory Coast, Africa. *Clinical Microbiology & Infection*. 15: 251-252.

Bouyer, D.H., Stenos, J., Crocquet-Valdes, P., Moron, C.G., Popov, V.L., Zavala-Velazquez, J.E., Foil, L.D., Stothard, D.R., Azad, A.F. & Walker, D.H. (2001). *Rickettsia felis*: molecular characterization of a new member of the spotted fever group. *International Journal of Systematic Bacteriology*. 51: 339-347.

Breitschwerdt, E.B., Hegarty, B.C. & Hancock, S.I. (1998). Sequential evaluation of dogs naturally infected with *Ehrlichia canis, Ehrlichia chaffeensis, Ehrlichia equi, Ehrlichia ewingii*, or *Bartonella vinsonii*. *Journal of Clinical Microbiology*. 36:2645-2651.

Brouqui, P. & Dumler, J.S. (2000). Serologic evidence of human monocytic and granulocytic ehrlichiosis in Israel. *Emerging Infectious Diseases*. 6:314-315.

Brouqui, P., Le, C.C., Kelly, P.J., Laurens, R., Tounkara, A., Sawadogo, S., Velo, M., Gondao, L., Faugere, B., Delmont, J., et al. (1994). Serologic evidence for human ehrlichiosis in Africa. *European Journal of Epidemiology*. 10:695-698.

Brouqui, P. & Raoult, D. (1994). Human ehrlichiosis. *New England Journal of Medicine.* 330:1760-1761.

Calic, S.B., Galvao, M.A., Bacellar, F., Rocha, C.M., Mafra, C.L., Leite, R.C. & Walker, D.H. (2004). Human ehrlichioses in Brazil: first suspect cases. *Brazilian Journal of Infectious Diseases.* 8: 259-262.

Cao, W.C., Gao, Y.M., Zhang, P.H., Zhang, X.T., Dai, Q.H., Dumler, J.S., Fang, L.Q. & Yang, H. (2000). Identification of *Ehrlichia chaffeensis* by nested PCR in ticks from Southern China. *Journal of Clinical Microbiology.* 38: 2778-2780.

Cardenas, A.M., Doyle, C.K., Zhang, X., Nethery, K., Corstvet, R.E., Walker, D.H. & McBride, J.W. (2007). Enzyme-linked immunosorbent assay with conserved immunoreactive glycoproteins gp36 and gp19 has enhanced sensitivity and provides species-specific immunodiagnosis of *Ehrlichia canis* infection. *Clinical &Vaccine Immunology.* 14:123-128.

Chapman, A.S., Bakken, J.S., Folk, S.M., Paddock, C.D., Bloch, K.C., Krusell, A., Sexton, D.J., Buckingham, S.C., Marshall, G.S., Storch, G.A., Dasch, G.A., McQuiston, J.H., Swerdlow, D.L., Dumler, S.J., Nicholson, W.L., Walker, D.H., Eremeeva, M.E. & Ohl, C.A. (2006). Diagnosis and management of tickborne rickettsial diseases: Rocky Mountain spotted fever, ehrlichioses, and anaplasmosis--United States: a practical guide for physicians and other health-care and public health professionals. *MMWR Recommended Report.* 55: (RR-4) 1-27.

Dawson, J.E., Anderson, B.E., Fishbein, D.B., Sanchez, J.L., Goldsmith, C.S., Wilson, K.H. & Duntley, C.W. (1991). Isolation and characterization of an *Ehrlichia* sp. from a patient diagnosed with human ehrlichiosis. *Journal of Clinical Microbiology.* 29:2741-2745.

Doyle, C.K., Labruna, M.B., Breitschwerdt, E.B., Tang, Y.W., Corstvet, R.E., Hegarty, B.C., Bloch, K.C., Li, P., Walker, D.H. & McBride, J.W. (2005). Detection of medically important *Ehrlichia* by quantitative multicolor TaqMan real-time polymerase chain reaction of the *dsb* gene. *Journal of Molecular Diagnostics.* 7: 504-510.

Dugan, V.G., Little, S.E., Stallknecht, D.E., & Beall, A.D. (2000). Natural infection of domestic goats with *Ehrlichia chaffeensis. Journal of Clinical Microbiology.* 38: 448-449.

Dumler, J.S., Barbet, A.F., Bekker, C.P., Dasch, G.A., Palmer, G.H., Ray, S.C., Rikihisa, Y. & Rurangirwa, F.R. (2001). Reorganization of genera in the families Rickettsiaceae and Anaplasmataceae in the order Rickettsiales: unification of some species of *Ehrlichia* with *Anaplasma, Cowdria* with *Ehrlichia* and *Ehrlichia* with Neorickettsia, descriptions of six new species combinations and designation of *Ehrlichia equi* and 'HGE agent' as subjective synonyms of *Ehrlichia phagocytophila. International Journal of Systematic Bacteriology.* 51:2145-2165.

Dumler, J.S., Madigan, J.E., Pusterla, N. & Bakken, J.S. (2007). Ehrlichioses in humans: epidemiology, clinical presentation, diagnosis, and treatment. *Clinical InfectiousDiseases.* 45:S45-S51.

Dumler, J.S., Sutker, W.L. & Walker, D.H. (1993). Persistent infection with *Ehrlichia chaffeensis. Clinical Infectious Diseases.* 17:903-905.

Dunning Hotopp, J.C., Lin, M., Madupu, R., Crabtree, J., Angiuoli, S.V., Eisen, J.A., Seshadri, R., Ren, Q., Wu, M., Utterback, T.R., Smith, S., Lewis, M., Khouri, H., Zhang, C., Niu, H., Lin, Q., Ohashi, N., Zhi, N., Nelson, W., Brinkac, L.M., Dodson, R.J., Rosovitz, M.J., Sundaram, J., Daugherty, S.C., Davidsen, T., Durkin, A.S., Gwinn,

M., Haft, D.H., Selengut, J.D., Sullivan, S.A., Zafar, N., Zhou, L., Benahmed, F., Forberger, H., Halpin, R., Mulligan, S., Robinson, J., White, O., Rikihisa, Y. & Tettelin, H. (2006). Comparative genomics of emerging human ehrlichiosis agents. *PLoS.Genetics.* 2 (2): e21.

Dupont, H.T., Cornet, J.P. & Raoult, D. (1994). Identification of rickettsiae from ticks collected in the Central African Republic using the polymerase chain reaction. *American Journal of Tropical Medicine &Hygiene.* 50:373-380.

Edwards, M.S. (1991). Human ehrlichiosis. *Advances in Pediatric Infectious Diseases.* 6:163-178.

Fishbein, D.B., Dawson, J.E. & Robinson, L.E. (1994). Human ehrlichiosis in the United States, 1985 to 1990. *Annals of Internal Medicine.* 120:736-743.

Font, C.B. & Segura, P.F. (1983). Mediterranean boutonneuse fever. *Medicina Clinica (Barcelona).* 80:182-186.

Fournier, P.E., Gouriet, F., Brouqui, P., Lucht, F. & Raoult, D. (2005). Lymphangitis-associated rickettsiosis, a new rickettsiosis caused by *Rickettsia sibirica mongolotimonae*: seven new cases and review of the literature. *Clinical Infectious Diseases.* 40:1435-1444.

Fournier, P.E., Roux, V. & Raoult, D. (1998). Phylogenetic analysis of spotted fever group rickettsiae by study of the outer surface protein rOmpA. *International Journal of Systematic Bacteriology.* 48:839-849.

Fournier, P.E., Xeridat, B. & Raoult, D. (2003). Isolation of a rickettsia related to Astrakhan fever rickettsia from a patient in Chad. *Annals of the New York Academy of Sciences.* 990: 152-157.

Ganta, R.R., Peddireddi, L., Seo, G.M., Dedonder, S.E., Cheng, C. & Chapes, S.K. (2009). Molecular characterization of *Ehrlichia* interactions with tick cells and macrophages. *Frontiers in Bioscience.* 14: 3259-3273.

Gongora-Biachi, R.A., Zavala-Velazquez, J., Castro-Sansores, C.J. & Gonzalez-Martinez, P. (1999). First case of human ehrlichiosis in Mexico. *Emerging Infectious Diseases.* 5:481.

Hechemy, K.E., Raoult, D., Fox, J., Han, Y., Elliott, L.B. & Rawlings, J. (1989). Cross-reaction of immune sera from patients with rickettsial diseases. *Journal of Medical Microbiology.* 29:199-202.

Heo, E.J., Park, J.H., Koo, J.R., Park, M.S., Park, M.Y., Dumler, J.S. & Chae, J.S. (2002). Serologic and molecular detection of *Ehrlichia chaffeensis* and *Anaplasma phagocytophila* (human granulocytic ehrlichiosis agent) in Korean patients. *Journal of Clinical Microbiology.* 40:3082-3085.

Heppner, D.G., Wongsrichanalai, C., Walsh, D.S., McDaniel, P., Eamsila, C., Hanson, B. & Paxton, H. (1997). Human ehrlichiosis in Thailand. *The Lancet.* 350:785-786.

Huang, H., Lin, M., Wang, X., Kikuchi, T., Mottaz, H., Norbeck, A. & Rikihisa, Y. (2008). Proteomic analysis of and immune responses to *Ehrlichia chaffeensis* lipoproteins. *Infection & Immunity.* 76:3405-3414.

Ismail, N., Bloch, K.C. & McBride, J.W. (2010). Human ehrlichiosis and anaplasmosis. *Clinical Laboratory Medicine.* 30:261-292.

Jacobs, R.F. & Schutze, G.E. (1997). Ehrlichiosis in children. *Journal of Pediatrics.* 131:184-192.

Jensenius, M., Fournier, P.E., Vene, S., Hoel, T., Hasle, G., Henriksen, A.Z., Hellum, K.B., Raoult, D. & Myrvang, B. (2003). African tick bite fever in travelers to rural sub-Equatorial Africa. *Clinical Infectious Diseases.* 36:1411-1417.

Jensenius, M., Hasle, G., Henriksen, A.Z., Vene, S., Raoult, D., Bruu, A.L. & Myrvang, B. (1999). African tick-bite fever imported into Norway: presentation of 8 cases. *Scandinavian Journal of Infectious Diseases*. 31:131-133.

Kelly, P., Matthewman, L., Beati, L., Raoult, D., Mason, P., Dreary, M. & Makombe, R. (1992). African tick-bite fever: a new spotted fever group rickettsiosis under an old name. *The Lancet*. 340: 982-983.

Kelly, P.J. (2001). *Amblyomma hebraeum* is a vector of *Rickettsia africae* and not *R. conorii*. *Journal of South African Veterinary Association*. 72:182.

Kelly, P.J., Beati, L., Mason, P.R., Matthewman, L.A., Roux, V. & Raoult, D. (1996). *Rickettsia africae* sp. nov., the etiological agent of African tick bite fever. *International Journal Systematic Bacteriology*. 46:611-614.

Kelly, P.J., Beati, L., Matthewman, L.A., Mason, P.R., Dasch, G.A. & Raoult, D. (1994). A new pathogenic spotted fever group rickettsia from Africa. *Journal of Tropical Medicine & Hygiene*. 97:129-137.

Kelly, P.J. & Mason, P.R. (1991). Transmission of a spotted fever group rickettsia by *Amblyomma hebraeum* (Acari: Ixodidae). *Journal of Medical Entomology*. 28:598-600.

Kelly, P.J., Raoult, D. & Mason, P.R. (1991). Isolation of spotted fever group rickettsias from triturated ticks using a modification of the centrifugation-shell vial technique. *Transactions of the Royal Society of Tropical Medicine & Hygiene*. 85:397-398.

Keysary, A., Amram, L., Keren, G., Sthoeger, Z., Potasman, I., Jacob, A., Strenger, C., Dawson, J.E. & Waner, T. (1999). Serologic evidence of human monocytic and granulocytic ehrlichiosis in Israel. *Emerging Infectious Diseases*. 5:775-778.

Kim, C.M., Kim, M.S., Park, M.S., Park, J.H. & Chae, J.S. (2003). Identification of *Ehrlichia chaffeensis, Anaplasma phagocytophilum,* and *A. bovis* in *Haemaphysalis longicornis* and *Ixodes persulcatus* ticks from Korea. *Vector Borne & Zoonotic Diseases*. 3:17-26.

Kocan, A.A., Levesque, G.C., Whitworth, L.C., Murphy, G.L., Ewing, S.A. & Barker, R.W. (2000). Naturally occurring *Ehrlichia chaffeensis* infection in coyotes from Oklahoma. *Emerging Infectious Diseases*. 6: 477-480.

Kramer, V.L., Randolph, M.P., Hui, L.T., Irwin, W.E., Gutierrez, A.G., & Vugia, D.J. (1999). Detection of the agents of human ehrlichioses in ixodid ticks from California. *American Journal of Tropical Medicine & Hygiene*. 60:62-65.

Le, N.P., Rickenbach, A., Ravisse, P. & Le, N.D. (1977). Serological survey of animal rickettsioses in Cameroon. II. Results of the survey. *Bulletin de la Societe de Pathologie Exotique et de ses Filiales*. 70: 410-421.

Lee, J.H., Park, H.S., Jung, K.D., Jang, W.J., Koh, S.E., Kang, S.S., Lee, I.Y., Lee, W.J., Kim, B.J., Kook, Y.H., Park, K.H. & Lee, S.H. (2003). Identification of the spotted fever group rickettsiae detected from *Haemaphysalis longicornis* in Korea. *Microbiology & Immunology*. 47:301-304.

Lee, M.J. & Chae, J.S. (2010). Molecular detection of *Ehrlichia chaffeensis* and *Anaplasma bovis* in the salivary glands from *Haemaphysalis longicornis* ticks. *Vector Borne Zoonotic Diseases*. 10:411-413.

Lin, M. & Rikihisa, Y. (2003). *Ehrlichia chaffeensis* and *Anaplasma phagocytophilum* lack genes for lipid A biosynthesis and incorporate cholesterol for their survival. *Infection & Immunity*. 71: 5324-5331.

Luo, T., Zhang, X., Nicholson, W.L., Zhu, B. & McBride, J.W. (2010). Molecular characterization of antibody epitopes of *Ehrlichia chaffeensis* ankyrin protein 200 and tandem repeat protein 47 and evaluation of synthetic immunodeterminants for serodiagnosis of human monocytotropic ehrlichiosis. *Clinical & Vaccine Immunology*. 17: 87-97 .

Maeda, K., Markowitz, N., Hawley, R.C., Ristic, M., Cox, D., & McDade, J.E. (1987). Human infection with *Ehrlichia canis*, a leukocytic rickettsia. *New England Journal of Medicine*. 316:853-856.

Mahan, S.M. (1995). Review of the molecular biology of *Cowdria ruminantium*. *Veterinary Parasitology*. 57:51-56.

Maurice, Y., Fernagut, R., & Gerome, R. (1968). Rickettsial diseases of North Cameroon; epidemiological study. *Revue d Elevage et de Medecine Veterinaire des Pays Tropicaux*. 21:341-349.

McBride, J.W., Comer, J.E. & Walker, D.H. (2003). Novel immunoreactive glycoprotein orthologs of *Ehrlichia spp*. *Annals of the New York Academy of Sciences*. 990:678-684.

McBride, J.W., Doyle, C.K., Zhang, X., Cardenas, A.M., Popov, V.L., Nethery, K.A. & Woods, M.E. (2007). Identification of a glycosylated *Ehrlichia canis* 19-kilodalton major immunoreactive protein with a species-specific serine-rich glycopeptide epitope. *Infection & Immunity*. 75:74-82.

McBride, J.W. & Walker, D.H. (2010). Progress and obstacles in vaccine development for the ehrlichioses. *Expert Review onVaccines*. 9:1071-1082 .

McQuiston, J.H., McCall, C.L. & Nicholson, W.L. (2003). Ehrlichiosis and related infections. *Journal of the American Veterinary Medical Association*. 223:1750-1756.

McQuiston, J.H., Paddock, C.D., Singleton, J., Jr., Wheeling, J.T., Zaki, S.R. & Childs, J.E. (2004). Imported spotted fever rickettsioses in United States travelers returning from Africa: a summary of cases confirmed by laboratory testing at the Centers for Disease Control and Prevention, 1999-2002. *American Journal of Tropical Medicine & Hygiene*. 70:98-101.

Mediannikov, O., Trape, J.F., Diatta, G., Parola, P., Fournier, P.E. & Raoult, D. (2010). *Rickettsia africae*, Western Africa. *Emerging Infectious Diseases*. 16:571-573.

Ndip, L.M., Bouyer, D.H., Travassos Da Rosa, A.P., Titanji, V.P., Tesh, R.B. & Walker, D.H. (2004a). Acute spotted fever rickettsiosis among febrile patients, Cameroon. *Emerging Infectious Diseases*. 10:432-437.

Ndip, L.M., Fokam, E.B., Bouyer, D.H., Ndip, R.N., Titanji, V.P., Walker, D.H. & McBride, J.W. (2004b). Detection of *Rickettsia africae* in patients and ticks along the coastal region of Cameroon. *American Journal of Tropical Medicine & Hygiene*. 71:363-366.

Ndip, L.M., Ndip, R.N., Esemu, S.N., Dickmu, V.L., Fokam, E.B., Walker, D.H. & McBride, J.W. (2005). Ehrlichial infection in Cameroonian canines by *Ehrlichia canis* and *Ehrlichia ewingii*. *Veterinary Microbiology*. 111:59-66.

Ndip, L.M., Ndip, R.N., Ndive, V.E., Awuh, J.A., Walker, D.H. & McBride, J.W. (2007). *Ehrlichia* species in *Rhipicephalus sanguineus* ticks in Cameroon. *Vector Borne & Zoonotic Diseases*. 7:221-227.

Ndip, L.M., Labruna, M., Ndip, R.N., Walker, D.H. & McBride, J.W. (2009). Molecular and clinical evidence of *Ehrlichia chaffeensis* infection in Cameroonian patients with undifferentiated febrile illness. *Annals of Tropical Medicine & Parasitology*. 103:19-725.

Ndip, L.M., Ndip, R.N., Esemu, S.N., Walker, D.H. & McBride, J.W. (2010). Predominance of *Ehrlichia chaffeensis* in *Rhipicephalus sanguineus* ticks from kennel-confined dogs in Limbe, Cameroon. *Experimental & Applied Acarology.* 50:163-168.

Ndip, L.M., Biswas, H.H., Nfonsam, L.E., LeBreton, M., Ndip, R.N., Bissong, M.A., Mpoudi-Ngole, E., Djoko, C., Tamoufe, U., Prosser, A.T., Burke, D.S. & Wolfe, N.D. (2011). Risk factors for African tick-bite fever in rural central Africa. *American Journal of Tropical Medicine &Hygiene.* 84:608-613.

Nutt, A.K. & Raufman, J. (1999). Gastrointestinal and hepatic manifestations of human ehrlichiosis: 8 cases and a review of the literature. *Digestive Diseases.* 17:37-43.

O'Connor, T.P., Saucier, J.M., Daniluk, D., Stillman, B.A., Krah, R., Rikihisa, Y., Xiong, Q., Yabsley, M.J., Adams, D.S., Diniz, P.P., Breitschwerdt, E.B., Gaunt, S.D. & Chandrashekar, R. (2010). Evaluation of peptide- and recombinant protein-based assays for detection of anti-*Ehrlichia ewingii* antibodies in experimentally and naturally infected dogs. *American Journal Veterinary Research.* 71: 1195-1200.

Ohashi, N., Zhi, N., Zhang, Y. & Rikihisa, Y. (1998). Immunodominant major outer membrane proteins of *Ehrlichia chaffeensis* are encoded by a polymorphic multigene family. *Infection & Immunity.* 66:132-139.

Olano, J.P. & Walker, D.H. (2002). Human ehrlichioses. *Medical Clinics of North America.* 86: 375-392.

Olano, J.P., Hogrefe, W., Seaton, B. & Walker, D.H. (2003). Clinical manifestations, epidemiology, and laboratory diagnosis of human monocytotropic ehrlichiosis in a commercial laboratory setting. *Clinical Diagnostic & Laboratory Immunology.* 10: 891-896.

Paddock, C.D., Sumner, J.W., Shore, G.M., Bartley, D.C., Elie, R.C., McQuade, J.G., Martin, C.R., Goldsmith, C.S. & Childs, J.E. (1997). Isolation and characterization of *Ehrlichia chaffeensis* strains from patients with fatal ehrlichiosis. *Journal of Clinical Microbiology.* 35:2496-2502.

Paddock, C.D., Folk, S.M., Shore, G.M., Machado, L.J., Huycke, M.M., Slater, L.N., Liddell, A.M., Buller, R.S., Storch, G.A., Monson, T.P., Rimland, D., Sumner, J.W., Singleton, J., Bloch, K.C., Tang, Y.W., Standaert, S.M. & Childs, J.E. (2001). Infections with *Ehrlichia chaffeensis* and *Ehrlichia ewingii* in persons coinfected with human immunodeficiency virus. *Clinical Infectious Diseases.* 33:1586-1594.

Paddock, C.D. & Childs, J.E. (2003). *Ehrlichia chaffeensis*: a prototypical emerging pathogen. *Clinical Microbiology Reviews.* 16: 37-64.

Park, J.H., Heo, E.J., Choi, K.S., Dumler, J.S. & Chae, J.S. (2003). Detection of antibodies to *Anaplasma phagocytophilum* and *Ehrlichia chaffeensis* antigens in sera of Korean patients by western immunoblotting and indirect immunofluorescence assays. *Clinical & Diagnostic Laboratory Immunology.* 10:1059-1064.

Parola, P., Inokuma, H., Camicas, J.L., Brouqui, P. & Raoult, D. (2001). Detection and identification of spotted fever group Rickettsiae and Ehrlichiae in African ticks. *Emerging Infectious Diseases.* 7:1014-1017.

Parola, P., Paddock, C.D. & Raoult, D. (2005). Tick-borne rickettsioses around the world: emerging diseases challenging old concepts. *Clinical Microbiology Reviews.* 18:719-756.

Peddireddi, L., Cheng, C. & Ganta, R.R. (2009). Promoter analysis of macrophage- and tick cell-specific differentially expressed *Ehrlichia chaffeensis p28-Omp* genes. *BMC Microbiology*. 9:99.

Perez, M., Bodor, M., Zhang, C., Xiong, Q. & Rikihisa, Y. (2006). Human infection with *Ehrlichia canis* accompanied by clinical signs in Venezuela. *Annals of the New York Academy of Sciences*. 1078:110-117.

Perez, M., Rikihisa, Y. & Wen, B. (1996). *Ehrlichia canis*-like agent isolated from a man in Venezuela: antigenic and genetic characterization. *Journal of Clinical Microbiology*. 34:2133-2139.

Popov, V.L., Chen, S.M., Feng, H.M. & Walker, D.H. (1995). Ultrastructural variation of cultured *Ehrlichia chaffeensis*. *Journal of Medical Microbiology*. 43:411-421.

Pretorius, A.M. & Birtles, R.J. (2004). *Rickettsia mongolotimonae* infection in South Africa. *Emerging Infectious Diseases*. 10:125-126.

Raoult, D., Fournier, P.E., Fenollar, F., Jensenius, M., Prioe, T., de Pina, J.J., Caruso, G., Jones, N., Laferl, H., Rosenblatt, J.E. & Marrie, T.J. (2001). *Rickettsia africae*, a tick-borne pathogen in travelers to sub-Saharan Africa. *New England Journal of Medicine*. 344: 504-1510.

Raoult, D. & Roux, V. (1997). Rickettsioses as paradigms of new or emerging infectious diseases. *Clinical Microbiology Reviews*. 10:694-719.

Rapmund, G. (1984). Rickettsial diseases of the Far East: new perspectives. *Journal of Infectious Diseases*. 149:330-338.

Richards, A.L., Jiang, J., Omulo, S., Dare, R., Abdirahman, K., Ali, A., Sharif, S.K., Feikin, D.R., Breiman, R.F. & Njenga, M.K. (2010). Human infection with *Rickettsia felis*, Kenya. *Emerging Infectious Diseases*. 16:1081-1086.

Rikihisa, Y. (1991). The tribe Ehrlichieae and ehrlichial diseases. *Clinical Microbiology Reviews*. 4:286-308.

Rikihisa, Y. (1999). Clinical and biological aspects of infection caused by *Ehrlichia chaffeensis*. *Microbes & Infection*. 1:367-376.

Rolain, J.M., Maurin, M., Vestris, G. & Raoult, D. (1998). *In vitro* susceptibilities of 27 rickettsiae to 13 antimicrobials. *Antimicrobial Agents & Chemotherapy*. 42:1537-1541.

Roland, W.E., Everett, E.D., Cyr, T.L., Hasan, S.Z., Dommaraju, C.B. & McDonald, G.A. (1998). *Ehrlichia chaffeensis* in Missouri ticks. *American Journal of Tropical Medicine & Hygiene*. 59:641-643.

Romdhane, F.B., Loussaief, C., Toumi, A., Yahia, S.B., Khaiyrallah, M., Bouzouaia, N. & Chakroun, M. (2009). Mediterranean spotted fever: a report of 200 cases in Tunisia. *Clinical Microbiology & Infection*. 15(S2):209-210.

Roux, V., Fournier, P.E. & Raoult, D. (1996). Differentiation of spotted fever group rickettsiae by sequencing and analysis of restriction fragment length polymorphism of PCR-amplified DNA of the gene encoding the protein rOmpA. *Journal of Clinical Microbiology*. 34:2058-2065.

Roux, V. & Raoult, D. (2000). Phylogenetic analysis of members of the genus Rickettsia using the gene encoding the outer-membrane protein rOmpB (*ompB*). *International Journal of Systematic and Evolutionary Microbiology*. 50:1449-1455.

Sfar, N., Kaabia, N., Letaief, A., Rolain, J.M., Parola, P., Bouattour, A. & Raoult, D. (2009). First molecular detection of *R. conorii* subsp. *conorii* 99 years after the Conor description of Mediterranean spotted fever, in Tunisia. *Clinical Microbiology & Infection*. 15(S2):309-310 .

Socolovschi, C., Barbarot, S., Lefebvre, M., Parola, P. & Raoult, D. (2010). *Rickettsia sibirica mongolitimonae* in traveler from Egypt. *Emerging Infectious Diseases*. 16:1495-1496.

Socolovschi, C., Mediannikov, O., Sokhna, C., Tall, A., Diatta, G., Bassene, H., Trape, J.F. & Raoult, D. (2010). *Rickettsia felis*-associated uneruptive fever, Senegal. *Emerging Infectious Diseases*. 16:1140-1142 .

Standaert, S.M., Yu, T., Scott, M.A., Childs, J.E., Paddock, C.D., Nicholson, W.L., Singleton, J., Jr. & Blaser, M.J. (2000). Primary isolation of *Ehrlichia chaffeensis* from patients with febrile illnesses: clinical and molecular characteristics. *Journal of Infectious Diseases*. 181:1082-1088.

Stephany, D., Buffet, P., Rolain, J.M., Raoult, D. & Consigny, P.H. (2009). *Rickettsia africae* infection in man after travel to Ethiopia. *Emerging Infectious Diseases*. 15:1867-1870.

Sumner, J.W., Childs, J.E. & Paddock, C.D. (1999). Molecular cloning and characterization of the *Ehrlichia chaffeensis* variable-length PCR target: an antigen-expressing gene that exhibits interstrain variation. *Journal of Clinical Microbiology*. 37:1447-1453.

Toutous-Trellu, L., Peter, O., Chavaz, P. & Saurat, J.H. (2003). African tick bite fever: not a spotless rickettsiosis! *Journal of the American Academy of Dermatology*. 48(2S):S18-S19.

Uhaa, I.J., MacLean, J.D., Greene, C.R. & Fishbein, D.B. (1992). A case of human ehrlichiosis acquired in Mali: clinical and laboratory findings. *American Journal of Tropical Medicine & Hygiene*. 46:161-164.

Uilenberg, G. (1983). Heartwater (*Cowdria ruminantium* infection): current status. *Advances in Veterinary Science & Comparative Medicine*. 27:427-480.

Yu, X.J., Crocquet-Valdes, P. & Walker, D.H. (1997). Cloning and sequencing of the gene for a 120-kDa immunodominant protein of *Ehrlichia chaffeensis*. *Gene*. 184:149-154.

Yu, X.J., McBride, J.W. & Walker, D.H. (1999). Genetic diversity of the 28-kilodalton outer membrane protein gene in human isolates of *Ehrlichia chaffeensis*. *Journal of Clinical Microbiology*. 37:1137-1143.

Yu, X., McBride, J.W., Zhang, X. & Walker, D.H. (2000). Characterization of the complete transcriptionally active *Ehrlichia chaffeensis* 28 kDa outer membrane protein multigene family. *Gene*. 2481-2):59-68.

Znazen, A., Hammami, B., Lahiani, D., Ben, J.M. & Hammami, A. (2011). Israeli spotted Fever, Tunisia. *Emerging Infectious Diseases*. 17:1328-1330.

6

Bartonella Infections in Rodents and Bats in Tropics

Ying Bai and Michael Kosoy
*Division of Vector-Borne Diseases, National Center for Emerging and
Zoonotic Infectious Diseases, Centers for Disease Control and Prevention
USA*

1. Introduction

Bacteria of genus *Bartonella* are mainly hemotropic, intracellular gram-negative bacteria associated with erythrocytes and endothelial cells of mammals and other vertebrates (Anderson & Neuman, 1997; Schülein et al., 2001). Members within the genus have been expanded during last three decades with over 30 species or subspecies having been described. In addition to the well-known human pathogens *B. bacilliformis* (agent of Carrión's disease), *B. quintana* (agent of trench fever), and *B. henselae* (agent of cat-scratch disease), a growing number of *Bartonella* species, such as *B. alsatica*, *B. elizabethae*, *B. grahamii*, *B. koehlerae*, *B. clarridgeiae*, *B. washoensis*, *B. vinsonii* subsp. *berkhoffii*, *B. vinsonii* subsp. *arupensis*, *B. tamiae*, and *B. rochalimae*, have been identified as human pathogens (Kordick et al., 1997; Margileth & Baehren, 1998; Kerkhoff et al., 1999; Welch et al., 1999; Roux et al., 2000; Sander et al., 2000; Kosoy et al., 2003 & 2008; Raoult et al., 2006; Eremeeva et al., 2007). Infections caused by these microorganisms have been encountered in vertebrates of virtually all species surveyed, which to date have extended to members of at least eight different orders of mammals, including Artiodactyla, Cetacea, Carnivora, Chiroptera, Insectivora, Lagomorpha, Primates, and Rodentia (Boulouis et al., 2005; Concannon et al., 2005; Maggi et al., 2005). Results have demonstrated that the prevalence of bacteremia can range from 0 to almost 100% in vertebrate populations. Persistent infections in domestic and wild animals result in a substantial reservoir of bartonellae in nature. Several mammalian species, such as rodents, cats, and dogs are reservoir hosts of some of these pathogenic *Bartonella* species. However, animal reservoirs remain unknown for some newly identified human *Bartonella* species, such as *B. tamiae* and *B. rochalimae*. Knowledge of the transmission of *Bartonella* bacteria between mammalian hosts is incomplete. However, hematophagous arthropods, such as fleas, flies, lice, mites, and ticks, have been found naturally infected and are frequently implicated in transmitting *Bartonella* species (Baker, 1946; Garcia-Caceres & Garcia, 1991; Chomel et al., 1995& 1996; Higgins et al., 1996; Pappalardo et al., 1997; Roux & Raoult, 1999; Welch et al., 1999).

Bartonella infections can cause a wide spectrum of emerging and reemerging diseases, ranging from a short-term fever that resolves quickly on its own to potentially fatal diseases with cardiovascular, nervous system, or hepatosplenic involvement (Anderson & Neuman, 1997; Koehler, 1996). These findings have shown the emerging medical importance of bartonellae. In fact, bartonella infections have become a big world-wide issue. This review presents the current findings of bartonella infections in rodents and bats from tropics. We are proposing the urgent need to expand studies of bartonella infections in tropics for better understanding the ecology, reservoir potential, vector transmission, pathogenesis of bartonellosis, and their roles in tropical medicine.

2. Bartonella infections in rodents in tropics

The order Rodentia contains over 2,000 species and makes up the largest group of mammals. Rodents can carry many different zoonotic pathogens, such as *Leptospira, Yersinia pestis, Toxoplasma gondii, Campylobacter,* and *Bartonella* species. With their broad distribution and close contact with humans, rodents play an important role in serving as natural reservoir hosts of these zoonotic pathogens. The first *Bartonella* species found in rodents was isolated from the blood of the vole *Microtus pennsylvanicus.* Originally described as a rickettsial agent (Baker, 1946), this bacterium was later reclassified as *Bartonella vinsonii* (Weiss & Dasch, 1982). During the last three decades, numerous surveys have been conducted in a variety of rodent communities at many locations. These surveys demonstrated that bartonellae are widely distributed in rodents of numerous species in all continents (Birtles et al.,1994; Kosoy et al., 1997; Heller et al., 1998; Hofmeister et al., 1998; Laakkonen et al., 1998; Bermond et al., 2000; Fichet-Calvet et al., 2000; Bajer et al., 2001; Bown et al., 2002; Holmberg et al., 2003; Engbaek & Lawson, 2004; Gundi et al., 2004; Pawelczyk et al., 2004; Pretorius et al., 2004; Tea et al., 2004; Jardine et al., 2005; Kim et al., 2005; Telfer et al., 2005; Markov et al., 2006; Knap et al., 2007).

The very first investigation of bartonella infection in rodents from tropic areas was conducted in Yunnan, a province located in southwestern China (Ying et al., 2002). This study revealed the important finding that *Rattus* rats are the reservoir hosts of *B. elizabethae,* a bartonella strain associating with human diseases. With this discovery, more investigations of bartonella infections in rodents were later carried out in several other tropical countries, including Bangladesh, Thailand, Vietnam, Indonesia, Kenya, and others (Castle et al., 2004; Winoto et al., 2005; Bai et al., 2007b & 2009b; Kosoy et al., 2009 & unpublished data). In this section, we compare the composition of rodent community, bartonella prevalence, and genetic diversity of the *Bartonella* strains, mainly based on three most complete studies that were conducted in southwestern China, Bangladesh, and Thailand (Ying et al., 2002; Bai et al., 2007b & 2009b). We discuss the epidemiological significance of these findings.

2.1 Rodent community

As an environment with a moderate climate, ample food, and plenty of water, the tropics harbor highly diverse rodent communities. The rodents tested for bartonella infections from different regions of tropics represented over 20 species of 10 genera, including *Apodemus chevrieri, A. draco, A. peninsulae, Bandicota bengalensis, B. indica, B. savilei, Berylmys berdmorei, Eothenomys miletus, Lemniscomys striatus, Mastomys natalensis, Mus caroli, M. cervicolor, M. minutoides, M. musculus, Rattus argentiventer, R. exulans, R. losea, R. nitidus, R. norvegicus, R. rattus, R. remotes, R. surifer,* and *R. tanezumi* subsp. *flavipectus.* Among these, rats of the genus *Rattus* were the most widely distributed and prevalent, being found in all study areas. For example, in the survey of bartonella infections in rodents from 17 provinces of Thailand, the total number of *Rattus* rats accounted for more than 80% of the tested rodents (Bai et al., 2009b); in studies in southwestern China and Bangladesh, more than 50% rodents also were

Rattus rats (Ying et al., 2002; Bai et al., 2007b). Nevertheless, the most common *Rattus* species varied among the study sites. In Thailand, the *R. rattus*, *R. norvegicus*, and *R. exulans* were the most common species; in southwestern China, *R. norvegicus* and *R. tanezumi* subsp. *flavipectus* were the most common species; and *R. rattus* were the most common species in Bangladesh (Table 1). In addition to *Rattus* rats, rats of the genus *Bandicota* also were commonly distributed in Bangladesh and Thailand. *Bandicota bengalensis*, for example, accounted for 41% in the local rodent community in Dhaka, Bangladesh, and were actually the most common species; *Bandicota indica* and *Bandicota savilei* accounted for 16% of all rodents in Thailand (Table 1). In fact, *Bandicota indica* alone accounted for 78% of tested rodents in another study conducted in Chiang Rai, a northern province of Thailand (Castle et al., 2004), indicating that *Bandicota* rats could be more common than *Rattus* rats in some areas in Thailand. Mice of the genus *Apodemus* were found more popular in rural areas in southwestern China, and accounted for 35% of local rodents. Rodents of some other genera, including *Mus*, *Berylmys*, and *Eothenomys* were also found in different areas but in smaller numbers.

2.2 Bartonella prevalence in rodents

Ecologic and bacteriologic observations of rodents in different regions of the world have shown the wide spread of bartonella infection in rats and mice of various species. Nevertheless, large variations in prevalence of infection have been observed among different studies and rodents of different genera, or even species, ranging from 0 to >80% (Birtles et al., 1994; Kosoy et al., 1997; Bai et al., 2009a & 2011). A possible explanation for such variation is the different composition of rodent communities in which the biodiversity can affect the prevalence in a local community (Bai et al., 2009a).

Similar observations were reported from studies of bartonella infection in rodents conducted in tropical areas. A relatively low prevalence of bartonella infection in rodents was reported from Kenya (15%) (Kosoy et al., 2009), while high prevalence was demonstrated in studies conducted in several countries of Southeast Asia. More interestingly, the overall prevalence of bartonella infection in rodents reported from these countries was very similar, with 42.8%, 44.5%, and 41.5% in Bangladesh, southwestern China, and Thailand, respectively (Ying et al., 2002; Bai et al., 2007b & 2009b), although composition of the rodent communities differed among the study sites.

Nevertheless, the bartonella prevalence varied by rodent species. Generally, rats of the genus *Rattus* are highly infected with *Bartonella* species. In Thailand, bartonella prevalence in *Rattus* rats was 43% with a range of 0-86% among eight investigated species. *R. norvegicus* and *R. rattus*, as the most common species present, exhibited very high prevalence of bartonella infection with 86% and 65% in each, respectively, while only 3% of another common tropical species, *R. exulans*, were infected with *Bartonella* species. In one southwestern China study, *Rattus tanezumi* subsp. *flavipectus* was the predominant species among the local rodents and also highly infected by *Bartonella* species with 41% prevalence. In addition to the variation in prevalence between rodent species, the same rat species can exhibit different degrees of susceptibility to infection with *Bartonella* species at different locations. For example, the infection rate in *R. rattus* was 32% in Bangladesh, but 65% in Thailand; the infection rate in *R. norvegicus* was 43% in southwestern China, but 86% in Thailand (Table 1).

Rats of the genus *Bandicota* were also frequently infected with *Bartonella* species. In Bangladesh, 63% of *B. bengalensis* were infected; in Thailand, 33% and 57% of *B. indica* and *B. savilei* were infected with *Bartonella* species, respectively.

Mice of genus *Apodemus* were also highly susceptible to bartonella infection, with 33-71% prevalence in different species in southwestern China; in Kenya, 63% of *Mastomys natalensis* had bartonella infection; rodents of the genus *Mus* and several other genera seem to exhibit lower susceptibility to bartonella infection. In Bangladesh, none of the 12 tested *Mus musculus* had bartonella infection; but in Thailand, three of seven *Mus cervicolor* were infected with *Bartonella* species.

2.3 Diversity of *Bartonella* species in rodents

Studies from different regions of the world have demonstrated that rodents harbor extremely diverse *Bartonella* strains. Although many strains remain uncharacterized or were only partially characterized, quite a few novel rodent-associated *Bartonella* species and subspecies have been described, including *B. birtlesii, B. coopersplainensis, B. elizabethae, B. doshiae, B. grahamii, B. phoceensis, B. queenslandensis, B. rattimassiliensis, B. taylorii, B. tribocorum, B. vinsonii* subsp. *arupensis*, and *B. washoensis* (Daly et al., 1993; Birtles et al., 1995; Heller et al., 1998; Kosoy et al., 2003; Gundi et al., 2004 & 2009; Bai et al., 2011). Among these, *B. coopersplainensis, B. elizabethae, B. phoceensis, B. queenslandensis, B. rattimassiliensis*, and *B. tribocorum* were all associated with rats of the genus *Rattus*, and they are genetically closer to each other than to other *Bartonella* species that are associated with *Apodemus* spp., *Peromyscus* spp., *Spermophilus* spp., *Myodes* spp., and other rodent genera.

Comparative analyses of bartonella cultures obtained from the rodents in the tropics also revealed diverse assemblages of *Bartonella* strains, many of which appear to represent a variety of distinct species. These bartonella isolates clustered into different lineages that mostly had a close association with their host genus or species. In southwestern China, *Bartonella* isolates obtained from *Rattus norvegicus* and *R. tanazumi.* subsp. *flavipectus* were closely related to *B. elizabethae* or to the closely related *B. tribocorum*. In fact, isolates obtained from the *R. norvegicus* in Vietnam were identical to the type strain of *B. elizabethae* (Kosoy et al., unpublished). Subsequent studies from Bangladesh, Thailand, and Kenya showed that *B. elizabethae*-like bacteria are highly prevalent in a large portion of the local populations of *Rattus* rats. In addition to *B. elizabethae*, several more *Bartonella* species were identified, including *B. tribocorum, B. coopersplainensis, B. phoceensis, B. queenslandensis*, and *B. rattimassiliensis*, all of which were previously described from *Rattus* rats captured in France and Australia (Heller et al., 1998; Gundi et al., 2004 and 2009), as well as the tropics (Castle et al., 2004; Bai et al., 2007b & 2009b; Kosoy et al., 2009). These results suggested that these *Bartonella* species probably co-speciated with rats of the genus *Rattus*.

The spectrum of *Bartonella* species found in rats of the genus *Bandicota* from Bangladesh and Thailand were very similar to those of the genus *Rattus* (Bai et al., 2007b; Castle et al., 2004), demonstrating sharing of *Bartonella* strains among rodents of these species. In fact, *Bandicota* rats share the same habitat with *Rattus* rats and these rats are phylogenetically related as well. *Rattus* rats and *Bandicota* rats may play equally important roles in serving as reservoir hosts of these *Bartonella* strains.

Interestingly, in Kenya, all bartonella isolates obtained from rodents of *Mastomys natalensis* and *Lemniscomys striatus* were relatively closely related but not identical to *Bartonella tribocorum* and *B. elizabethae*. It is questionable whether these mice can also serve as reservoirs of these highly rat-associated *Bartonella* species.

Bartonella isolates obtained from rodents of other species, such as *Apodemus* mice, *Eothenomys* voles, and others, were distant from strains obtained from *Rattus* rats and *Bandicota* rats, and were classified into different phylogenetic groups of *Bartonella*. Further characterization is needed for fully description of these strains.

| Rodent species | Bangladesh | | China | | Thailand | |
	No. tested	Prevalence (%)	No. tested	Prevalence (%)	No. tested	Prevalence (%)
Apodemus chevrieri			32	62.5		
Apodemus draco			6	33.3		
Apodemus peninsulae			7	71.4		
Bandicota bengalensis	76	63.2				
Bandicota indica					46	32.6
Bandicota savilei					7	57.1
Berylmys berdmorei					1	100
Eothenomys miletus			16	18.8		
Mus caroli					3	0
Mus cervicolor					7	42.9
Mus musculus	12	0	1	0		
Rattus argentiventer					3	66.7
Rattus exulans					95	3.2
Rattus losea					4	0
Rattus nitidus					3	33.3
Rattus norvegicus			7	42.9	22	86.4
Rattus rattus	99	32.3			135	65.2
Rattus remotus					2	50
Rattus surifer					2	0
Rattus tanezumi subsp. *flavipectus*			58	41.4		
Total	187	42.8	127	44.2	330	41.5

Table 1. Bartonella in rodents from Bangladesh, China, and Thailand

2.4 Host-specificity relationships between *Bartonella* spp. and rodents

Studies from different regions of the world have shown controversial relationships between *Bartonella* species and their natural rodent hosts. A study of bartonella infection in rodents from the United Kingdoms by Birtles and his colleagues (1994), questioned host-specificity of *Bartonella* species by finding that three *Bartonella* species (*B. grahamii, B taylorii,* and *B. doshiae*) were circulating among woodland mammals of all dominant rodent species (*Apodemus sylvaticus, A. flavicollis, Myomys glareolus, Microtus agrestis* and *Neomys fodiens*). Subsequent investigations of bartonella infections in rodent communities in central Sweden reported similar results, demonstrating that *Bartonella grahamii* frequently infected *Microtus* voles (*M. glareolus*), *Apodemus* mice (*A. flavicollis, A. sylvaticus*) and house mice (*Mus musculus*) (Holmberg et al., 2003). By contrast, investigations from North America suggested a completely different picture of *Bartonella* species - rodent relationships from those found in Europe. In these North American studies, *Bartonella* species specific to a particular rodent species have been reported, such as those found in mice of the genus *Peromyscus*, rats of the genus *Neotoma*, chipmunks of the genus *Tamias*, ground squirrels of the genus *Spermopnilus*, prairie dogs of the genus *Cynomys*, and other rodents (Kosoy et al., 1997 & 2003; Stevenson et al., 2003; Jardine et al., 2006; Bai et al., 2008), indicating definite host-specific relationships exist between these *Bartonella* strains and their rodent hosts.

Observations of the studies of rodent-borne bartonella infections in the tropics showed some different views in regards to a relationship between *Bartonella* species and rodents. In southwestern China and Vietnam, *Barotnella* isolates obtained from *Rattus* rats were all classified as *B. elizabethae* and/or genetically very closely related to *B. tribocorum*, showing a very specific relationship (Ying et al., 2002; Kosoy et al., unpublished data); in Bangladesh and Thailand, all isolates obtained from the *Rattus* rats also fell within the cluster of *Rattus* rats-associated *Bartonella* species, including *B. elizabethae*, *B. tribocorum*, *B. coopersplainensis*, *B. phoceensis*, *B. queenslandensis*, and *B. rattimassiliensis*. However, all of these strains were also frequently harbored by *Bandicota* rats in these same regions. Sharing of the same *Bartonella* strains by rats of two genera might suggest a lower level of host-specificity in these areas or reflect a phylogenetic relatedness between rats belonging to both genera. In Kenya, *B. elizabethae*-like bartonellae were even more widely spread, being found not only in *Rattus* rats, but also in *Mastomys natalensis* and *Lemniscomys striatus*, both which are taxonomically much further from *Rattus* rats than *Bandicota* rats are from *Rattus* rats. Such results implied that *B. elizabethae* and related *Bartonella* species, as the dominant species, may have extended the range of their animal reservoir hosts because long periods of coexistence have provided numerous opportunities to infect local rodent.

2.5 *Rattus* rats as reservoir hosts of zoonotic bartonellae

Bartonella species usually do not cause diseases or pathologic changes to their natural animal hosts. However, some *Bartonella* species can become opportunistic pathogens following a host switch, such as could occur when a strain of rodent bartonella infects humans. During recent years, more and more evidence has accumulated showing that bartonella infections are indeed associated with human illnesses and can be considered as emerging infections. This has raised public health concern and drawn the attention of scientists studying zoonotic diseases. Some rodents often live with or near humans. Close contact between rodents and humans throughout the world makes the study of rodent-borne *Bartonella* essential in order to determine the extent to which rodents may serve as sources of human infections. The epidemiological importance of rodent-borne bartonellae as causes of disease in animals and humans is emerging. Rodents of some species have been found to be reservoir hosts of some *Bartonella* species that are human pathogens, such as *B. elizabethae*, *B. grahamii*, *B. vinsonii* subsp. *arupensis*, and *B. washoensis* (Daly et al., 1993; Birtles et al., 1995; Ellis et al., 1999; Kerkhoff et al., 1999; Welch et al., 1999; Kosoy et al., 2003; Iralu et al., 2006). It is likely that new rodent-borne bartonellae will be identified in the near future, and some of these possibly can be proven to be as zoonotic pathogens.

The most intriguing result of studying bartonella infection in rodents in tropics was the finding of a large number of *Bartonella* strains that are genetically related to the recognized human pathogen *B. elizabethae*. These strains widely infect rats of genera *Rattus* and *Bandicota* in Bangladesh, southwestern China, Thailand, Kenya, and other areas (Ying et al., 2002; Castle et al., 2004; Bai et al., 2007b & 2009b; Kosoy et al., 2009). *B. elizabethae* was originally isolated from the blood of a patient with endocarditis in Massachusetts, USA (Daly et al., 1993). Subsequent studies have implicated *B. elizabethae* as a cause of additional cases of endocarditis, as well as a case of Leber's neuroretinitis, and some have shown the presence of *B. elizabethae*-reactive antibodies in a high proportion of intravenous drug users (O'Halloran et al., 1998; Comer et al., 1996).

In Thailand, researchers have reported that febrile illnesses in human patients were associated with infections of several *Bartonella* species, including *B. elizabethae*, *B.*

rattimassiliensis, B. tribocorum, B. vinsonii subsp. *arupensis, B. tamiae,* and others (Kosoy et al., 2010). Homologous sequences comparison indicated that the *Bartonella* genotypes identified as *B. elizabethae, B. rattimassiliensis,* and *B. tribocorum* in the patients were completely identical or very close to *Bartonella* strains that were derived from black rats, bandicoot rats, Norway rats, and other rodents from Bangladesh, China, Thailand, and other Asian countries. These results suggested that the rodents are the potential source of the infection. Very recently, a serological survey studying source of undiagnosed febrile illness conducted in Nepal also reported antibodies specific to *B. elizabethae, B. tamiae, B. vinsonii* supsp. *arupensis,* and other *Bartonella* species (Myint et al., 2.11).

A natural reservoir for *B. elizabethae* was not implicated until 1996 when Birtles & Raoult identified a strain of *Bartonella* obtained in Peru from a *R. norvegicus* that had *gltA* and 16SrRNA gene sequences that matched the sequences for the respective genes of *B. elizabethae* (Birtles & Raoult, 1996). Numerous isolates were later obtained from *R. norvegicus* in United States and from *R. rattus* in Portugal. Genetic analyses demonstrated that these isolates formed a phylogenetic group along with the genotypes of *B. elizabethae* and the *Bartonella* strains found in rats from Peru (Ellis et al., 1999). *Rattus* rats occupy many different ecologic niches in the sites in Southeast Asia where these animals initially evolved (Eisenberg, 1981). These rats were introduced into other continents through the aid of humans and have become common and widespread in urban and rural environments in Europe, North America, and South America. The findings of *B. elizabethae* in *Rattus* rats from Peru, United States, Portugal, France, and other areas have led to the hypothesis of an Old World origin of *B. elizabethae* and related *Bartonella* bacteria (Childs, et al., 1999; Ellis et al., 1999). These bacteria could have spread from the Old World to other parts of the world through infected rats traveling by ship. Investigations conducted in southwestern China, Bangladesh, Thailand, and Kenya provided evidence in support of the Old World origin hypothesis. The finding of *B. elizabethae*-like agents in a high proportion of the rats raised potential public health concerns of humans acquiring the bartonella infection and the need to study whether these agents are responsible for cases of non-culturable bacterial endocarditis and febrile illnesses of unknown etiology in tropics.

B. vinsonii supsp. *arupensis* was first isolated from a bacteremic cattle rancher in USA (Welch et al., 1999). This bacterium is highly prevalent among deer mice (*Peromyscus maniculatus*), a strict North American rodent species, and has never been detected in any rodents from elsewhere, including tropics. However, the strain was found in stray dogs in Thailand (Bai et al., 2010). It is logical to suggest that this bacterium was acquired by dogs from wild rodents in North America and then, relocated to other continents through the translocation of infected dogs. Regardless, further investigations are needed to define the role of domestic animals as potential sources for human bartonellosis in Thailand and other tropical areas.

3. Bartonella infections in bats in tropics

Like rodents, bats (Order: Chiroptera) are another group of very abundant, diverse, and geographically dispersed vertebrates on the earth (Simmons, 2005; Calisher et al., 2006). Multiple studies have highlighted that bats may play an important role in serving as natural reservoirs to a variety of pathogens (Schneider et al., 2009). Transmission of pathogenic bat-borne viruses capable of causing disease with high human mortality has been demonstrated for a number of viruses, including rabies virus and related lyssaviruses, Nipah and Hendra viruses, Marburg virus, Ebola viruses, and the very recently emerged inferred for SARS-CoV-like virus and other coronaviruses and others (Halpin et al., 2000; Li et al., 2005; Williams, 2005; Tang et al., 2006). The high mobility, broad distribution, social behavior (communal roosting, fission-fusion social structure) and longevity of bats make them ideal reservoir hosts and sources of infection for various etiologic agents.

There is very limited information regarding *Bartonella* infections in bats. In England, detection of *Bartonella* DNA in bats was reported recently (Concannon et al., 2005). A few studies from Egypt and United States reported presence of *Bartonella* species in ectoparasites collected from bats (Loftis et al., 2005; Reeves et al., 2005, 2006, & 2007).

From tropic areas, two studies of bartonella infections in bats were conducted in Kenya and Guatemala very recently (Kosoy et al., 2010; Bai et al., 2011). These studies brought large information regarding distribution of bartonellae in bats. Here we present the findings from these two studies. We compare the composition of bat communities, prevalence of bartonella infections in bat populations, genetic diversity of *Bartonella* strains circulating among the bat populations. We also discuss the epidemiological significance of these findings.

3.1 Bat community

Belonging to 28 species, bats collected from these two studies showed large diversity. Species composition was completely different in the two studies. Bats collected from Kenya represented 13 species of 9 genera (Table 2), including *Chaerephon* sp., *Coleura afra*, *Eidolon helvum*, *Epomophorus* spp., *Hipposideros commersoni*, *Miniopterus* spp., *Rhinolophus* spp., *Rousettus aegyptiacus*, and *Triaenops persicus*. Accounted for 32% of all bats, *Rousettus aegyptiacus* was the most prevalent species in Kenya. The other common species included *Eidolon helvum* (27%) and *Miniopterus* spp. (26). Other species only accounted for a very small portion (Table 2).

Bat species	No. tested	No. pos	Prevalence (%)
Chaerephon sp.	1	0	0
Coleura afra	9	4	44.4
Eidolon helvum	88	23	26.1
Epomophorus spp.	23	0	0
Hipposideros commersoni	4	1	25
Miniopterus spp.	87	49	56.3
Rhinolophus spp.	6	0	0
Rousettus aegyptiacus	105	22	20.9
Triaenops persicus	8	7	87.5
Total	331	106	32

Table 2. Bartonella in bats, Kenya

Bats collected from Guatemala represented 15 species of 10 genera (Table 3), including *Artibeus jamaicensis, Artibeus lituratus, Artibeus toltecus, Carollia castanea, Carollia perspicillata, Desmodus rotundus, Glossophaga soricina, Micronycteris microtis, Myotis elegans, Myotis nigricans, Phyllostomus discolor, Platyrrhinus helleri, Pteronotus davyi, Sturnira lilium*, and *Sturnira ludovici. Desmodus rotundus* comprised 26% of all bats and was the most prevalent species. *Glossophaga soricina, Carollia perspicillata, Artibeus jamaicensis*, and *Sturnira lilium* comprised 13%, 12%, 11%, and 10%, respectively, also were frequently found. The other six species comprised a smaller portion (Table 3).

3.2 Bartonella prevalence in bats

Although composition of bat species was completely different in the Kenya and Guatemala, interestingly, the overall prevalence of bartonella infection in bats was quite similar: 32% in Kenya and 33% in Guatemala. Such high prevalence may suggest persistent infection of long-lived bats with *Bartonella* species, similar to their infection with some viruses (Sulkin & Allen, 1974). Nevertheless, large variations of bartonella prevalence were observed among the bat specie. *Bartonella* species exhibit high, low, or no infectivity depending on the bat species. In Kenya, the bartonella prevalence was 88%, 56%, 44%, 26%, 25%, and 21% for *Triaenops persicus* bats, *Miniopterus* spp. bats, *Coleura afra* bats, *Eidolon helvum* bats, *Hipposideros commersoni* bats, and *Rousettus aegyptiacus* bats, respectively. In Guatemala, *Phyllostomus discolor* bats, *Pteronotus davyi* bats, and *Desmodus rotundus* bats were highly infected with *Bartonella* species, with prevalence of 89%, 70%, and 48% in each, respectively. Bartonella prevalence was relatively low in *Sturnira lilium* bats (8%) and *Glossophaga soricina* bats (13%), and no bartonellae were discovered in some bat species, such as *Epomophorus* spp., *Rhinolophus* spp., and *Artibeus jamaicensis* (Table 2 & Table 3).

3.3 Bartonella genetic heterogeneity and relationships with bat species

Genetic analyses of a portion of citrate synthase gene (*glt*A) demonstrated that the *Bartonella* strains obtained from bats in both Kenya and Guatemala represent a variety of distinct phylogroups, including 11 from Kenya and 13 from Guatemala. Further characterization is necessary to verify whether the *Bartonella* strains represent novel *Bartonella* species.

In Kenya, a definite host-specificity was observed for *Bartonella* strains in bat species. All *Bartonella* isolates obtained from *Rousettus aegyptiacus* bats are similar to each other (>96%) and clustered in a monophyletic genogroup that is distant from all other *Bartonella* species; similarly, *Bartonella* cultures obtained from *Coleura afra* bats, *Triaenops persicus* bats also clearly belonged to the specific *Bartonella* species group found exclusively in the particular bat species. By contrast, *Bartonella* cultures obtained from *Eidolon helvum* bats and *Miniopterus* bats showed great variation, clustering into three or four clades, each representing a distinct *Bartonella* phylogroup. Nevertheless, all strains of *Bartonella* species recovered from *Eidolon helvum* bats were typical for this species of bats only. Similarly, the *glt*A sequences from all strains obtained from *Miniopterus* spp. bats have not been found in bats of other bat genera.

Unlike the discovery in bats in Kenya, host specificity of *Bartonella* species was not found in bats in Guatemala. In some instances, bats of two or more species may share the same *Bartonella* strains. For example, one *Bartonella* strain recovered in *Desmodus rotundus* bats was also found in *Carollia perspicillata* bats. Similarly, same *Bartonella* strain was found in both *Glossophaga soricina* bats and *Pteronotus davyi* bats, or both *Carollia perspicillata* bats and *Phyllostomus discolor* bats. On the other hand, co-infection with multiple *Bartonella* strains in the same bat species was observed. For example, *Desmodus rotundus* bats and *Carollia perspicillata* bats each were infected with two *Bartonella* strains; while *Pteronotus davyi* bats and *Phyllostomus discolor* bats were infected with four *Bartonella* strains, respectively. The tendency of some bat species to share roosts, reach large population densities, and roost crowded together creates the potential for dynamic intraspecies and interspecies transmission of infections (Streicker et al., 2010). The observations in the Guatemala study suggested active interspecies transmission of *Bartonella* species likely occurs among bats in Guatemala, which may have contributed to the lack of host-specificity. Arthropod vectors that parasitize bats may also be partly associated with none host-specificity.

Bat species	No. cultured	No. positive	Prevalence (%)
Artibeus jamaicensis	13	0	0
Artibeus lituratus	3	0	0
Artibeus toltecus	1	1	100
Carollia castanea	1	0	0
Carollia perspicillata	14	4	28.6
Desmodus rotundus	31	15	48.4
Glossophaga soricina	15	2	13.3
Micronycteris microtis	3	1	33.3
Myotis elegans	2	0	0
Myotis nigricans	1	0	0
Phyllostomus discolor	9	8	88.9
Platyrrhinus helleri	1	0	0
Pteronotus davyi	10	7	70
Sturnira lilium	12	1	8.3
Sturnira ludovici	2	0	0
Total	118	39	33.1

Table 3. Bartonella in bats, Guatemala

3.4 Epidemiology significance

Bartonellae were virtually unrecognized as pathogens of humans until 1990s. Identifications of bartonellae as agents of cat-scratch disease, bacillary angiomatosis, urban trench fever, and recent outbreaks of Carrión's disease have left no doubt about the emerging medical importance of these bacteria. Within the last two decades, new bacteria of the genus of *Bartonella* were isolated from large number of several mammalian reservoirs, including rodents, cats, dogs, and rabbits, and recognized as emerging zoonotic agents. At least 13 *Bartonella* species or subspecies have been recognized as emerging human pathogens or zoonotic agents, causing a wide range of syndromes, from a self-limiting to life-threaten endocarditis, myocarditis, and meningoencephalitis. All of these emphasize the concept that inadvertent transmission of known or currently uncharacterized *Bartonella* spp. from both wild animals and domestic animals occurs in nature.

Although evidence of overt disease in bats caused by *Bartonella* species has not been demonstrated to date, high incidence of bartonella infection in bats from the studies carried out in Guatemala, Kenya, and other regions suggested that bats may be natural reservoirs in maintaining circulation of *Bartonella* species in nature. Bats have very long life spans compared to other mammals of similar body size, such as rodents. This may make them serve as reservoirs contributing to the maintenance and transmission of *Bartonella* to other animals and/or humans. Some bat species have been known to directly transmit infections to humans. For example, the common vampire bat (*Desmodus rotundus*) has been long recognized to transmit rabies virus to humans by biting throughout Latin America (Schneider et al., 2009). These bats typically feed on the blood of mammals, including domestic animals, such as cattle, horses, pigs, dogs, but also feed on the blood of humans (Turner & Bateson, 1975). Predation of vampire bats on humans is a major problem in Latin America (Schneider et al., 2009). If *Bartonella* species can be transmitted to humans through the bite of bats, the need for further studies with vampire bats is imperative. Findings of bartonella in bats highlight the need to study whether the bat-originated *Bartonella* species are responsible for the etiology of local undiagnosed illnesses in humans and domestic animals in tropics.

In addition to the large number of documented reservoir hosts, an increasing number of arthropos vectors, includingbiting flies, fleas, keds, lice, sandflies, and ticks have been confirmed or suspected to be associated with the transmission of *Barotella* spp. among animal populations (Billeter et al., 2008). *Bartonella* species–specific DNA has been detected in ectoparasites collected from bats (Loftis et al., 2005; Reeves et al., 2005 & 2007). Presumably, if *Bartonella* species are transmitted through a bat ectoparasite vector, some, if not all, bat-associated *Bartonella* species could be transmitted to humans because bats are frequent hosts to a wide variety of ectoparasites, including bat flies, fleas, soft ticks, and mites.

Very recently, two novel *Bartonella* species, *B. tamiae*, isolated from febrile Thai patients (Kosoy et al., in press), and *B. rochalimae*, isolated from an American patient who traveled in Peru and developed fever and splenomegaly after return (Eremeeva et al., 2007). However, the reservoir remains unknown as do the mode of transmission, pathogenesis, and many other characteristics of these organisms. There is the need to identify the animal reservoirs of these novel *Bartonella* species and to understand their disease ecology. These studies of *Bartonella* species in bats have enlarged the scope of this zoonotic potential as we search for the reservoirs that harbor novel and known *Bartonella* species.

4. References

Anderson, B. & Neuman, M. (1997). *Bartonella* spp. as emerging human pathogens. Clin. Microbiol. Rev. 10:203-219.

Bai, Y., Kosoy M. Y., Cully, J. F., Bala, T., Ray, C., & Collinge, S. K. (2007a). Acquisition of nonspecific Bartonella strains by the northern grasshopper mouse (*Onychomys leucogaster*). FEMS Microbiol. Ecol. 61:438-448.

Bai, Y., Montgomery, S. P., Sheff, K. W., Chowdhury, M. A., Breiman, R. F., Kabeya, H., et al. (2007b.) *Bartonella* strains in small mammals from Dhaka, Bangladesh, related to *Bartonella* in America and Europe. Am. J. Trop. Med. Hyg. 77:567-570.

Bai, Y., Kosoy, M. Y., Martin, A., Ray, C., Sheff, K., Chalcraft, L., et al. (2008). Characterization of *Bartonella* strains isolated from black-tailed prairie dogs (*Cynomys ludovicianus*). Vector Borne Zoonotic Dis. 8:1-5.

Bai, Y., Kosoy, M. Y., Calisher, C. H., Cully, J. F. Jr, & Collinge, S. K. (2009a). Effects of rodent community diversity and composition on prevalence of an endemic bacterial pathogen – Bartonella. Biodiversity. 10:3-11.

Bai, Y., Kosoy, M. Y., Lerdthusnee, K., Peruski, L. F., & Richardson, J. H. (2009b). Prevalence and Genetic Heterogeneity of *Bartonella* Strains Cultured from Rodents from 17 Provinces in Thailand. Am. J. Trop. Med. Hyg. 81:811-816.

Bai, Y., Calisher, C., Kosoy, M., Root, J., & Doty, J. (2011). Persistent Infection or Successive Reinfection of Deer Mice with *Bartonella vinsonii* subsp. *arupensis*. Appl. Environ. Microbiol. 77:1728-1731. doi:10.1128/AEM.02203-10.

Bai, Y., Kosoy, M. Y., Boonmar, S., Sawatwong, P., Sangmaneedet, S., & Peruski, L. F. (2010). Enrichment culture and molecular identification of diverse *Bartonella* species in stray dogs. Vet. Microbiol. 146:314-319.

Bai, Y., Kosoy, M., Recuenco, S., Alvarez, D., Moran, D., Turmelle, A., et al. (2011). *Bartonella* spp. in Bats, Guatemala. Emerg. Infects. Dis. 17:1269-1271.

Bajer, A., Pawelczyk, A., Behnke, J. M., Gilbert, F. S., & Sinski, F. (2001). Factors affecting the component community structure of haemoparasites in bank voles (*Clethrionomys glareolus*) from the Mazury Lake District region of Poland. Parasitology 122:43-54.

Baker, J. A. 1946. A rickettsial infection in Canadian voles. J. Exp. Med. 84:37- 51.

Bermond, D., Heller, R., Barrat, F., Delacour, G., Dehio, C., Alliot, A., et al. (2000). *Bartonella birtlesii* sp. nov., isolated from small mammals (*Apodemus* spp.). Int. J. Syst. Evol. Microbiol. 50:1973-1979.

Billeter, S. A., Levy, M. G., Chomel, B. B., & Breitschwerdt, E. B. (2008). Vector transmission of *Bartonella* species with emphasis on the potential for tick transmission. Med. Vet. Entomol. 22:1-15.

Birtles, R. J., Harrison, T. G., & Molyneux, D. H. (1994). *Grahamella* in small woodland mammals in the UK - isolation, prevalence and host-specificity. Ann. Trop. Med. Parasitol. 88:317-327.

Birtles, R. J., Harrison, T. G., Saunders, N. A., & Molyneux, D. H. (1995). Proposals to unify the genera *Grahamella* and *Bartonella*, with descriptions of *Bartonella talpae* comb. nov., *Bartonella peromysci* comb. nov., and three new species, *Bartonella grahamii* sp. nov., *Bartonella taylorii* sp. nov., and *Bartonella doshiae* sp. nov. Int. J. Syst. Bacteriol. 45:1-8.

Birtles, R. J., & D. Raoult. (1996). Comparison of partial citrate synthase gene (*gltA*) sequences for phylogenetic analysis of *Bartonella* species. Int. J. Syst. Bacteriol. 46: 891-897.

Boulouis, H. J., C. C. Chang, J. B. Henn, R. W. Kasten, et al. 2005. Factors associated with the rapid emergence of zoonotic Bartonella infections. Vet. Res. 36:383-410.

Bown, K. J., Ellis, B. A., Birtles, R. J., Durden, L. A., Lelllo, J., Begon, M., et al. (2002). New world origins for haemoparasites infecting United Kingdom grey squirrels (*Sciurus carolinensis*), as revealed by phylogenetic analysis of bartonella infecting squirrel populations in England and the United States. Epidemiol. Infect. 129:647-653.

Calisher, C. H., Childs, J. E., Field, H. E., Holmes, K. V., & Schountz, T. (2006).Bats: important reservoir hosts of emerging viruses. Clin. Microbiol. Rev.19:531–545. doi:10.1128/CMR.00017-06.

Castle, K., Kosoy, M., Lerdthusnee, K., Phelan, L., Bai, Y., Gage, K. L., et al. (2004). Prevalence and diversity of *Bartonella* in rodents of Northern Thailand: A comparison with *Bartonella* in rodents from southern China. Am. J. Trop. Med. Hyg. 70:429-433.

Childs, J. E., Ellis, B. A., Nicholson, W. L., Kosoy, M. Y., & Sumner, J. W. (1999). Shared vector-borne zoonoses of the Old World and New World: home grown or translocated? Schweiz Med. Wochenschr.129:1099-1105.

Chomel, B. B., Abbott, R. C., Kasten, R. W., Floyd-Hawkins, K. A., Kass, P. H., Glaser, C. A., et al. (1995). *Bartonella henselae* prevalence in domestic cats in California: Risk factors and association between bacteremia and antibody titers. J. Clin. Microbiol. 33:2445-2450.

Chomel, B. B., Kasten, R. W., Floyd-Hawkins, K. A., Chi, B., Yamamoto, K., Roberts-Wilson, J., et al. (1996) Experimental transmission of *Bartonella henselae* by the cat flea. J. Clin. Microbiol. 34:1952-1956.

Comer, J. A., Flynn, C., Regnery, R. L., Vlahov, D., & Childs, J. E. (1996). Antibodies to *Bartonella* species in inner-city intravenous drug users in Baltimore, MD. Arch. Intern. Med. 156:2491-2495.

Concannon, R., Wynn-Owen, K., Simpson, V. R., & Birtles, R. J. (2005). Molecular characterisation of haemoparasites infecting bats (Microchiroptera) in Cornwall, United Kingdom. Parasitology. 131:489-496.

Daly, J. S., Worthington, M. G., Brenner, D. J., Moss, C. W., Hollis, D. G., Weyant, R. S., et al. (1993). *Rochalimaea elizabethae* sp. nov. isolated from a patient with endocarditis. J. Clin. Microbiol. 31: 872–881.

Eisenberg, J. F., (1981). The Mammalian Radiations: An Analysis of Trends in Evolution, Adaptation, and Behavior. Chicago: The University of Chicago Press.

Ellis, B. A., Regnery, R. L., Beati, L., Bacellar, F., Rood, M., Glass, G. G., et al. (1999). Rats of the genus *Rattus* are reservoir hosts for pathogenic *Bartonella* species: an Old World origin for a New World disease? J. Infect. Dis.180: 220-224.

Engbaek, K., & Lawson, P. A. (2004). Identification of *Bartonella* species in rodents, shrews and cats in Denmark: detection of two *B. henselae* variants, one in cats and the other in the long-tailed field mouse. APMIS. 112:336-341.

Eremeeva, M. E., Gerns, H. L., Lydy, S. L., Goo, J. S., Ryan, E. T., Mathew, S. S., et al. (2007). Bacteremia, fever, and splenomegaly caused by a newly recognized *Bartonella* species. N. Engl. J. Med. 356:2381-2387.

Fichet-Calvet, E., Jomaa, I., Ben Ismail, R., & Ashford, R. W. (2000). Pattern of infection of haemoparasites in the fat sand rat, *Psammomys obesus*, in Tunisia, and effect on the host. Ann. Trop. Med. Parasitol. 94:55-68.

Garcia-Caceres, U., & Garcia, F. U. (1991). Bartonellosis: an immunodepressive disease and the life of Daniel Alcides Carrion. J. Clin. Pathol .95 (Suppl): 58-66.

Gundi, V. A., Davoust, B., Khamis, A., Boni, M., Raoult, D., & La Scola, B. (2004). Isolation of *Bartonella rattimassiliensis* sp. nov. and *Bartonella phoceensis* sp. nov. from European Rattus norvegicus. J. Clin. Microbiol.42:3816-3818.

Gundi, V. A., Taylor, C., Raoult, D., & La Scola, B. (2009). *Bartonella rattaustraliani* sp. nov., *Bartonella queenslandensis* sp. nov. and *Bartonella coopersplainsensis* sp. nov., identified in Australian rats. Int. J. Syst. Evol. Microbiol. 59:2956-2961.

Halpin, K., Young, P. L., Field, H. E., & Mackenzie, J. S. (2000). Isolation of Hendra virus from pteropid bats: a natural reservoir of Hendra virus. J. Gen. Virol. 81:1927-1932.

Heller, R., Riegler, P., Hansmann, Y., Delacour, G., Bermound, D., Dehio, C., et al. (1998). *Bartonella tribocorum* sp. nov., a new *Bartonella* species isolated from the blood of wild rats. Int. J. Syst. Bacteriol. 48: 1333-1339.

Higgins, J. A., Radulovic, S., Jaworski, D. C., & Azad, A. F. (1996). Acquisition of the cat scratch disease agent *Bartonella henselae* by cat fleas (Siphonaptera: Pulicidae). J. Med. Entomol. 33:490-495.

Hofmeister, E. K., Kolbert, C. P., Abdulkarim, A. S., Magera, J. M., Hopkins, M. K., Uhl, J. R., et al. (1998). Cosegregation of a novel *Bartonella* species with *Borrelia burgdorferi* and *Babesia microti* in *Peromyscus leucopus*. J. Infect. Dis. 177:409-416.

Holmberg, M., Mills, J. N., McGill, S., Benjamin, G., & Ellis, B. A. (2003). *Bartonella* infection in sylvatic small mammals of central Sweden. Epidemiol Infect 130:149-157.

Iralu, J., Bai, Y., Crook, L., Tempest, B., Simpson, G., Mckenzie, T., et al. (2006). Rodent-associated bartonella febrile illness, southwestern United States. Emerg. Infect. Dis. 12:1081-1086.

Jardine, C., Appleyard, G., Kosoy, M. Y., McColl, D., Chirino-Trejo, M., Wobeser, G., et al. (2005). Rodent-associated *Bartonella* in Saskatchewan, Canada. Vector Borne Zoonotic Dis. 5:402-409.

Jardine, C., McColl, D., Wobeser, G., & Leighton, F. A. (2006). Diversity of *Bartonella* genotypes in Richardson's ground squirrel populations. Vector Borne Zoonotic Dis. 6:395-403.

Kerkhoff, F.T., Bergmans, A. M., van Der Zee, A., & Rothova, A. (1999). Demonstration of *Bartonella grahamii* DNA in ocular fluids of a patient with neuroretinitis. J. Clin. Microbiol. 37: 4034-4038.

Kim, C. M., Kim, J. Y., Yi, Y. H., Lee, M. J., Cho, M. R., Shah, D. H., et al. (2005). Detection of *Bartonella* species from ticks, mites and small mammals in Korea. J. Vet. Sci. 6:327-334.

Knap, N., Duh, D., Birtles, R., Trilar, T., Petrovec, M., & Avsic-Zupanc, T. (2007). Molecular detection of *Bartonella* species infecting rodents in Slovenia. FEMS Immunol. Med. Microbiol. 50:45-50.

Koehler, J. E. (1996). Bartonella infections. Adv. Pediatr. Infect. Dis. 11:1-27.

Kordick, D. L., Hilyard, E. J., Hadfield, T. L., Wilson, K. H., Steigerwalt, A. G., Brenner, D. J., et al. (1997). *Bartonella clarridgeiae*, a newly recognized zoonotic pathogen causing inoculation papules, fever, and lymphadenopathy (cat scratch disease). J. Clin. Microbiol. 35:1813-1818.

Kosoy, M. Y., Regnery, R. L., Tzianabos, T., Marston, E. L., Jones, D. C., Green, D., et al. (1997). Distribution, diversity, and host specificity of *Bartonella* in rodents from the Southeastern United States. Am. J. Trop. Med. Hyg. 57:578-588.

Kosoy, M., Murray, Gilmore, M., R., Bai, Y., & Gage, K. (2003). *Bartonella* strains obtained from ground squirrels in Nevada are identical by sequencing of three genes to *Bartonella washoensis* isolated from a patient with cardiac disease. J. Clin. Microbiol. 41: 645-650.

Kosoy, M., Morway, C., Sheff, K. W., Bai, Y., Colborn, J., Chalcraft, L., et al., (2008). *Bartonella tamiae* sp. nov., a Newly recognized pathogen isolated from three human patients from Thailand. J. Clin. Microbiol. 46:772-775.

Kosoy, M., Iverson. J., Bai. Y., Knobel. D., Halliday J., Agwanda B., et al. (2009). Identification of *Bartonella* species in small mammals from urban and sylvatic foci in Kenya. The International Conference on Emerging Infectious Diseases.

Kosoy M., Bai, Y., Sheff, K., Morway, C., Baggett, H., Maloney S. A., et al. (2010). Identification of *Bartonella* Infections in Febrile Human Patients from Thailand and Their Potential Animal Reservoirs. Am. J. Trop. Med. Hyg. 82:1140-1145.

Kosoy, M., Bai, Y., Lunch, T., Kuzmin, I., Niezgoda, M., Franka, R., et al. (2010). *Bartonella* spp. in bats, Kenya. Emerg. Infects. Dis. 16:1875-1881.

Laakkonen, J., Haukisalmi ,V., & Merritt. J. F. (1998). Blood parasites of shrews from Pennsylvania. J. Parasitol. 84:1300-1303.

Li, W., Shi, Z., Yu, M., Ren, W., Smith, C., Epstein, J. H., et al. (2005). Bats are natural reservoirs of SARS-like coronaviruses. Science. 310:676-679.

Loftis, A. D., Gill, J. S., Schriefer, M. E., Levin, M. L., Eremeeva, M. E., Gilchrist, M. J., et al. (2005). Detection of *Rickettsia, Borrelia,* and *Bartonella* in *Carios kelleyi* (Acari: Aragasidae). J. Med. Entomol. 42:473-480.

Maggi, R. G., Harms, C. A., Hohn, A. A., Pabst, D. A., McLellan, W. A., Walton, W.J., et al. (2005). *Bartonella henselae* in porpoise blood. Emerg. Infect. Dis. 11:1894-1898.

Margileth, A. M., & Baehren, D. F. (1998). Chest-wall abscess due to cat-scratch disease (CSD) in an adult with antibodies to *Bartonella clarridgeiae*: case report and review of the thoracopulmonary manifestations of CSD. Clin. Infect. Dis. 27:353-357.

Markov, A. P., Lopyrev, I. V., Irkhin, A. I., Khliap, L. A., Levitskii, S. A., Kinillov, M., et al. (2006). Wild small mammals are the reservoir hosts of the *Bartonella* genus bacteria in the south of Moscow region. Mol. Gen. Mikrobiol. Virusol. 4:8-13.

Myint, K. S. A., Gibbons, R. V., Iverson, J., Shrestha, S. K., Pavlin, J. A., Mongkolsirichaikul, D., et al. Serological response to *Bartonella* species in febrile patients from Nepal. Trans. R. Soc. Trop. Med. Hyg. *In press.*

O'Halloran, H. S., Draud, K., Minix, M., Rivard, A. K., & Pearson, P. A. (1998). Leber's neuroretinitis in a atient with serologic evidence of *Bartonella elizabethae*. Retina 18: 276-278.

Pappalardo, B. L., Correa, M. T., York, C. C., Peat, C. Y., & Breitschwerdt, E. B. (1997). Epidemiologic evaluation of the risk factors associated with exposure and seroreactivity to *Bartonella vinsonii* in dogs. Am. J. Vet. Res. 58:467-471.

Pawelczyk, A., Bajer, A., Behnke, J. M., Gilbert, F. S., & Sinski, E. (2004). Factors affecting the component community structure of haemoparasites in common voles (*Microtus arvalis*) from the Mazury Lake District region of Poland. Parasitol. Res. 92:270-284.

Pretorius, A. M., Beati, L., & Birtles, R. J. (2004). Diversity of bartonellae associated with small mammals inhabiting Free State Province, South Africa. Int. J. Syst. Evol. Microbiol .54:1959-1967.

Reeves, W. K., Loftis, A. D., Gore, J. A., & Dasch, G. A. (2005). Molecular evidence for novel *Bartonella* species in *Trichobius major* (Diptera: Streblidae) and *Cimex adjunctus* (Hemiptera: Cimicidae) from two southeastern bat caves, U.S.A. J. Vector. Ecol. 30:339-341.

Reeves, W. K., Streicker, D. G., Loftis, A. D., &Dasch, G. A. (2006). Serologic survey of *Eptesicus fuscus* from Georgia, U.S.A. for *Rickettsia* and *Borrelia* and laboratory transmission of a *Rickettsia* by bat ticks. J. Vector. Ecol. 31:386-389.

Reeves, W. K., Rogers, T. E., Durden, L. A., & Dasch, G. A. (2007). Association of *Bartonella* with the fleas (Siphonaptera) of rodents and bats using molecular techniques. J. Vector. Ecol. 32:118-122.

Roux, V., & D. Raoult. (1999). Body lice as tools for diagnosis and surveillance of reemerging diseases. J. Clin. Microbiol. 37:596-599.

Roux, V., Eykyn, S. J., Wyllie, S., & Raoult, D. (2000). *Bartonella vinsonii* subsp. *berkhoffii* as an agent of afebrile blood culture-negative endocarditis in a human. J. Clin. Microbiol. 38:1698-1700.

Raoult, D., Roblot, F., Rolain, J. M., Besnier, J. M., Loulergue, J., Bastides, F., et al. (2006). First isolation of *Bartonella alsatica* from a valve of a patient with endocarditis. J. Clin. Microbiol. 44:278-279.

Sander, A., Zagrosek, A., Bredt, W., Schiltz, E., Piemont, Y., Lanz, C., et al. (2000). Characterization of *Bartonella clarridgeiae* flagellin (FlaA) and detection of antiflagellin antibodies in patients with lymphadenopathy. J. Clin. Microbiol. 38:2943-2948.

Schneider, M. C., Romijn, P. C., Uieda, W., Tamayo, H., da Silva, D. F., Belotto, A., et al. (2009). Rabies transmitted by vampire bats to humans: an emerging zoonotic disease in Latin America? Rev. Panam. Salud. Publica. 25:260–269. doi:10.1590/S1020-49892009000300010

Schülein, R., Seubert, A., Gille, C., Lanz, C., Hansmann, Y., Piemont, Y., et al. (2001). Invasion and persistent intracellular colonization of erythrocytes: a unique parasitic strategy of the emerging pathogen bartonella. J. Exp. Med. 193:1077-1086.

Simmons, N. B. (2005). Order Chiroptera, p. 312-529. *In* D. E. Wilson and D. M. Reeder (ed.), Mammal species of the world: a taxonomic and geographic reference, 3rd ed. Johns Hopkins University Press, Baltimore, Md.

Stevenson, H., Bai, Y., Kosoy, M., Montenieri, J., Lowell, J., Chu, M., et al. (2003). Detection of novel *Bartonella* strains and *Yersinia pestis* in prairie dogs and their fleas (*Siphonaptera:* Ceratophyllidae and *Pulicidae*) using multiplex PCR. J. Med. Entomol. 40:329-337.

Streicker, D. G., Turmelle, A. S., Vonhof, M. J., Kuzmin, I. V., McCracken, G. F., & Rupprecht, C. E. (2010). Host phylogeny constrains cross-species emergence and establishment of rabies virus in bats. Science. 329:676–379. doi:10.1126/science.1188836

Sulkin, S. E., & Allen, R. (1974). Virus infections in bats. Monogr. Virol.8:1–103.

Tang, X. C., Zhang, J. X., Zhang, S. Y., Wang, P., Fan, X. H., Li, L. et al. (2006). Prevalence and genetic diversity of coronaviruses in bats from China. J. Virol. 80:7481-7490.

Tea, A., Alexiou-Daniel, S., Papoutsi, A., Papa, A., & Antoniadis, A. (2004). *Bartonella* species isolated from rodents, Greece. Emerg. Infect. Dis. 10: 963-964.

Telfer, S., Bown, K. J., Sekules, R., Begon, M., Hayden, T., & Birtles, R. (2005). Disruption of a host-parasite system following the introduction of an exotic host species. Parasitology. 130:661-668.

Turner, D. C., & Bateson, P. (1975).The vampire bat: a fi eld study in behavior and ecology. Baltimore: Johns Hopkins University Press; p. 1–7.

Welch, D. F., Carroll, K. C., Hofmeister, E. K., Persing, D. H., Robison, D. A., Steigerwalt, A. G., et al. (1999). Isolation of a new subspecies, *Bartonella vinsonii* subsp. *arupensis* , from a cattle rancher: identity with isolates found in conjunction with *Borrelia burgdorferi* and *Babesia microti* among naturally infected mice. J. Clin. Microbiol. 37: 2598-2601.

Weiss, E., & Dasch, G. (1982). Differential characteristics of strains of *Rochalimae: Rochalimae vinsonii* sp. nov., the Canadian vole agent. Int. J. Syst. Bacteriol. 32: 305-314.

Williams, C. J. 2005. Bats as the reservoir for outbreaks of emerging infectious diseases. Erup. Serveill. 10:E051110.4.

Winoto, I. L., Goethert, H., Ibrahim, I. N., Yuniherlina, I., Stoops, C., Susanti, I., et al. (2005). *Bartonella* species in rodents and shrews in the greater Jakarta area. Southeast Asian J. Trop. Med. Public Health 36:1523-1529.

Ying, B., Kosoy, M., Maupin, G., Tsuchiya, K., & Gage, K. (2002). Genetic and ecological characteristics of *Bartonella* communities in rodents in southern China. Am. J. Trop. Med. Hyg. 66:622-627.

7

Leptospirosis: Epidemiologic Factors, Pathophysiological and Immunopathogenic

Marcia Marinho

Laboratory of Microbiology, Department of Support, Animal Production and Health Course for Veterinary Medicine of UNESP, Campus Araçatuba, São Paulo Brazil

1. Introduction

Leptospirosis is a disease of worldwide distribution present on all continents except Antarctica (Adler & Montezuma, 2010) affecting wildlife, domestic and man. Leading consequently serious socio-economic and public health. It is currently the highest incidence of zoonosis in the world, also considers as an occupational disease, and reemerging infectious disease, occurring endemic and epidemic in developing countries with tropical and subtropical (Levett, 2001; Bharti et al., 2003, Ko et al , 2009). more frequently in tropical and developing countries (Bharti et al, 2003), acarrretando with this serious social and economic problems. The disease is an acute infection caused by a spirochete *Leptospiraceae* family, consisting of two genera, *Leptospira* and *Leptonema*. Recently, the genus *Leptospira* was divided into 17 species based on molecular classification (DNA), saprophytic and pathogenic species (Brazil 2002; Bharti et al. 2003). The pathogenic species are: *L. interrogans, L. alexanderi, L. fanei, L. inadai, L. kirschineri, L. meyeri, L. borgetersenii, L. weil, L. noguchi, L. santarosai,* Genomospecie 1, Genomospecie 4, 5 Genomospecie. The serotypes of *Leptospira* are interrogans Australis, Bratislava, Bataviae, Canicola, Hebdomadis, Icterohaemorrhagiae Copenhageni, Lai, Pomonoa, Pyrogenes, Hardjo and divided into serogroups (Ribeiro, 2006). The reservoir animals, mainly rats, are the most frequent disseminators, by eliminating spirochetes in the urine. *Leptospira* spp. can enter the body through intact skin or not, the oral mucosa, nasal and conjunctival (Kobayashi, 2001). The clinical manifestations of leptospirosis vary according to species, individual susceptibility, the pathogenicity and virulence of the serovar involved (Venugopal, 1990, Macedo 1991). After penetration of the bacteria likely, the organism spreads to the bloodstream to all organs (Hüttner et al, 2002). The incubation period is usually around 5-14 days, but have been described as short or long periods in some cases, such as 72 hours a month or more (Jezior, 2005). Leptospirosis is characterized by a vasculitis. The damage to capillary endothelial cells to the underlying cause of clinical manifestations such as renal tubular dysfunction, liver disease, myocarditis and pulmonary hemorrhage (Hill, 1997).

The clinical features are: a) kidneys: interstitial nephritis, tubular necrosis, decreased capillary permeability, and the combination of hypovolemia resulting in renal failure, b) in the liver: necrosis with central lobular proliferation of Kupffer cells and hepatocellular dysfunction c) in the lung, the lesions were secondary to vascular damage resulting in interstitial hemorrhage d) in the skin, the lesions occur as a result of vascular epithelial injury, and) in skeletal muscle: the lesions were secondary to edema, vacuolation of the myofibril and damage of blood vessels, lesions of the vascular system in general, would result in capillary rupture, hypovolemia and shock (Jezior, 2005). In humans and dogs the most frequent clinical symptoms are severe hepatitis and nephritis (Mosier, 1957; Hagiwara et al., 1975). In dogs the most obvious symptom is jaundice (Greene et al. 1998; Sonrie et al., 2001), fever, myalgia, prostration and the evolution of the process, can present anuria, oliguria or polyuria, indicating different degrees of commitment renal (Masuzawa et al. 1991; Mcdonough, 2003). In cattle, the symptoms are related to the reproductive sphere as abortion and agalactia (Bercovich, 1989) and may have episodes of mastitis caused by serovar hardjo when determining the drop syndrome milk or "milk drop syndrome" (Higgins et al. , 1980, Pearson et al., 1980). In pigs, sheep and goats are seen sporadic reproductive disorders and, possibly, nervous and respiratory systems framework (Andre-Fontaine, 1985; Giles, 1993). Horses can be no abortion (Shapiro & Prescott, 1999) and ocular lesions (Jungherr 1944; Bohl and Ferguson 1952; Kemenes et al., 1985), such as recurrent uveitis, which have been observed after infection, particularly, by L. interrogans serovar pomona (Nick et al., 2000). The cats have to be refractory (Find and Szyfres, 1989). However, seroepidemiologic study in this species, conducted by different authors report seroconversion to multiple *Leptospira* spp (Langoni et al. 1998; Alves et al., 2003). From the epidemiological point of view, it is important to know the species of animals that act as reservoirs, and what the serovars prevalent in a given area. Some serovars have right choice for some species, so called primary hosts, in which cause mild disease with little damage. These can still host the leptospira in their renal tubules, where they remain free from the action of antibodies, and eliminate them through urine intermittently for long periods (Lamb et al., 1981), thus acting as a source of infection for man and other animals. The impact of leptospirosis in terms of public health is reflected in the high cost of treatment of humans afflicted with a fatality rate of about 5% to 20%. However, with regard to animal health, the consequences of infection are particularly the economic sphere, in view of the involvement of cattle, horses, pigs, goats and sheep, food producing animal species noble as meat, milk, and still products of industrial interest, such as wool and leather (Badke, 2001).

The disease course can vary from common symptomatic infection in endemic regions (Ashford et al., 2000), undifferentiated febrile illness, or syndrome to the presence of aseptic meningitis with low morbidity (Berman et al., 1973) or fulminant disease similar to toxic shock syndrome (Vernel-Pauillac and Merien, 2006) with jaundice, myocarditis, renal failure and cardiac hemorrhage, meningitis and death (Levett, 2001) have been described as epidemic in regions of severe leptospirosis in urban areas of Brazil (Ko et. al., 1999) The Jarisch-Herxheimer reaction is not an uncommon complication, when investigated (McBriede et al., 2005). The lung is a target organ that during leptospira infection, presents a hemorrhagic pneumonitis with varying degrees of severity. Under electron microscopy it is observed that the primary lesion is found in endothelial cells of capillaries (Huttner et al., 2002). Seijo et al (2002) classified the respiratory impairment present in leptospirosis in three groups: a) mild to moderate (20 to 70% of patients), pulmonary infiltrates frequently associated with jaundice and a slight alteration of renal function, b) with jaundice severe kidney disease and bleeding (Weill syndrome) occasionally death from kidney failure and myocarditis or cardiovascular collapse with extensive hemorrhage, c) pulmonary hemorrhage, often fatal, without the occurrence of jaundice, kidney disease or other bleeding.

Over the past year has been a frequent higher prevalence of leptospirosis with the observation of episodes of hemoptysis associated with pulmonary respiratory distress syndrome and death (Gill et al., 1992). The same authors, after review, mentioning that the death in Brazil is primarily linked with renal failure, 76.2% of cases, while 3.5% are related to pulmonary hemorrhage. In an outbreak of leptospirosis occurred in Nicaragua in 1995, 40% of fatal cases were associated with pulmonary hemorrhage (Trevejo et al. 1998).

The lung injury during inflammatory processes has been linked to excess stimulated cells in the lung, including alveolar macrophages, polymorphonuclear cells and production of reactive intermediates of oxygen and nitrogen, or other inflammatory mediators. The etiology of respiratory bleeding is unknown, however Nally et al. (2004) verified by immunofluorescence, the presence of immunoglobulins IgM, IgG, IgA and complement factor C3 deposited along the alveolar basement membrane, thus suggesting the existence of autoimmune process associated with the immunopathogenesis of pulmonary hemorrhage observed in fatal cases of leptospirosis.

The involvement of toxins or toxic factors in the pathogenesis of leptospirosis has long been contemplated, since the absence of the microorganism at the site of tissue injury is a factor that strengthens this hypothesis (Knight et al., 1973). Vinh et al. (1986) extracted a glycoprotein (GLP) present in cell walls of a strain of serovar L.interrogans copenhageni that had cytotoxic effect against the fibroblasts of mice (L929). Later it was demonstrated that GLP induced the production of cytokines, TNF-α and IL-10 by peripheral blood monocytes of healthy volunteers (Diament, et al. 2002). The mechanism by which leptospira activate the immune system has been the main focus of many studies, especially regarding the involvement of cytokines (Yang et al., 2000, Maragoni et al., 2004). High levels of TNF-α in serum of patients with leptospirosis were observed by Estavoyer et al. (1991) and Tajiki and Solomon (1996), and in the culture supernatant of macrophages from mice genetically selected Marinho et al. (2005, 2006) who also associated the severity of infection. Vernel-Pauillac and Merien (2006), tested using the technique of quantitative real-time PCR, found elevated levels of inflammatory cytokines, IL-4 and IL-10 in the late stage of infection with Leptospira interrogans icterohaemorrhagiae establishing a profile of involvement of cytokines in type 1 cellular immunity. It is believed that the naturally acquired immunity may result from humoral-mediated response (Adler and Faine, 1977, Adler et al., 1980), which in turn serovar-specific (Adler and Faine, 1977). The development of the humoral response is related to activation-dependent mechanism Recetor Tool-like type 2 (TLR-2), via the innate immune system that would be activated by LPS leptospiral (Werts et al., 2001). Klimpel et al. (2003), demonstrated that Leptospira can activate T cell proliferation and γ-δ α-β, suggesting therefore the involvement of these cell populations in host defense or in the pathology of leptospirosis.

The humoral immune response, compared to the exposure to leptospires, is demonstrated by serological tests, where there is an increased activity of immunoglobulins IgG and IgM after natural infection or immunization. In men there was a greater prevalence of immunoglobulin class IgM (Adler et al, 1980; Petchclai et al. 1991; and Ribeiro et al, 1992), in all the patients, but not all produce agglutinins IgG, after infection. The cause of this individual variation is unknown, however it is observed more frequently in patients afflicted with Weill syndrome (Adler et al., 1980).

Other factors such as hemolysins (Lee et al., 2002), hyaluronidases, phospholipases and glycoproteins (Yang et al. 2001; Sitprija et al., 1980) are implicated in the pathogenesis of leptospirosis. The spiral movement itself would facilitate adherence to renal tubular epithelial cells by lipoproteins wall as Lip41, Lip 36 and LPS (Dobrin et al. 1995). Pathogenic Leptospira present several surface proteins that mediate the interactions between the bacteria with the extracellular matrix and host cells, proteins that facilitate adhesion and invasion of host cell proteins that allow motility in connective tissue, secreted proteins such as enzymes degradation (collagenase, hemolysins, phospholipids and sphingomyelin) and pore-forming proteins. No leptospires in protein secretion of type III and IV, as used by Gram-negative bacteria for introducing proteins into host cells (Ko et al, 2009). The cell apoptosis, or programmed cell death plays an important role in modulating the pathogenesis of many infectious processes. The occurrence of apoptosis in the mechanism of tissue injury is a well known event in renal disease processes (Wong et al., 2001). Cell death by an apoptotic process would regulate the number of cells during induction and resolution of renal injury (Savill, 1994, Ortiz et al., 2002). Leptospira interrogans has been considered as an agent inductor of apoptosis of macrophages (Merian et al. 1997) and guinea pig hepatocytes (Merien et al., 1998) However, the mechanism responsible for cell death remains desconheciso. Jin (2009) showed that L. interrogans induces apoptosis in cell line J774A.1 via dependent on caspase 3 and 8. Caspases (*cysteine-dependent aspartate-specific proteases*) signal for apoptosis and cleave substrates leading to condensation and nuclear fragmentation, externalization of membrane phospholipids that will signal to these cells were engulfed by macrophages (Nicholson et al. 1997, Boatright et al ., 2003).

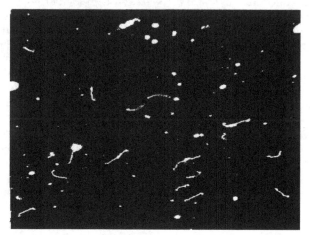

Fig. 1. *Leptospira* spp in dark field microscopy100 increased Microbiology Laboratory, Unesp Brazil Dr. Márcia Marinho /2011

The actual mechanisms that involve the immune response to leptospiral remain controversial and complex. The importance of understanding better the complexity of the mechanisms involved in leptospirosis, such as the virulence of the serovar, the immunocompetence of the host to the agent, the form of clinical manifestations presented, represents a major paradigm in the understanding of infectious diseases and factors related to imunofisiologia leptospirosis, foster the development of preventive and therapeutic strategies aimed at curbing the infection, contributing directly to reducing the prevalence of the disease. New studies are needed to determine the role of apotpose cell in the immunopathogenesis of leptospirosis and the mechanisms that underlie and induce infection. Understanding these mechanisms and kinetics of their occurrence in the future will develop treatment strategies

2. References

Acha, P.N., Syfres, B. Leptospiroses. Publ. Cient. Org. Panam. De La Salud, 503, p.112-120, 1989.

Adler, B., De La Peña Moctezuma, A., 2010. Leptospira and leptospirosis. Vet. Microbiol. 140, 2010 287-296.

Adler, B., Faine,S. Host immunological mechanisms in the resistence of mice to leptospiral infections. Infect Immun. v.17, p.67-72, 1977.

Adler, B., Murphy, K.H., Locarnini,S.A., Faine,S. Detection of specific anti-leptospiral immunoglobulin M and immunoglobulin G in human serum by solid phase enzyme-linked immunosorbent assay. J Clin Microbiol v.11, p.452-457, 1980.

Alves, C.J., Vasconcellos, S.A., Morais Z.M., Andrade J.S.L., Clementino, I. J.,Azevedo, S.S., Santos, F.A. Avaliação dos níveis de aglutininas antileptospiras em gatos no município de Patos - PB Clínica Veterinária, v.46, p.48-54, 2003.

André – Fontaine,G., Caniere, J.P. Donnés actuelles sur la leptospirose des animaux d`élevage. NOTE I. Ëtiologie, Symptones et epidemiologie. Rev. Med. Vet., v. 136, p.627-637, 1985.

Ashford, D. A., Kaiser, R.M., Spiegel, R.A., Perkins, B.A., Weyant R.S., Bragg, S.L., Plikavtis, B., Jarquin, C., Reys, De J.H.L., Amador, I.J. Asymptomatic infection and risk factors for leptospirosis in Nicaragua. Am. J. Trop. Med. Hyg v.63, p.249, 2000.

Badke M. R. T Leptospirose 2001 Disponível em [www.cnpsa.embrapa.br/abraves-sc/pdf/Memorias2001/1_manoelrenato.pdf] Acesso em 13 /10 /2007.

Bercovich, Z., Taaijk E., Kokhout, B.A. Evaluation of an ELISA for the diagnosis of experimentally induced and naturally occurring Leptospira hardjo infections cattle. Vet. Microbiol v. 21,p. 255-262, 1989.

Berman, S.J.; Tsai, C.C.; Holmes, K.; Fresh, J.W.; Watten, R.H. Sporadic anicteric leptospirosis in South Vietnam. A study in 150 patients. Am. Intern. Med v. 79, p.167, 1973.

Bharti, A.R., Nally Je, Ricaldi Jn, Matthias Ma, Diaz Mm, Lovett M, Lovett Pn, Gilman Rh, Willig Mr, Gotuzzo E, Vinetz Jm. Leptospirosis: a zoonotic disease of global importance Lancet Infect Dis v.3, p.757-771, 2003.

Boatright KM, Salvesen GS. Mechanisms of caspase activation. Curr Opin Cell Biol. 2003;15:725-31.

Bohl, E.H., Ferguson, L.C. Leptospirosis in domestic animals. J. Am. Vet. Med. Assoc v.121, p.421-423, 1952.

Brasil. Ministério Da Saúde. Secretaria Nacional de Ações Básicas de Saúde Manual de controle da Leptospirose. Ministério da Saúde. Divisão Nacional de Zoonoses – Brasília: Centro de Documentação do Ministério da Saúde, 2002. 726p. (Série A: Normas e manuais técnicos).

Cordeiro, F., Sulzer, C.R., Ramos, A.A. Leptospira interrogans in several wildlife species in Southeast,Brazil. Pesquisa Agropecuária Brasileira, Série Veterinária, v. 1, p.19-29, 1981.

Diament, D., Karina M., Brunialti, C., Romero E.C., Kallas E.G., Salomao R. Peripheral blood mononuclear cell activation induced by *Leptospira interrogans* glycoliprotein. Infection and Immun v.70, p.1677-1687, 2002.

Dobrina A., Nardon E., Vecicle E., Cinco M. & Patriarca P. 1995. *Leptospira* Icterohaemorrhagiae and *Leptospira peptideoglicans* induce endothelial cell adhesiveness for polymorphonuclear leukocytes. Infect. Immun. 63:2995-2999.

Estavouyer, J.M.; Rcadot, E.; Couetdic, G.; Lerroy, J.; Grosperrin, L. Tumor necrosis factor in patiens with leptospirosis [letter]. Rev. Infect. Dis v.13 p.1245-1246, 1991.

Faber, N.C., Crawford, M., .Lefebvre, R.B.,Buyukmihci, N.C., Madigan, J.E., Willits, N.H. Detection of *Leptospira* spp. In the aqueous humor of horses with naturally acquired recurrent uveitis J. Clin. Microbiol v.38, p.2731-2733, 2000.

Giles,N., Hataway,S.C., StevenS, A.E. Isolation of Leptospira interrognas serovar hardjo from a viable premature calf. Vet. Rec v. 113, p.153-154, 1993.

Gonçalves, A.J, De Carvalho, M., Guedes, J.B.S, Rozembaum, R., Riera, A.R.M. Hemoptise e síndrome de angustia respiratória do adulto como causas da morte na leptospirose: mudanças de padrões clínicos e anatomopatologicos. Rev Bras Med Trop v.25, p.261. 1992.

Greene, C. E.; Miller, M. A.; Brown, C. A. Leptospirosis. In: Infectious Diseases of the Dog and Cat. 2 ed. W. B. Saunders, Philadelphia, 1998. p. 273-281.

Hagiwara, M. K.; Santa Rosa, C. A. Leptospirose canina em São Paulo. Arq Inst Biol São Paulo. v. 42, p. 111-118, 1975.

Higgins, R.J.; Harbourne, J.F.; Little, T.W.A.; Stevens, A.E. Mastitis and abortion in dairy cattle associated with *Leptospira* serotype *hardjo*. Vet. Rec v.107, p. 307-10, 1980.

Hill, M.K, Sanders, C.V. Leptospiral pneumonia. Semin Respir Infect v.12, p.44-49. 1997.

Huttner, M.D., Pereira, H.C.P., Tanaka, R.M. Pneumonia por Leptospirose J Pneumol v.28, p.229-232, 2002

Jezior, M. R. Leptospirosis. 2005 Disponível em [URL: http://www.emedicine.com/med/topic1283.htm] Acesso em 28 de abril de 2006

Jin D. (2009)Leptospira interrogans induces apoptosis in macrophages via caspase-8- and caspase-3-dependent pathways. Inf Immun 77:799

Jungherr, W. Bovine Leptospirosis. J. Am. Vet. Med. Assoc v. 105, p.276-281, 1944.

Kemenes, F., Surjan, J., Kasza, L. Studies on equine leptospirosis with emphasis on eye-lesions (equine periodic ophthalmia) Ann. Immunol. Hung. v.24, p.345-355, 1985.

Klimpel G.R., Mathias M.A., Vinetz, J. *Leptospira interrogans* activation of human peripheral blood mononuclaer cells: preferential expacion of TCR gamma delta + cells vs TCR alpha beta + T cells J. Immunol. v .171 p.1447-1455, 2003.

Knight, L.L., Miller, N.G., White, R.J. Cytotoxic factor in the blood and plasma of animals during Leptospirosis Infect. Immunity v.8 p.401-405, 1973.

Ko, 2009 Leptospirosis: a zoonotic disease of global importance. Lancet Infect. Dis. 3, 757-

Ko, A. I. M., Reis, G., Dourado, C.M.R., Johnson, W.D., Rielly,L. W. Urban Epidemic of severe leptospirosis in Brazil. Lancet v .354, p.820, 1999.

Kobayashi ,Y. Clinical observation and treatment of leptospirosis. J Infect Chemother. v. 7 p. 59-68, 2001.

Langoni, H., Cabral, K.G., Kronfly, C.S. Pesquisa de aglutininas anti-leptospíricas em gatos Clínica Veterinária n.17, p.24-6, 1998.

Lee, S.H.; Kim, S.; Park, S.C.; Kim,M. J., Cytotoxic activies of Leptospira interrogans hemolysin SphH as a pore: foirming protein on mammalian cells. Infect. Immun., v. 70, nn1, p., 315-322,2002.

Levett, P.N. Leptospirosis Clin. Microbiol v. 14, p.296, 2001.

Macedo, N.A. Influência da via de inoculação sobre o estabelecimento e a evolução da leptospirose em hamster (Mesocricetus auratus) experimentalmente infectados com L. interrogans sorovar Pomona. São Paulo, 1991, 45 p. Dissertação (Mestrado) – Faculdade de Medicina Veterinária e Zootecnia, Universidade de São Paulo.

Marangoni, A. R. Aldini, V., Sambri, L., Giacani, K., Di Leo, Cevenini R. Production of tumor necrosis factor alpha by Treponema pallidum, Borrelia burgdorferi, s.l., and Leptospira interrogans in isolated rat Kupffer cells. FEMS Immunol. Med. Microbiol v.40, p.187-191, 2004.

Marinho, M., Langoni, H., Oliveira S.L., Lima V.M.F.., Peiró J.R., Perri, S.H.V., Carreira, R. Role of cytokines, NO, and H_2O_2 on the immunopathology of Leptospirosis in genetically selected mice. J. Venom. Anim. Toxins incl. Trop. Dis. v. 11, p.198-212, 2005.

Marinho, M., Silva, C., Lima, V.M.F, Peiró, J.R., Perri, S.H.V. Citokine and antibody production during murine leptospirosis. J. Venom. Anim. Toxins incl. Trop. Dis.v 12 , p.595-603, 2006.

Masuzawa, T.; Suzuki, R.; Yanagihara, Y.Comparison of protective effects with tetravalentglicolipid antigens and whole cell inactivated vaccine inexperimental infection of Leptospira. Microbiol Immunol v. 35, p. 199-208, 1991.

Mcbried, A.J.A, ATHANAZIO, D.A, REIS, M. G., KO A.I. Leptospirosis Curr Opin Infect Dis v.18 p. 595-603, 2005

Mcdonough, P. L. Leptospirosis in dogs – Currentstatus. In: CARMICHAEL, L. Recent Advances in Canine Infectious Diseases. International Veterinary Information Service (www.ivis.org). Ithaca. 2001. Último acesso em julho 2003.

Merien, F., Baranton, G., Perolat, P. (1997). Invasion of Vero cells and induction of apoptosis in macrophages by pathogenic Leptospira interrogans are correlated with virulence. Infection and Immunity 65, 729–738

Merien, F., Truccolo, J, Rougier Y (1998). In vivo apoptosis of hepatocytes in guinea pigs infected with Leptopira interrogans serovar Icterohaemorrhagiae. FEMS Microb Letters, 169:95-102.

Mosier,J.E. Leptospirosis of pet animals. Vet. Med v. 52, p. 537-539, 1957.

Nally, J.E., Chantranuwat, C., Wu, X-Yang, Fishbein, M.C., Pereira, M.M., Silva, J. J. Pereira, Blanco D.R., Lovett, M.A. Alveolar septal deposition of immunoglobulin and complement parallels pulmonary hemorrhage in guinea pig model of severe pulmonary leptospirosis. Am J Pathol. v.164 p.1115-1127. 2004.

Nicholson Dw, Thornberry NA. Caspases: killer proteases. Trends Biochem Sci.1997;22:299-306.

Ortiz A, Justo P, Catalán Mp (2002). Apoptotic cell death in renal injury: the rationale for intervention. Curr Drug Targ- Imm Endoc Metabo Disords 2: 181-192.

Pearson, J.K.L., Mackie, D.P., Ellis, W.A. Milk drop syndrome resulting from Leptospira Hardjo. Vet. Rec v.107, p. 135-37, 1980.

Petchclai, B., Hiranra, S. S., Potha,U. Gold immunoblot analysis of IgM-specific antibody in the diagnosis of human leptospirosis. Am J Trop Med Hyg v. 45, p.672-675, 1991.

Ribeiro, A.F. Leptospirose, avaliação de fatores prognósticos da doença, município de São Paulo Boletim Epidemiológico Paulista BEPA, v.3, n.28, 2006. Disponível em:[hhtp://www.cve.saude.sp.gov.br/gencia/bepa28_lepto.htm]. Acesso em: 7 jun.2007.

Ribeiro, M.A., Sakata, E.E., Silva, M.V., Camargo, E.D., Vaz,A.J. De Brito,T. Antigens involvrd in the human antibody response to natural infections with *Leptospira interrogans* serovar Copenhageni J Trop Med Hyg v.95 p.239-245, 1992.

Savill J (1994) Apoptosis and kidney. J Am Soc Nephrol 5:12-21.

Seijo, A, Coto H., San Juan J., Videla J., Deodato, B., Cernigoi B et al. Lethal leptospirosis pulmonary hemorrhage: Na emerging disease in Buenos Aires, Argentina Emerg Infect Dis v.8 p.491-499, 2002.

Shapiro, J.L., Prescott, J.F., Equine abortions in eastern Ontario due to leptospirosis. Can Vet J. v.40 p. 350-351, 1999.

Sitprija V, Pipatanagul V, Mertowidjojo K (1980) Pathogenesis of renal disease in leptospirosis:clinical and experimental studies. Kidney Intern,17:827-6.

Sonrier, C.; Branger, C.; Michel, V.; Ruvoënclouet,N.; Ganière, J. P.; André-Fontaine, G.Evidence of cross-protection within *Leptospira interrogans* in an experimental model. Vaccine. v. 19, p. 86-94, 2001.

Tajiki, M.H., Salomao, R. Association of plasma levels of tumor necrosis factor α with severity of diseases and mortality among patients with leptospirosis. CID v.23 p.1177-1178, 1996.

Trevejo, R.T., Rigau-Perz, J.G., Ashford D.A., Zaki, S.R., Shieh, W.J., Peters, C.U.J. et al. Epidemic Leptospirosis associated with pulmonary hemorrhage-Nicaragua, 1995 J infect Dis v.178, p.1457-1463, 1998.

Venugopal, K. Ratnam, S. Lesions and immune responses produced in hamsters and guinea pigs inoculated with some strains of *Leptospira* Indian J. Exp. Biol., v.28, p.1075-1077, 1990.

Vernel-Pauillac, F; Merien F. Proinflammatory and immunomodulatory cytokine mRNA Time Course Profiles in Hamsters Infected with a virulent Variant of *Leptospira interrogns* Infect. Immun v.6 p.4172-4179, 2006.

Vinh,T., Adler,B., Faine, S. Glycolipoprotein Cytotoxin from *Leptospira interrogans serovar copenhageni J. Gen. Micob.* v. 132 p.111-123, 1986.

Werts, C.,R.,I., Tapping, J.C., Mathinson, T. H., Chuang, V., Kravchenko, I. Saint Giron, D.A., Haake, P.J., Godowski, F., Hayashi,A.,Ozinsky, D.M., Underhill,C.J., Kirsching, H,. Wagner, A. Aderem, P. S., Tobias A.N.D., Ulevitch, R.J. Leptospiral lipopolysaccharid activates cells through a TLR-2 dependent mechanism. Nat. Immunol. v. 2 p.346-452, 2001.

Wong Vy,Keller Pm, Nuttall Me(2001). Role of caspases in human renal proximal tubular epithelial cell apoptosis. Eur J Pharmacol, 433:135-140.

Yang Cw,Wu Ms, Pan Mj. (2001) Leptospirosis renal disease, Nephrol Dial Transplant, 16 (Suppl 5):73-77.

Yang, C.W., Wu, M.S., Pan, M.J., Hong, J.J., Yu, C.C., Vandewalle, A., Huang, C.C. Leptospira outer membrane protein actives NF-kappa B and downstream genes expressed in medullary thick ascending limb cells. J.Am. Soc. Nephrol. v.11, p.2017-2026, 2000.

8

Social Networking in Tuberculosis: Experience in Colombia

Diana M. Castañeda-Hernández and Alfonso J. Rodriguez-Morales
[1]*Tuberculosis Control Program, Health and Social Security Secretary,
Pereira and Fundación Universitaria del Área Andina, Pereira*
[2]*Instituto José Witremundo Torrealba, Universidad de Los Andes, Trujillo; Faculty of
Health Sciences, Universidad Tecnológica de Pereira, Pereira and Office of Scientific
Research, Cooperativa de Entidades de Salud de Risaralda (COODESURIS), Pereira*
[1,2]*Colombia*
[2]*Venezuela*

1. Introduction

Tuberculosis (TB) is an infectious disease caused by different species of *Mycobacteria*. Human disease is usually caused by *Mycobacterium tuberculosis*, also know as the Koch's bacilli, which can affect any organ or tissue in the body. Although this, pulmonary disease, with their particular hallmarks such as occurrence of cough with expectoration lasting more than 15 days, is the main corporal area affected by this mainly tropical pathogen (Rodríguez-Morales et al. 2008). In such cases, previous to a microbiological diagnosis, individuals in such state are so-called respiratory symptomatic.

Besides those symptoms/signs, disease can be manifested with hemoptisis, fever, night sweating, general malaise, thoracic pain, anorexia and weight lost. This disease is still a significant public heal problem due to is highly transmissibility, but is highly potentially preventable and treatable condition (Curto et al. 2010, Dim et al. 2011, Orcau et al. 2011, Marais & Schaaf 2010, Glaziou et al. 2009). Even more, in the context of HIV and newer immunosuppressive conditions mycobacterial diseases emerge as public health threat in the World (Vargas et al. 2005).

According to the World Health Organization (WHO), in 2010, there were 8.8 million (range, 8.5–9.2 million) incident cases of TB, 1.1 million (range, 0.9–1.2 million) deaths from TB among HIV-negative people and an additional 0.35 million (range, 0.32–0.39 million) deaths from HIV-associated TB. Important new findings at the global level are: a) the absolute number of TB cases has been falling since 2006 (rather than rising slowly as indicated in previous global reports); b) TB incidence rates have been falling since 2002 (two years earlier than previously suggested); c) Estimates of the number of deaths from TB each year have been revised downwards; d) In 2009 there were almost 10 million children who were orphans as a result of parental deaths caused by TB (World Health Organization 2011).

Beyond its epidemiology, particularly mostly due to pulmonary disease, other important forms of disease represent also a significant burden in thee World. When the infection affects organ other than the lung is called extrapulmonary TB. The most common form of this disease is at the pleura, followed by the lymphatic nodes. Extrapulmonary TB includes various manifestations according to the affected organ. Prognosis and time to develop disease also can vary according to the affected organ.

Disease can ranges a spectrum that can begin from a latent infection or reactivation slowly evolving into a focal or whole spread and involvement of multiple organs, which makes it difficult to diagnosis by clinicians and health care workers, who many times could not identify it timely (Castañeda-Hernández et al. 2012a). One of the most severe forms of extrapulmonary TB is the meningitis (TB meningitis), which occurs as a result of hematogenous spread of bacilli into the subarachnoid space. This is known as a complication of primary TB and may occur years later as an endogenous reactivation of a latent tuberculosis or as a result of exogenous reinfection (Glaziou et al. 2009, Hoek et al. 2011, Galimi 2011, Garcia-Rodriguez et al. 2011).

Tuberculosis is a complex disease in terms of the multiple factors that are involved in its occurrence and persistence in the human societies. In first place there are factors associated with the bacillus (viability, transmissibility and virulence), with the host as a biological individual (immune status, genetic susceptibility, duration and intensity of exposure) as well, at the bacillus-host interaction (place of affection, severity of illness).

At a second, clinical level, the occurrence of pulmonary tuberculosis undiagnosed or untreated, overcrowding, malnutrition, immunosuppresion from any cause (HIV infection, use of immunosuppressive drugs, diabetes, cancer, chronic renal failure, silicosis, alcoholism and drug addiction), are also important factors.

At community public health interventional level, protective factors include the BCG (Bacille Calmette Guerin) vaccine, applied in developing countries, which provides protection before exposure and prevent severe infection forms, especially in infants and young children, reaching up to 80% of protection against the development of forms of the disease such as meningeal and miliary TB (Garcia-Rodriguez et al. 2011, Garg 2010, Black et al. 2003, Francis et al. 2002, Arbelaez et al. 2000, Ginsberg 2000).

Additional to those clinical implications, changes in the susceptibility of the etiological agent to the therapy used drugs has imposed more challenges in the management of TB. The magnitude of problem with TB now lies in the fact that one third of the world population is infected by *Mycobacterium tuberculosis*. Even in the 21st century, TB kills more people than any other infective agent. This, then, occurs in part as a result of a progressive decrease in its susceptibility to anti-TB drugs or resistance emergence. Cases of resistant TB, defined by the recommendations of the World Health Organization (WHO) as primary, initial, acquired multidrug resistant (MDR-TB) or extensively drug resistant TB (XDR-TB) are emerging in different areas of the World.

The development of resistance TB may result from the administration of mono-therapy or inadequate combinations of anti-TB drugs. A possible role of health care workers in the development of multi drug-resistant TB is very important. Actually, multi drug-resistant TB is a direct consequence of mistakes in prescribing chemotherapy, provision of anti-tuberculosis drugs, surveillance of the patient and decision-making regarding further treatment as well as in a wrong way of administration of anti-TB drugs. The problem of XDR-TB in the world has become very alarming. Only adequate treatment according to directly supervised short regiment for correctly categorized cases of TB can stop the escalation of MDR-TB or XDR-TB, which is actually, in large magnitude, a global threat in the 21st century (Torres et al. 2011, Solari et al. 2011, Chadha et al. 2011, Arenas-Suarez et al. 2010, Ferro et al. 2011, Martins 2011).

Another important issue in TB is the social component, related to a complex background and multiple interacting factors that internally and externally affect individuals affected by the disease, which still represents a significant stigma in many communities in the World. Given this setting, TB approach is complex and requires not only medical but also psychological and especially sociological approaches in order to improve its management from a collective medicine perspective as well better acceptability by non-affected people surrounding infected individuals at their communities or neighborhoods. In this way, programs approaching taking all these considerations in count will benefit with better strategies that allow good interactions between social actors involve in the complex social matrix in which sometimes TB can be present at societies. Taking advantage from this, regular activities, such as proper diagnosis and treatment would be achieve in a more efficient way (Murray et al. 2011, Santin & Navas 2011, Juniarti & Evans 2011).

This chapter will cover how using social networks in the context of tuberculosis control program would achieve a better management of cases at individual and at a collective level in a western area of Colombia, where TB is a highly prevalent condition and where available resources for disease management and program are still limited in multiple aspects.

2. Social networking

Human societies can be regarded as large numbers of locally interacting agents, connected by a broad range of social and economic relationships. These relational ties are highly diverse in nature and can represent, e.g., the feeling a person has for another (friendship, enmity, love), communication, exchange of goods (trade), or behavioral interactions (cooperation or punishment). Each type of relation spans a social network of its own. A systemic understanding of a whole society can only be achieved by understanding these individual networks and how they influence and co-construct each other. The shape of one network influences the topologies of the others, as networks of one type may act as a constraint, an inhibitor, or a catalyst on networks of another type of relation.

For instance, the network of communications poses constraints on the network of friendships, trading networks are usually constrained to positively connoted interactions such as trust, and networks representing hostile actions may serve as a catalyst for the network of punishments. A society is therefore characterized by the superposition of its constitutive socioeconomic networks, all defined on the same set of nodes. This superposition is usually called multiplex, multirelational, multimodal, or multivariate network (Szell et al. 2010). Summarizing, a social network is a social structure made up of individuals (or organizations) called "nodes", which are tied (connected) by one or more specific types of interdependency, such as friendship, kinship, common interest, financial exchange, dislike, sexual relationships, or relationships of beliefs, knowledge or prestige (Palinkas et al. 2011, Szell et al. 2010).

Understanding and modeling network structures have been a focus of attention in a number of diverse fields, including physics, biology, computer science, statistics, and social sciences. Applications of network analysis include friendship and social networks, marketing and recommender systems, the World Wide Web, disease models, and food webs, among others (Zhao et al. 2011). Social network analysis (SNA) is the study of structure. It involves relational datasets. That is, structure is derived from the regularities in the patterning of relationships among social entities, which might be people, groups, or organizations. Social network analysis is quantitative, but qualitative interpretation also its necessary. It has a long history in sociology and mathematics and it is creeping into health research as its analytical methods become more accessible with user friendly software (Hawe et al. 2004). SNA views social relationships in terms of network theory consisting of nodes and ties (also called edges, links, or connections).

Nodes are the individual actors within the networks, and ties are the relationships between the actors. The resulting graph-based structures are often very complex. There can be many kinds of ties between the nodes. Research in a number of academic fields has shown that social networks operate on many levels, from families up to the level of nations, and play a critical role in determining the way problems are solved, organizations are run, and the degree to which individuals succeed in achieving their goals (McGrath 1988, Palinkas et al. 2011, Szell et al. 2010, Zhao et al. 2011, Hawe et al. 2004).

In its simplest form, a social network is a map of specified ties, such as friendship, between the nodes being studied. The nodes to which an individual is thus connected are the social contacts of that individual. The network can also be used to measure social capital – the value that an individual gets from the social network. These concepts are often displayed in a social network diagram, where nodes are the points and ties are the lines.

Its use in health (Bhardwaj et al. 2010, Lawrence & Fudge 2009), and more on in infectious diseases (Klovdahl et al. 2002), has been recently highlighted, including sexually transmitted infections (Perisse & Costa Nery 2007), as well in TB (Boffa et al. 2011, Waisbord 2007, Curto et al. 2010, Burlandy & Labra 2007, Santos Filho & Santos Gomes 2007, Freudenberg 1995, Murray et al. 2011).

3. Tuberculosis as a social issue

Multiple studies have evidenced links between social, economic and biologic determinants to TB, recently using modeling approaches that have been used to understand their contribution to the epidemic dynamics of TB (Murray et al. 2011). Specifically, different authors have evidence for associations between smoking, indoor air pollution, diabetes mellitus, alcohol, nutritional status, crowding, migration, aging and economic trends, and the occurrence of TB infection and/or disease. We outline some methodological problems inherent to the study of these associations; these include study design issues, reverse causality and misclassification of both exposure and outcomes. From a social perspective, multiple analyses can be useful and approaches to modeling the impact of determinants and the effect of interventions as the follow will help: the population attributable fraction model, which estimates the proportion of the TB burden that would be averted if exposure to a risk factor were eliminated from the population, and deterministic epidemic models that capture transmission dynamics and the indirect effects of interventions. Can be stated that by defining research priorities in both the study of specific determinants and the development of appropriate models to assess the impact of addressing these determinants (Murray et al. 2011, Santin & Navas 2011, Juniarti & Evans 2011).

Although not considered neglected, TB disproportionally affect resource-constrained areas of the World, including Latin America. In tropical and subtropical areas of this region, the vicious cycle of poverty, disease and underdevelopment is widespread, including TB as one of the significant pathologies involved. The burden of disease associated to TB in this region is highly significant in some countries (eg. Bolivia, Haiti, Brazil, among others). TB has burdened Latin America throughout centuries and has directly influenced their ability to develop and become competitive societies in the current climate of globalization.

Therefore, the need for a new paradigm that integrates various public health policies, programs, and a strategy with the collaboration of all responsible sectors is long overdue. In this regard, innovative approaches are required to ensure the availability of low-cost, simple, sustainable, and locally acceptable strategies to improve the health of neglected populations to prevent, control, and potentially eliminate poverty diseases, such as TB. Improving the health of these forgotten populations will place them in an environment more conducive to development and will likely contribute significantly to the achievement of the Millennium Development Goals in this area of the globe (Franco-Paredes et al. 2007). For example in Colombia, TB is still a significant public health problem. Figure 1 shows the WHO profile for TB in Colombia for 2010.

4. Social networks in tuberculosis

Multiple studies have evidenced links between social, economic and biologic determinants to TB, recently using modeling approaches (Guzzetta et al. 2011, Drewe et al. 2011, Wilson et al. 2011, Bohm et al. 2008, Cook et al. 2007, Cohen et al. 2007, Ayala & Kroeger 2002). Tuberculosis is the archetypal disease of poverty, and social inequalities undermine TB control (Rocha et al. 2011, Lonnroth et al. 2010). Poverty predisposes individuals to TB through multiple mechanisms, such as malnutrition (Rocha et al. 2011, Lonnroth et al. 2010, Cegielski & McMurray 2004), and TB worsens poverty as it increases expenses and reduces income (Rocha et al. 2011, Pantoja et al. 2009, Pantoja et al. 2009, Kemp et al. 2007, Lonnroth et al. 2007, Rajeswari et al. 1999).

Furthermore, poor TB-affected households often experience stigmatization; adding barriers to TB control (Rocha et al. 2011, Atre et al. 2011, Dhingra & Khan 2010, Pungrassami et al. 2010, Jittimanee et al. 2009). Poor people at the greatest risk of TB are therefore, in many settings, also the least able to access TB care (Rocha et al. 2011). Then, socio-economic interventions adapted to the needs of TB-affected households living in impoverished peri-urban shantytowns and other demographical settings.

The socio-economic interventions can successfully engaged most TB-affected households in an active civil society that was associated with marked improvements in uptake of TB prevention, diagnosis and treatment, resulting in strengthened TB control (Rocha et al. 2011). The development of social networks and SNA, however, has been mostly approached only for investigation of TB outbreaks (Fitzpatrick et al. 2001, Sterling et al. 2000) and fewly in the support with the strategies of the WHO for TB Control (World Health Organization 2011).

The WHO Stop TB Strategy, recently revised (World Health Organization 2011), stated a vision for a TB-free world, with a goal of to dramatically reduce the global burden of TB by 2015 in line with the Stop TB Partnership targets and the Millennium Development Goals (MDGs) which pursue the significant reduction in endemic diseases, such as TB and others, even regional diseases (e.g. Chagas disease), that can represent an impediment in achieving the MDGs (Franco-Paredes et al. 2007). In their components, it is included Empower people with TB, and communities through partnership through: a. Pursue advocacy, communication and social mobilization; b. Foster community participation in TB care, prevention and health promotion; and c. Promote use of the Patients' Charter for Tuberculosis Care (World Health Organization 2011).

In Brazil, one of the countries in Latin America where TB is a major public health problem, recent experiences suggest the importance of networking and civil society participation for TB control (Santos Filho & Santos Gomes 2007). In that country, until 2003, the presence of civil society in the fight against TB took place by means of several initiatives from researchers, healthcare professionals and medicine students, especially from the Sociedade Brasileira de Pneumologia e Tisiologia (Brazilian Thoracic and Tuberculosis Society), Rede

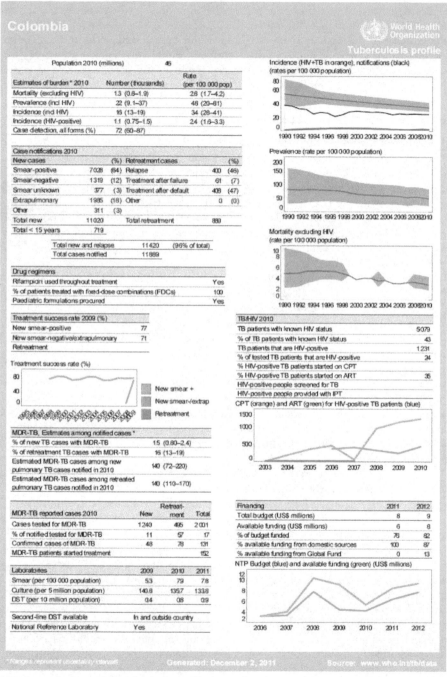

Fig. 1. Tuberculosis epidemiological profile for Colombia according to the World Health Organization, 2010.

TB (TB Network) and Liga Científica contra a Tuberculose (Scientific League against Tuberculosis). Since their creation, these entities have been constituted by people who are committed to TB control, though lacking the "community" component represented by people who are affected by and live with the disease (Santos Filho & Santos Gomes 2007). After that in recent years more organizations were involved in the fight against TB in the country.

The actions by the community entities in the fight against tuberculosis have been particularly concentrated on the networking among diverse social and govern mental actors; plus, on making the problem noticeable to their target populations or the general population, aiming their sensitization (Santos Filho & Santos Gomes 2007). For some relevant social actors, such as the Rede TB (TB Network) and the Liga Científi ca (Scientific League), the participation of the community sector in their activities aims at contributing to greater efficacy of their actions and responses to certain problems that are presented. Without the user's voice and perspective, there is the risk of repeating mistakes of not evaluating correctly the efficacy of actions such as applied methods and methodologies in health services (Santos Filho & Santos Gomes 2007). Then, multiple strategies are important in this context of development of new alternatives in the control of TB. The practice of participation, networking, advocacy and multi-sector cooperation will provide the necessary conditions for an effective control of tuberculosis in Brazil, as well in other countries where they would be applied (Santos Filho & Santos Gomes 2007).

5. Social networks in tuberculosis in Pereira, Colombia

Taking in account general epidemiology of TB in Colombia and particularly at a municipality where this strategy of social networking was developed, social conditions were analyzed (Collazos et al. 2010, Jalil-Paier & Donado 2010, Ascuntar et al. 2010, Mateus-Solarte & Carvajal-Barona 2008, Jaramillo 1999). Also, in the scenarios were considered the recent impacts of the health sector reform (Carvajal et al. 2004, Ayala & Kroeger 2002), that also have influenced the TB control programs from a national to a local perspective. Pereira is the capital municipality of the Department of Risaralda (Figure 2). It stands in the center of the western region of the country, located in a small valley that descends from a part of the western Andes mountain chain. Its strategic location in the coffee producing area makes the city an urban center in Colombia, as does its proximity to Bogotá, Cali and Medellín.

For 2011, Pereira municipality has an estimated population of 459,690. Official reported records for TB in Risaralda registered a disease incidence for 2011 of 66 cases per 100,000 pop (as 15 December) (which is above the national average rate of 24 cases per 100,000 pop). Pereira is divided into 19 urban submunicipalities: Ferrocarril, Olímpica, San Joaquín, Cuba, Del Café, El oso, Perla del Otún, Consota, El Rocío, El poblado, El jardín, San Nicolás, Centro, Río Otún, Boston, Universidad, Villavicencio, Oriente y Villasantana. Additionally also has rural townships which include Altagracia, Arabia, Caimalito, Cerritos, La Florida, Puerto Caldas, Combia Alta, Combia Baja, La Bella, Estrella- La Palmilla, Morelia, Tribunas. The municipality of Pereira has a diversified economy: the primary sector accounts for 5.7% of domestic product, the secondary sector shows a relative weight of 26.2%, while the tertiary sector is the most representative with a 68.1%. The GDP of Pereira grew by 3.7% in 2004. For 2010, Pereira reported 301 cases of TB (incidence rate of 65.85 cases per 100,000pop). In Pereira, previously reported interventions have been developed and working intersectorially with the academia in order to increase the impact of activities in TB control (Castañeda-Hernández et al. 2012b).

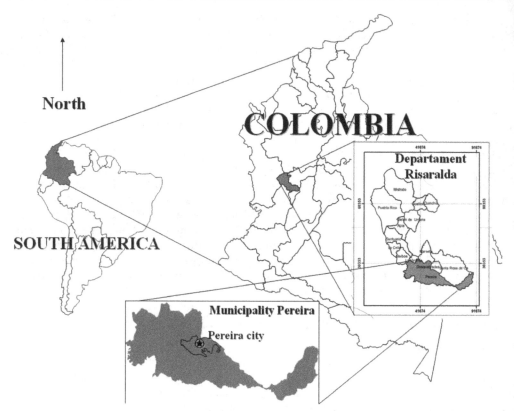

Fig. 2. Relative location of Pereira, Risaralda, Colombia, South America.

In the country, the strategic plan "*Colombia Libre de Tuberculosis para la Expansión y Fortalecimiento de la Estrategia Alto a la TB, 2010-2015*" (Colombia Free of TB for the Expansion and Enhancement of the Strategy Stop TB, 2010-2015), define as goal the achievement of notifications of new positive baciloscopy cases in more than 70% and a curation rate of at least 85%. In this context the routine surveillance allow to follow management and measurement of the impact of the realized actions by the control programs at municipal, departmental and national level, in order to generate interventions that contribute to achievement of the established goals to stop the advance of TB in the country.

Those considered strategies in the referred plan include the previously mentioned pursue advocacy, communication and social mobilization (ACMS), from the WHO Global Plan to STOP TB (World Health Organization 2011). In the context of wide-ranging partnerships for TB control, advocacy, communication and social mobilization (ACSM) embrace: advocacy to influence policy changes and sustain political and financial commitment; two-way communication between the care providers and people with TB as well as communities to improve knowledge of TB control policies, programmes and services; and social mobilization to engage society, especially the poor, and all allies and partners in the campaign to Stop TB. Each of these activities can help build greater commitment to fighting TB.

Advocacy is intended to secure the support of key constituencies in relevant local, national and international policy discussions and is expected to prompt greater accountability from governmental and international actors. Communication is concerned with informing, and enhancing knowledge among, the general public and people with TB and empowering them to express their needs and take action. Equally, encouraging providers to be more receptive to the expressed wants and views of people with TB and community members will make TB services more responsive to community needs. Social mobilization is the process of bringing together all feasible and practical intersectoral allies to raise people's knowledge of and demand for good-quality TB care and health care in general, assist in the delivery of resources and services and strengthen community participation for sustainability. Thus, ACSM is essential for achieving a world free of TB and is relevant to all aspects of the Stop TB Strategy. ACSM efforts in TB control should be linked with overarching efforts to promote public health and social development (World Health Organization 2011).

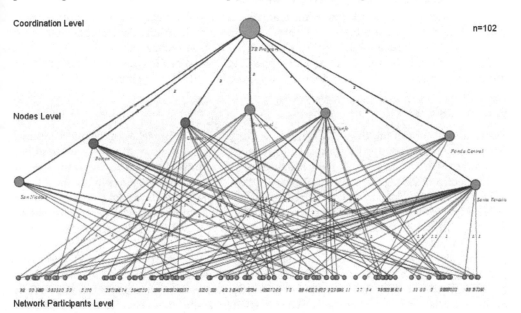

Fig. 3. SNA for Tuberculosis Network in Pereira, Colombia (developed with the Software SocNETV 0.81).

With these considerations in mind, in Pereira a social network for TB was developed. This network include the participation of ex-patients with TB, also healthy general population participated. All of them through the creation of nodes of the network, which were considered for this purposes as communitarian organizations constituted for a common objective and which are present regularly at neighborhoods in the municipality. Nodes were located at the 7 most highly prevalent areas of the municipality, previous to epidemiological analyses of those areas. Then, these locations were oriented to focalize the actions through the impact that, once established, this network would have on the control activities for TB in the areas of the municipality where most cases are concentrated.

In Pereira, with coordination of the TB control program on the top of the organization, a social network was developed with 7 strategically located and voluntary participation nodes

(Figure 3). This social network included more than 100 people supporting the program of TB in the municipality, then strengthening the control and surveillance activities necessary to reduce and to impact more the actions against the disease.

The nodes were constituted as communitarian organization, recognized by the communities and by the different related institutions, seen as long-lasting entities, with clear objectives and work plans for continued activity at the community. In all cases the participation was completely voluntary and non-profit.

As one of the key aspects of this network, multiple programmed activities were developed, including regularly meetings for discussions and for education on TB, giving multiple and different type of incentives in order to increase the interest on participation, helding workshops and different age-oriented designed activities that include games and handy-craft works, but in every case taking in consideration an structured and varied programation to include activities for TB education.

With this social TB network the municipal TB control program pursue to improve case detection and treatment adherence, combat stigma and discrimination, empower people affected by TB and mobilize political commitment and resources for TB.

Further implications of this social network, however, should be analyzed in the long term in order to measure its impact of epidemiological indicators of TB in the municipality.

6. Conclusions

Tuberculosis control in the XXI century requires new approaches and interventions, particularly those based in education and prevention with a community-based orientation. Programs such as the social network developed in Pereira TB control program, should performed in other highly endemic places. As the WHO recommends to pursue the ACMS (advocacy, communication and social mobilization), strategies as the social network allow to enhance particularly the communication and social mobilization components. Unfortunately at many national plans of TB control, how translate the ACMS in specific actions is not well defined in most occasions.

As has been previously stated, in the establishment of a social network for TB, previous diagnosis, including geo-referenced characterization, it is necessary to select the areas where the nodes will be established, taking also in consideration the suitability as the willingness of the potential participants of the network in each area and node. Finally, with the mining of the activities described, but also beginning with the idea of raise the awareness about the disease, taking in consideration a high level of diversity on the activities, as has been stated in order to warrant the continuous interest and participation of the network members on it.

In the future, in order to enhance the function and structure of the whole social network, further meetings between the nodes are expected. As now, only nodes interact internally, but the idea for the future activities in this setting is increase the links internally, but also between the main nodes in order to potentially increase the participation in the whole network.

Activities such as the development of social network of TB in Pereira will enhance the prevention, education and surveillance in the community, allowing a better integrated approach to the TB control in these scenarios and increasing the health profile in the community decreasing the lost opportunities for diagnosis and treatment of TB cases, finally leading to an improvement of the TB prevention and control.

7. References

Arbelaez MP, Nelson KE, Munoz A. 2000. BCG vaccine effectiveness in preventing tuberculosis and its interaction with human immunodeficiency virus infection. *Int. J Epidemiol.* 29(6):1085-91

Ascuntar JM, Gaviria MB, Uribe L, Ochoa J. 2010. Fear, infection and compassion: social representations of tuberculosis in Medellin, Colombia, 2007. *Int. J Tuberc. Lung Dis.* 14(10):1323-9

Atre S, Kudale A, Morankar S, Gosoniu D, Weiss MG. 2011. Gender and community views of stigma and tuberculosis in rural Maharashtra, India. *Glob. Public Health* 6(1):56-71

Ayala CC, Kroeger A. 2002. Health sector reform in Colombia and its effects on tuberculosis control and immunization programs. *Cad. Saude Publica* 18(6):1771-81

Bhardwaj N, Yan KK, Gerstein MB. 2010. Analysis of diverse regulatory networks in a hierarchical context shows consistent tendencies for collaboration in the middle levels. *Proceedings of the National Academy of Sciences of the United States of America* 107(15):6841-6

Black GF, Weir RE, Chaguluka SD, Warndorff D, Crampin AC et al. 2003. Gamma interferon responses induced by a panel of recombinant and purified mycobacterial antigens in healthy, non-mycobacterium bovis BCG-vaccinated Malawian young adults. *Clin. Diagn. Lab Immunol.* 10(4):602-11

Bohm M, Palphramand KL, Newton-Cross G, Hutchings MR, White PC. 2008. Dynamic interactions among badgers: implications for sociality and disease transmission. *J Anim Ecol.* 77(4):735-45

Carvajal R, Cabrera GA, Mateus JC. 2004. Effects of the health sector reform upon tuberculosis control interventions in Valle del Cauca, Colombia. *Biomedica.* 24 Supp 1:138-48

Castañeda-Hernández DM, Rodríguez-Morales AJ, Sepulveda-Arias JC. 2012a Importancia del uso de pruebas de medicion de la liberacion de interferon-gamma en la vigilancia epidemiologica de la tuberculosis. *Rev Med Chile* 140:(1)in press

Castañeda-Hernández DM, Mondragón-Cardona A, Campo-Betancourth CF, Tobón-García D, Alzate-Carvajal V, Jiménez-Canizales CE, Rodríguez Morales AJ. 2012b. Impacto de una Actividad Formativa en los Conocimientos, Actitudes y Percepciones (CAP) sobre Tuberculosis (TB) de Estudiantes de Medicina de una Universidad de Risaralda, Colombia. *Gaceta Médica de Caracas* 120(1):40-47

Cegielski JP, McMurray DN. 2004. The relationship between malnutrition and tuberculosis: evidence from studies in humans and experimental animals. *Int. J Tuberc. Lung Dis.* 8(3):286-98

Cohen T, Colijn C, Finklea B, Murray M. 2007. Exogenous re-infection and the dynamics of tuberculosis epidemics: local effects in a network model of transmission. *J R. Soc Interface* 4(14):523-31

Collazos C, Carrasquilla G, Ibanez M, Lopez LE. 2010. Prevalence of respiratory symptomatic in health institutions of Bogota, Colombia. *Biomedica.* 30(4):519-29

Cook VJ, Sun SJ, Tapia J, Muth SQ, Arguello DF et al. 2007. Transmission network analysis in tuberculosis contact investigations. *J Infect Dis.* 196(10):1517-27

Curto M, Scatena LM, de Paula Andrade RL, Palha PF, de Assis EG et al. 2010. Tuberculosis control: patient perception regarding orientation for the community and community participation. *Rev. Lat. Am. Enfermagem.* 18(5):983-9

Dhingra VK, Khan S. 2010. A sociological study on stigma among TB patients in Delhi. *Indian J Tuberc.* 57(1):12-8

Dim CC, Dim NR, Morkve O. 2011. Tuberculosis: a review of current concepts and control programme in Nigeria. *Niger. J Med* 20(2):200-6

Drewe JA, Eames KT, Madden JR, Pearce GP. 2011. Integrating contact network structure into tuberculosis epidemiology in meerkats in South Africa: Implications for control. *Prev. Vet. Med* 101(1-2):113-20

Fitzpatrick LK, Hardacker JA, Heirendt W, Agerton T, Streicher A et al. 2001. A preventable outbreak of tuberculosis investigated through an intricate social network. *Clin. Infect Dis.* 33(11):1801-6

Francis J, Reed A, Yohannes F, Dodard M, Fournier AM. 2002. Screening for tuberculosis among orphans in a developing country. *Am. J Prev. Med* 22(2):117-9

Franco-Paredes C, Jones D, Rodriguez-Morales AJ, Santos-Preciado JI. 2007. Commentary: improving the health of neglected populations in Latin America. *BMC Public Health* 7:11

Franco-Paredes C, Von A, Hidron A, Rodriguez-Morales AJ, Tellez I et al. 2007. Chagas disease: an impediment in achieving the Millennium Development Goals in Latin America. *BMC Int. Health Hum. Rights* 7:7

Galimi R. 2011. Extrapulmonary tuberculosis: tuberculous meningitis new developments. *Eur. Rev Med Pharmacol. Sci* 15(4):365-86

Garcia-Rodriguez JF, Alvarez-Diaz H, Lorenzo-Garcia MV, Marino-Callejo A, Fernandez-Rial A, Sesma-Sanchez P. 2011. Extrapulmonary tuberculosis: epidemiology and risk factors. *Enferm. Infecc. Microbiol. Clin.* 29(7):502-9

Garg RK. 2010. Tuberculous meningitis. *Acta Neurol. Scand.* 122(2):75-90

Ginsberg AM. 2000. A proposed national strategy for tuberculosis vaccine development. *Clin. Infect Dis.* 30 Suppl 3:S233-S242

Glaziou P, Floyd K, Raviglione M. 2009. Global burden and epidemiology of tuberculosis. *Clin. Chest Med* 30(4):621-36, vii

Guzzetta G, Ajelli M, Yang Z, Merler S, Furanello C, Kirschner D. 2011. Modeling socio-demography to capture tuberculosis transmission dynamics in a low burden setting. *J Theor. Biol.* 289:197-205

Hawe P, Webster C, Shiell A. 2004. A glossary of terms for navigating the field of social network analysis. *J Epidemiol. Community Health* 58(12):971-5

Hoek KG, Van RA, van Helden PD, Warren RM, Victor TC. 2011. Detecting drug-resistant tuberculosis: the importance of rapid testing. *Mol. Diagn. Ther.* 15(4):189-94

Jalil-Paier H, Donado G. 2010. Socio-political implications of the fight against alcoholism and tuberculosis in Colombia, 1910-1925. *Rev Salud Publica (Bogota.)* 12(3):486-96

Jaramillo E. 1999. Tuberculosis and stigma: predictors of prejudice against people with tuberculosis. *J Health Psychol.* 4(1):71-9

Jittimanee SX, Nateniyom S, Kittikraisak W, Burapat C, Akksilp S et al. 2009. Social stigma and knowledge of tuberculosis and HIV among patients with both diseases in Thailand. *PLoS. One.* 4(7):e6360

Kemp JR, Mann G, Simwaka BN, Salaniponi FM, Squire SB. 2007. Can Malawi's poor afford free tuberculosis services? Patient and household costs associated with a tuberculosis diagnosis in Lilongwe. *Bull. World Health Organ* 85(8):580-5

Klovdahl AS, Graviss EA, Musser JM. Infectious disease control: combining molecular biological and network methods. 8, 73-99. 2002.

Lawrence RJ, Fudge C. 2009. Healthy Cities in a global and regional context. *Health promotion international* 24 Suppl 1:i11-i18

Lonnroth K, Aung T, Maung W, Kluge H, Uplekar M. 2007. Social franchising of TB care through private GPs in Myanmar: an assessment of treatment results, access, equity and financial protection. *Health Policy Plan.* 22(3):156-66

Lonnroth K, Castro KG, Chakaya JM, Chauhan LS, Floyd K et al. 2010. Tuberculosis control and elimination 2010-50: cure, care, and social development. *Lancet* 375(9728):1814-29

Lonnroth K, Williams BG, Cegielski P, Dye C. 2010. A consistent log-linear relationship between tuberculosis incidence and body mass index. *Int. J Epidemiol.* 39(1):149-55

Marais BJ, Schaaf HS. 2010. Childhood tuberculosis: an emerging and previously neglected problem. *Infect Dis. Clin. North Am.* 24(3):727-49

Mateus-Solarte JC, Carvajal-Barona R. 2008. Factors predictive of adherence to tuberculosis treatment, Valle del Cauca, Colombia. *Int. J Tuberc. Lung Dis.* 12(5):520-6

Murray M, Oxlade O, Lin HH. 2011. Modeling social, environmental and biological determinants of tuberculosis. *Int. J Tuberc. Lung Dis.* 15 Suppl 2:S64-S70

Orcau A, Cayla JA, Martinez JA. 2011. Present epidemiology of tuberculosis. Prevention and control programs. *Enferm. Infecc. Microbiol. Clin.* 29 Suppl 1:2-7

Palinkas LA, Holloway IW, Rice E, Fuentes D, Wu Q, Chamberlain P. 2011. Social networks and implementation of evidence-based practices in public youth-serving systems: a mixed-methods study. *Implement. Sci* 6.113

Pantoja A, Floyd K, Unnikrishnan KP, Jitendra R, Padma MR et al. 2009. Economic evaluation of public-private mix for tuberculosis care and control, India. Part I. Socio-economic profile and costs among tuberculosis patients. *Int. J Tuberc. Lung Dis.* 13(6):698-704

Pantoja A, Lonnroth K, Lal SS, Chauhan LS, Uplekar M et al. 2009. Economic evaluation of public-private mix for tuberculosis care and control, India. Part II. Cost and cost-effectiveness. *Int. J Tuberc. Lung Dis.* 13(6):705-12

Perisse AR, Costa Nery JA. 2007. The relevance of social network analysis on the epidemiology and prevention of sexually transmitted diseases. *Cad. Saude Publica* 23 Suppl 3:S361-S369

Pungrassami P, Kipp AM, Stewart PW, Chongsuvivatwong V, Strauss RP, Van RA. 2010. Tuberculosis and AIDS stigma among patients who delay seeking care for tuberculosis symptoms. *Int. J Tuberc. Lung Dis.* 14(2):181-7

Rajeswari R, Balasubramanian R, Muniyandi M, Geetharamani S, Thresa X, Venkatesan P. 1999. Socio-economic impact of tuberculosis on patients and family in India. *Int. J Tuberc. Lung Dis.* 3(10):869-77

Rocha C, Montoya R, Zevallos K, Curatola A, Ynga W et al. 2011. The Innovative Socio-economic Interventions Against Tuberculosis (ISIAT) project: an operational assessment. *Int. J Tuberc. Lung Dis.* 15 Suppl 2:S50-S57

Rodríguez Morales AJ, Lorizio W, Vargas J, Fernández L, Durán B, Husband G, Rondón A, Vargas K, Barbella RA, Dickson SM. 2008. Malaria, Tuberculosis, VIH/SIDA e Influenza Aviar: ¿Asesinos de la Humanidad? *Rev Soc Med Quir Hosp Emerg Perez de Leon* 39(1):52-76

Santos Filho ET, Santos Gomes ZM. 2007. Strategies for tuberculosis control in Brazil: networking and civil society participation. *Rev. Saude Publica* 41 Suppl 1:111-6

Sterling TR, Thompson D, Stanley RL, McElroy PD, Madison A et al. 2000. A multi-state outbreak of tuberculosis among members of a highly mobile social network: implications for tuberculosis elimination. *Int. J Tuberc. Lung Dis.* 4(11):1066-73

Szell M, Lambiotte R, Thurner S. 2010. Multirelational organization of large-scale social networks in an online world. *Proc. Natl. Acad. Sci U. S. A* 107(31):13636-41

Vargas J, Gamboa C, Negrin D, Correa M, Sandoval C et al. 2005. Disseminated Mycobacterium mucogenicum infection in a patient with idiopathic CD4+ T lymphocytopenia manifesting as fever of unknown origin. *Clin. Infect Dis.* 41(5):759-60

Wilson GJ, Carter SP, Delahay RJ. 2011. Advances and prospects for management of TB transmission between badgers and cattle. *Vet. Microbiol.* 151(1-2):43-50

World Health Organization. 2011. *2011 Global Tuberculosis Control,* Geneva: WHO.

Zhao Y, Levina E, Zhu J. 2011. Community extraction for social networks. *Proc. Natl. Acad. Sci U. S. A* 108(18):7321-6

9

Lassa Fever in the Tropics

Ute Inegbenebor
Department of Physiology
College of Medicine
Ambrose Alli University, Ekpoma
Nigeria

1. Introduction

Lassa fever is a frequently underestimated but socially and economically devastating disease. Lassa fever first came into limelight in 1969, when two nuns died as a result of complications of a hemorrhagic fever in Lassa town in the Borno State of Nigeria. Since then it has become endemic in many parts of West Africa. Out breaks of Lassa fever are usually associated with high mortality rates as the cases usually present late to the hospitals. Besides, many doctors find it difficult to diagnose Lassa fever until complications have set in because of the similarity of presentation to other more common febrile illnesses such as malaria and typhoid. In a study carried out in Sierra Leone in 1987, Lassa fever was found to be responsible for 10-16% of admissions and 30% of deaths in a major referral center. In another study of adult medical admissions in a special center for the management of Lassa fever in Nigeria in 2008, Lassa fever was responsible for 7% of admissions and 13% of deaths with a case fatality rate of 28%. However, the enlightenment campaign for the prevention of Lassa fever and diagnostic facilities are either lacking or rudimentary in most countries where Lassa fever is endemic. Compared to HIV/AIDS, Lassa fever is more infectious to close associates and it rapidly kills in dozens. However, Lassa fever does not get the global attention it deserves.

2. Etiology/pathogenesis-

Lassa fever is caused by Lassa fever virus, a member of the family Arenaviridae. It is an enveloped single stranded bi-segmented rna virus Replication for Lassa virus is very rapid, while also demonstrating temporal control in replication. There are two genome segments. The first replication step is transcription of messenger RNA copies of the negative- or minus sense genome. This ensures an adequate supply of viral proteins for subsequent steps of replication, as proteins known as N and L are translated from the mRNA. The positive- or plus-sense genome then makes viral complementary (vcRNA) copies of itself, which are + sense. The vcRNA is a template for producing minus sense progeny but mRNA is also synthesized from it. The mRNA synthesized from vcRNA are translated to make the G (spike) proteins and Z proteins. Thus, with this temporal control, the spike proteins, which are on the outside of the virus particle, are produced last, making the infection more difficult for the host immune system to detect. Nucleotide studies of the genome have shown that Lassa has four lineages: three found in Nigeria and the fourth in Guinea, Liberia, and Sierra

Leone. The Nigerian strains seem likely to have been ancestral to the others but further research is required to confirm this.

The Lassa virus gains entry into the host cell by means of the cell-surface receptor the alpha-dystroglycan (alpha-DG), a versatile receptor for proteins of the extracellular matrix. It shares this receptor with the prototypic arenavirus lymphocytic choriomeningitis virus. Receptor recognition depends on a specific sugar modification of alpha-dystroglycan by a group of glycosyltransferases known as the LARGE proteins. Specific variants of the genes encoding these proteins appear to be under positive selection in West Africa where Lassa is endemic. Alpha-dystroglycan is also used as a receptor by viruses of the New World clade C arenaviruses (Oliveros and Latino viruses). In contrast, the New World areanviruses of clades A and B, which include the important viruses Machupo, Guanarito, Junin, and Sabia in addition to the non pathogenic Amapari virus, use the transferrin receptor 1. A small aliphatic amino acid at the GP1 glycoprotein amino acid position 260 is required for high-affinity binding to alpha-DG. In addition, GP1 amino acid position 259 also appears to be important, since all arenaviruses showing high-affinity alpha-DG binding possess a bulky aromatic amino acid (tyrosine or phenylalanine) at this position.

Unlike most enveloped viruses which use clathrin coated pits for cellular entry and bind to their receptors in a pH dependent fashion, Lassa and lymphocytic choriomeningitis virus instead use an endocytotic pathway independent of clathrin, caveolin, dynamin and actin. Once within the cell the viruses are rapidly delivered to endosomes via vesicular trafficking albeit one that is largely independent of the small GTPases Rab5 and Rab7. On contact with the endosome pH-dependent membrane fusion occurs mediated by the envelope glycoprotein.

Lassa virus will infect almost every tissue in the human body. It starts with the mucosa, intestine, lungs and urinary system, and then progresses to the vascular system.

2.1 Predisposing factors

- Use of rat meat as a source of protein by people in some communities; contamination of exposed food by rat feces and urine;
- Traditional autopsy, where the operator may injure himself with scalpel and contaminate the injury with the blood of the deceased, who may have died of Lassa fever
- Forceful ingestion of water used in bathing a dead husband, by a widow suspected to be involved in his death. In many communities, family members may be forced to drink water used in bathing dead relatives in order to prove their innocence.
- Corrupt practices by staple food producers, which involve drying garri (cassava flour) in the open air in the daytime and sometimes at night. This enables all types of rat including mastomys natalensis to contaminate the flour with their excreta. This constitutes a public health hazard when the infected garri is sold to consumers in the market. The common habit of eating garri soaked in water may favor Lassa fever infection.
- Many other types of staple foods are also processed in the open sun, which is the major natural drier. These include rice, plantain chips, yam chips and cassava chips, which are processed into rice flour, plantain flour, yam flour, and raw cassava flour. Though these are also processed into staple foods such as tuwo shinkafa, plantain based amala, yam based amala and lafun respectively, the amount of heat involved in processing them into edible pastes, may be enough to denature lassa fever virus, which is heat labile.
- Bush burning of savannahs may be carried out by meat-hungry youths, during the dry season, in order to be able to have access to rodents and other animals. This habit often

drives mastomys natalensis, the reservoir of lassa fever virus, into peoples homes and may be responsible for outbreaks of lassa fever in the dry season.

3. Epidemiology

3.1 Distribution
Lassa fever is endemic in West Africa. However the world is now a global village and the previous geographical gap between the tropics and the developed world has been bridged by international travel. The 6 – 21 days incubation period indicates that a person who contacts Lassa fever in an endemic area in West Africa may travel to a developed country within the incubation period and cause an epidemic.

3.2 Prevalence
The prevalence of Lassa fever can be assesed by determining the prevalence of antibodies to Lassa fever in communities. The prevalence of Lassa fever in Nigeria, Guinea and Sierra Leone can be up to 21%, 55% and 52% respectively.

3.3 Reservoir
The reservoir of infection is mastomys natalensis. It is a species of rodent in the Muridae family. It is also known as the Natal multimammate rat, the common African rat, or the African soft-furred rat. It is found in Angola, Benin, Botswana, Burkina Faso, Burundi, Cameroon, Central African Republic, Chad, Republic of the Congo, Democratic Republic of the Congo, Ivory Coast, Equatorial Guinea, Ethiopia, Gabon, Ghana, Guinea, Guinea-Bissau, Kenya, Lesotho, Malawi, Mali, Mauritania, Mozambique, Namibia, Niger, Nigeria, Rwanda, Senegal, Sierra Leone, Somalia, South Africa, Sudan, Swaziland, Tanzania, Togo, Uganda, Zambia, and Zimbabwe. Its natural habitats are subtropical or tropical dry forests, subtropical or tropical moist lowland forests, dry savanna, moist savanna, subtropical or tropical dry shrubland, subtropical or tropical moist shrubland, arable land, pastureland, rural gardens, urban areas, irrigated land, and seasonally flooded agricultural land. In 1972, the Natal multimammate Mouse was found to be the natural host of the deadly Lassa fever virus.

3.4 Transmission
Lassa fever is transmitted to humans when they ingest food contaminated by the feces and urine of mastomys natalensis. Once humans are infected, transmission also occurs from human to human through contact with fluid and aerosol secretions in the form of sneezing, sputum, seminal fluid, stool, urine and blood. Vertical transmission through breast milk has been observed.

3.5 Host factors
Men are more commonly affected than women. However the case fatality rate is nearly two times higher in women. Men are more likely to buy food from food vendors especially at lunch time while women are more likely to eat personally cooked food. Contamination of food from this source may be responsible for the higher incidence of Lassa fever in men. Although the high case-fatality of Lassa fever is due to delayed cellular immunity, development of partial immunity as a result of frequent exposure to contaminated food may be responsible for the milder forms of the disease and lower case-fatality rate in men. Research is needed to find out whether Lassa fever infection confers partial or full immunity on affected people.

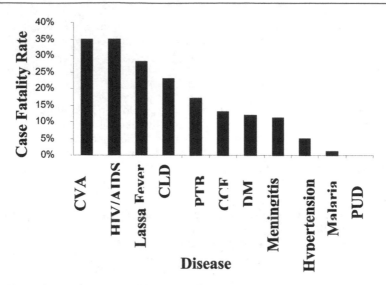

Fig. 1. Bar Chart showing Case Fatality Rates of Common Diseases of Medical Inpatients in Irrua Specialist Teaching Hospital (ISTH), Irrua, Nigeria in 2007

4. Clinical features

Signs and symptoms typically occur after an incubation period of 6 –21 days. The onset of illness is insidious, with fever and shivering accompanied by malaise, headache and generalized aching. Sore throat is a common early symptom. In some cases the tonsils and pharynx may be inflamed with patches of white or yellowish exudate and occasionally small vesicles or shallow ulcers. (Importantly, a similar appearance may be seen in cases of malignant tertian malaria). As the illness progresses the body temperature may rise to 41°C with daily fluctuations of 2-3°C. The duration and severity of fever is very variable. The average duration is 16 days but extremes of 6-30 days have been reported. A feature of severe attacks is lethargy or prostration disproportionate to the fever. During the second week of illness there may be edema of the head and neck, encephalopathy, pleural effusion and ascites. Vomiting and diarrhea may aggravate the effects of renal and circulatory failure. Severe cases develop significant hemorrhage and multi-organ failure with widespread edema and bleeding into the skin, mucosae and deeper tissues. In non-fatal cases, the fever subsides and the patient's condition improves rapidly although tiredness may persist for several weeks. There is usually a leucopenia early in the course, though a high polymorphonuclear leucocytosis may occur with severe tissue damage. Another common late complication is sensorineural deafness. Clinically, a Lassa fever infection is difficult to distinguish from other viral hemorrhagic fevers, such as Ebola and Marburg, and from more common febrile illnesses such as malaria and typhoid.

5. Complications of Lassa fever

Various complications may occur in the course of Lassa fever. These complications vary with duration of illness and sex of the victim. Thes complications include hypovolemic shock, Electrolyte imbalance, Disseminated intravascular coagulation, Renal failure, Sensorineural deafness, pregnancy complications.

5.1 Hypovolemic shock
Lassa fever viremia causes endothelial and platelet dysfunction with consequent leaky capillary syndrome. Bleeding occurs in all organs and from all mucosae leading to hypovolemic shock.

5.2 Electrolyte imbalance
Most Lassa fever victims lose fluid through vomiting and diarrhea and therefore develop electrolyte imbalance.

5.3 Renal failure
Renal tubular damage may also occur on Lassa fever and in conjunction with the hypovolemic shock predispose to renal failure

5.4 Complications of lassa fever in pregnancy
Lassa fever is especially dangerous in pregnant women. Abortion is common in early pregnancy and intrauterine fetal death is common in later pregnancies. Abortion reduces the mortality rate in affected pregnant women. Prognosis is very poor in pregnant women as mortality rate may be up to 80%.

5.5 Sensorineural deafness
This is the commonest complication of Lassa fever. It is not related to the severity of disease as it may occur with the same frequency in both mild and severe forms of the disease.

6. Laboratory diagnosis

Lassa fever is most often diagnosed using ELISAs. The virus can also be detected by reverse transcription PCR (RT-PCR) in all patients by the third day of illness, but immunofluorescence identifies only 52% of the patients.

6.1 Treatment
Ribavirin, an antiviral drug, is the current treatment of Lassa fever. The drug is to be administered in a volume of 50-100 ml of normal saline to be infused over 30-40 minutes.
- Loading dose: 33 mg/kg (maximum dose 2.64 g)
- Followed by a dose of 16 mg/kg (max dose 1.28 g) every 6 hours for the first 4 days
- Followed by a dose of 8 mg/kg (maximum dose 0.64 g) every 8 hours for the subsequent 6 days

Supportive treatment is usually carried out with intravenous fluids, and treatment of complications such as renal failure and infections may be necessary.

Although Lassa fever can be treated with ribavirin, early diagnosis and treatment is essential in all cases of Lassa fever. Ribavirin is most effective when given within 6 days of illness. Self-diagnosis and treatment is common in the tropics because of ignorance and poverty. It is only when there is no remission of fever that the patient seeks treatment in a health-care facility. However, many health-care providers are unable to make early

Disease	Number of Admissions			Laboratory Diagnosis	Treatment	Number of Deaths			Case Fatality Rate		
	Male	Female	Total			Male	Female	Total	Male	Female	General
Cerebrovascular accident (CVA)	44	35	79	Clinical diagnosis/ Occasional CT Scans.	Supportive Treatment: Aspirin 300mg daily Treatment for underlying problems e.g Hypertension, Diabetes Mellitus	18	10	28	41%	29%	35%
HIV/ AIDS	36	56	92	ELISA/ Confirmatory Test	Supportive treatment; Treatment for opportunistic infections followed by Combined therapy with AZT and lamivudine	13	19	32	36%	34%	35%
Lassa fever	48	16	64	Clinical triad of Pharygitis, Retrosternal pain and Proteinuria.; Confirmation wirh RT-PCR test	Supportive treatment Intravenous Ribavirin for 8 days	11	7	18	23%	44%	28%
Chronic liver disease (CLD)	13	9	22	Liver Function Tests	Supportive treatment, Interferon, Lipid clearing agents e.g . Litrison, Essentiale Lamivudine for chronic Hepatitis B infection	2	3	5	15%	33%	23%
Pulmonary Tuberculosis (PTB)	45	27	72	Clinical Diagnosis/ Chest X-Ray/ 3 early morning samples of Sputum for Ziehl Neelsen Stain and Microscopy for Acid Fast Bacilli	Supportive treatment; Rifampicin, Isoniazid, Ethambutol, Pyrazinimide	7	5	12	16%	19%	17%
Congestive Cardiac Failure(CCF)	52	41	93	Clinical Diagnosis/ Chest X Ray	Cardiac position, Oxygen therapy, Diuretic e.g. Furosemide ± Digoxin	6	6	12	12%	15%	13%
Diabetes Mellitus (DM)	73	84	157	Clinical Diagnosis Fasting Blood Sugar ≥8mmol/l Random Blood Sugar ≥11mmol/l	Soluble Insulin/ Lente Insulin (70:30) treatment	6	12	18	8%	14%	12%
Meningitis	23	23	46	Clinical Diagnosis Lumbar Puncture Cerebrospinal spinal fluid for Microscopy, culture & Sensitivity	Supportive therapy; Initial high dose Cephalosporins followed by Antimicrobial therapy based on sensitivity results	3	2	5	13%	9%	11%
Hypertension (HTN)	41	42	83	Blood Pressure ≥ 160/100mmHg	Anti hypertensive drugs e.g Nifedipine	2	2	4	5%	5%	5%
Malaria	82	76	158	Thick and Thin Blood Film for microscopy.	Supportive treatment; Intravenous Quinmine or Artesunate/ amodiaquine	1	0	1	1%	0%	<1%
Peptic Ulcer (PUD)	24	18	42	Clinical Diagnosis/ Barium meal	Supportive treatment; Ranitidine/ Proton inhibitors	0	0	0	0%	0%	0%
Total	481	427	908			69	66	135			

Table 1. Case fatality rates of common Diseases among Medical inpatients in ISTH, Irrua, Nigeria.

diagnosis, and are very likely to make a diagnosis of resistant malaria or typhoid. Besides most health care providers have no access to diagnostic facilities, which are only available in tertiary health centers. This allows the patient to get to terminal stages before they are transferred to a tertiary center. Sometimes the life of the health-care provider is claimed along with that of the patient.

7. Prognosis

Prognosis depends on how early a patient presents at the clinic. Most patients recover completely if diagnosed early and when treatment with ribavirin is commenced within 6 days of illness. In studies carried out in special referral centers in Nigeria and Sierra Leone, Lassa fever was responsible for 13% and 30% of adult deaths respectively. The death rates were in adult medical wards where only 7% and 10-16 % respectively of the total number of admissions were for Lassa fever. Prognosis is probably better in males who may acquire partial immunity due to the habit of patronizing food vendors. In a study done in Nigeria, the case fatality rate in males was 23% compared to women with 44%, though males were four times more commonly affected than females.

8. Control

8.1 The individual
The affected person should be admitted to a special center for the treatment of Lassa fever. Where this is not possible, the patient should be barrier-nursed. Health care providers and close associates of the patient should wear protective clothing, masks and gloves. Excrements from affected persons should be properly disposed.

8.2 The community
Legislation is needed to prevent widowhood rites, traditional autopsies, bush burning and unhygienic preparation of garri and other staple foods. Animal husbandry and fisheries should be encouraged in order to provide alternative sources of first-class proteins for rat eaters. Regular and sustainable environmental sanitation is needed to prevent rat breeding. The public should be made aware of the mode of contact of Lassa fever and its high case-fatality rate using print and electronic media. Community involvement and participation is necessary to provide sustainable Lassa fever control. Food vendors should be educated on the need to prevent food contamination with Lassa fever virus. Grains, flours and left-over foods should be adequately covered to prevent contamination by rats. Rodenticides should be used for the destruction of rats in homes, and development of Lassa fever vaccine should be facilitated. Regular seminars should be held for health-care providers on early diagnosis and treatment of Lassa fever, while diagnostic kits should be made available in district hospitals. Affected people should be referred early to the special center in order to prevent or limit disability, while those with disabilities should be rehabilitated functionally, socially and psychologically so that they can be gainfully employed.

9. Prospects

Though vaccines are not currently available for Lassa fever, there is evidence that they will be produced in the near future. Research done with non-human primates have revealed that survivors exhibit fewer lesions and a **lower** viral load than non-survivors.

Although all animals develop strong humoral responses, antibodies appear more rapidly in survivors and are directed against GP(1), GP(2), and NP. Activated T lymphocytes circulate in survivors, whereas T-cell activation is **low** and delayed in fatalities

A single injection of ML29 reassortant vaccine for **Lassa fever** induces **low**, transient viremia, and **low** or moderate levels of ML29 replication in tissues of common marmosets depending on the dose of the vaccination. The vaccination elicits specific immune responses and completely protects marmosets against fatal disease by induction of sterilizing cell-mediated immunity. DNA array analysis of human peripheral blood mononuclear cells from healthy donors exposed to ML29 revealed that gene expression patterns in ML29-exposed PBMC and **control**, media-exposed PBMC, clustered together confirming safety profile of the ML29 in non-human primates. The ML29 reassortant is a promising vaccine candidate for **Lassa fever**.

10. References

Baize S, Marianneau P, Loth P, et al. Early and strong immune responses are associated with control of viral replication and recovery in lassa virus-infected cynomolgus monkeys. J Virol (United States), Jun 2009, 83(11) p5890-903

Demby AH, Chamberlain J, Brown DW, Clegg CS. Early diagnosis of Lassa fever by reverse transcription PCR. J Clin Microbiol 1994; 32:2898–903

Donaldson, Ross I. (2009). The Lassa Ward:One Man's Fight Against One of the World's Deadliest Diseases. St. Martin's Press. ISBN 0312377002. ISBN 978-0312377007.

Frame JD, Baldwin JM, Gocke DJ, Troup JM. Lassa fever, a new virus disease of man from West Africa. I. Clinical description and pathological findings. Am J Trop Med Hyg 1970; 19:670–6.

Granjon, L., Lavrenchenko, L., Corti, M., Coetzee, N. & Rahman, E.A. Mastomys natalensis. 2006 IUCN Red List of Threatened Species. Accessed 09-06-2011.

Inegbenebor, U, Okosun, J, Inegbenebor, J. Prevention of Lassa fever in Nigeria. Trans R. Soc Trop Med Hyg, 2010; 4(1):51-54 PMID: 19712954

Lukashevich IS, Carrion R, Salvato MS, et al. Safety, immunogenicity, and efficacy of the ML29 reassortant vaccine for Lassa fever in small non-human primates. Vaccine (Netherlands), Sep 26 2008, 26(41) p5246-54

McCormick JB, King IJ, Webb PA, Johnson KM, O'Sullivan R, Smith ES. A case-control study of the clinical diagnosis and course of Lassa fever. J Infect Dis 1987;155:445–55.

McCormick JB, King IJ, Webb PA, Scribner CL, Craven RB, Johnson KM, et al. Lassa fever: effective therapy with ribavirin. N Engl J Med. 1986;314:20–6.

Ogbu O, Ajuluchukwu E, Uneke CJ. Lassa fever in West African subregion: an overview. J Vector Borne Dis 2007; 44:1–11.

Richmond JK, Baglole DJ. Lassa fever: epidemiology, clinical features,and social consequences. BMJ 2003;327:1271–5.

WHO. Lassa fever fact sheet no. 179. Geneva: World Health Organization; 2005.

Part 2

Other Tropical Infectious and Non-Infectious Conditions

10

Novel Molecular Diagnostic Platform for Tropical Infectious Diseases

Yasuyoshi Mori, Norihiro Tomita,
Hidetoshi Kanda and Tsugunori Notomi
Eiken Chemical Co., Ltd.
Japan

1. Introduction

Infectious disease is one of the most concerning health issues worldwide. To provide patients with effective medical treatment and prevent the spread of diseases and emergence of drug-resistant strains, quick and reliable diagnostic techniques are in high demand. However, lack of accessibility to such diagnostic systems has resulted in the deterioration of the situation in most developing countries, especially in sub-Saharan tropical countries (Rodrigues et al., 2010). Diagnostics using molecular technologies have emerged as a promising methodology because of their remarkable high sensitivity, and therefore, they have been applied as diagnostic tools for detecting various kinds of pathogens in clinical settings in developed countries. However, resources essential for molecular assays, such as bio-safety cabinets, a stable supply of electricity, and well-experienced technicians, are scarce in most of the peripheral laboratories in developing countries. In this chapter, we would like to describe a recently developed novel diagnostic platform and discuss its application for realizing molecular diagnostics for infectious diseases within resource-limited settings.

Molecular diagnostics comprise the following 3 steps: sample preparation, amplification, and detection. To develop a molecular diagnostic platform with the desired simplicity and performance, it is necessary to introduce element technologies for all the 3 steps, which are less complicated and can be used in peripheral laboratories with limited resources. Of the abovementioned 3 steps, amplification of target DNA/RNA is the most important. Therefore, the loop-mediated isothermal amplification (LAMP) method involving the calcein detection method has been applied to the platform as a key technology. LAMP, using the calcein method, enables recognition of small quantities of DNA/RNA of pathogens present in clinical specimens by means of the fluorescence emitted from the LAMP solutions after amplification.

The next important step is sample processing, for which we have developed a simple and easy-to-use technology, namely, procedure for ultra rapid extraction (PURE). The combination of both these technologies can be considered a novel platform for molecular diagnostics, which can be applied to resource-limited settings. The fundamental characteristics of these element technologies and application of the novel platform to diagnostics for evaluation of certain tropical diseases are discussed below.

2. Steps involved in molecular diagnostics

2.1 Amplification – LAMP

Since the publication of the first report regarding LAMP in 2000 (Notomi et al., 2000), LAMP has been used to detect different kinds of pathogens (Mori & Notomi, 2009), including viruses (Kubo et al., 2010), bacteria (Iwamoto et al., 2003), and protozoa (Spencer et al., 2010), and thus far, approximately 500 reports have been published regarding the application of LAMP. Because the LAMP method is simple and quick, it has been considered one of the most ideal nucleic acid amplification methods, which can be applied as an easy-to-use and cost-effective genetic test system (Parida et al., 2008).

2.1.1 Mechanism of LAMP

Although the reaction mechanism appears complicated, LAMP is simple to perform — it involves mixing primers (designed as depicted in figure 1-A), DNA polymerase with strand-displacement activity, and dNTPs, in a buffer containing magnesium ions, and maintaining the mixture at a constant temperature of 60–67 °C for 15–60 minutes. If template DNA molecules are present in the sample solution, large quantities of DNA with the target sequence (amplicon) are produced after incubation.

Figures 1-B and C show the schematic representation of the mechanism of LAMP. First, the forward inner primer (FIP) anneals to the template DNA at the F2c sequence and the extension reaction occurs by the enzymatic activity of *Bst* polymerase. Because *Bst* polymerase exhibits strand displacement activity, the product obtained from FIP is displaced by the other extension reaction associated with the F3 primer. Subsequently, the extension reaction occurs from the backward inner primer (BIP) on the product of the FIP, and not on the template DNA with a B2c sequence; the product obtained is also displaced by DNA synthesis associated with the B3 primer. These reactions result in a product with a dumbbell-like structure as shown in figure 1-B. The formation of the dumbbell-like product is essential for LAMP to establish isothermal amplification because the loop structures are always single stranded and can be annealed by FIP or BIP. Thus, formation of the loop structure can lead to the elimination of the denaturing step, which is otherwise essential in PCR for obtaining single-stranded DNA.

After the formation of the dumbbell-like structure, a cyclic reaction is spontaneously established between the dumbbell-like structure and its complementary product, as shown in figure 1-C. Furthermore, in the course of the cyclic reaction, elongated products with various copies of the target sequence are also produced.

The basic characteristics of the LAMP method are summarized below:

1.   The whole amplification reaction occurs continuously under isothermal conditions, thus eliminating the need to use a thermal cycler, which is commonly used for PCR.
2.   Because LAMP primers recognize 6 distinct regions, the specificity of LAMP is much higher than that of the other commonly used amplification techniques.
3.   Amplification can be performed using an RNA template only by the addition of reverse transcriptase to the reaction (one-step RT-LAMP).
4.   The LAMP reaction can be accelerated by using additional primers, called "loop primers," which are designed between F1c/B1c and F2c/B2c (Nagamine et al., 2002).

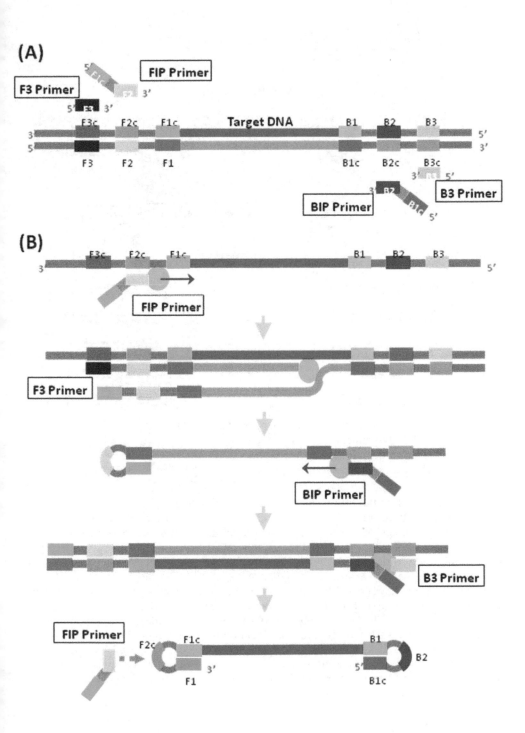

(C)

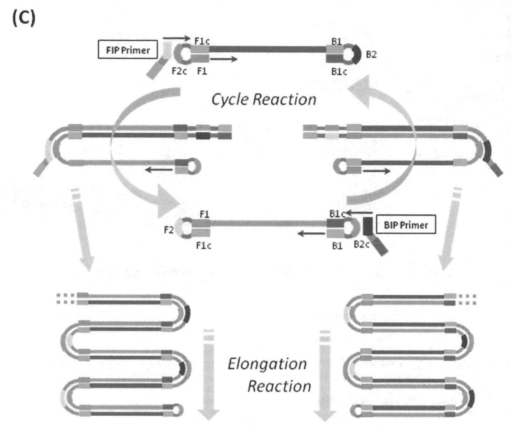

Fig. 1. Schematic representation of the mechanism of the LAMP assay
A) Design of the LAMP primers
B) Formation of a dumbbell-like structure
C) Cyclic and elongation reactions

2.1.2 Strategies that make LAMP simple and cost-effective

Conventional LAMP reagents are supplied in liquid form, and they have to be stored below -20 °C, similar to most PCR reagents. However, because of the lack of a freezer and cold chain transportation system in most of the peripheral laboratories in developing countries, it is essential to formulate LAMP reagents, which can be stably preserved at ambient temperatures (Jorgensen et al., 2006; Aziah et al., 2007). The newly formulated LAMP reagents are dried down into the lid of the reaction tubes, thus obtaining preservation stability at ambient temperatures for more than 12 months. The dried LAMP reagents can be reconstituted quite easily by shaking the tubes after the addition of the purified DNA solution. Because the LAMP reagent for each reaction is deposited on the individual tubes in advance, there is no longer a need to prepare and dispense master-mix solutions to the reaction tubes. Thus, liquid handling using micropipette, one of the most skillful steps, becomes unnecessary in the course of the assay. Moreover, this can contribute to reduced risk of carryover contamination during the assay.

2.2 Detection – Calcein method

The results of the LAMP assay can be detected visually by observing the strength of the green fluorescence emitted after the reaction. Figure 2 represents the mechanism of the calcein method (Tomita et al., 2008). Before LAMP amplification, the metalochrome indicator "calcein" is quenched by the effect of a manganese ion. After the LAMP reaction, pyrophosphate ions (PPi) are produced as a by-product of polymerase reaction; PPi subsequently forms a manganese pyrophosphate complex, causing the removal of the manganese ion from calcein, because the PPi are a stronger base than calcein. Next, free calcein combines with a magnesium ion to produce bright fluorescence. This technology enables the detection of LAMP reactions without the use of fluorescence detectors, which are usually expensive and difficult to manage in resource-limited settings. Other technologies for visual detection using LAMP have also been reported (Tao et al., 2011; Goto et al., 2009; Mori et al., 2006).

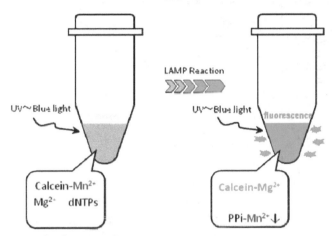

Fig. 2. Mechanism involved using calcein

2.3 Sample preparation – PURE

The sample processing method is the next important step in molecular diagnostics. Silica-based methods are well known and have been applied to a wide variety of samples, including blood and tissue (Bendall, 2002). However, these methods are unsuitable for resource-limited facilities due to the cumbersome procedures involved, including washing with organic solvents using high-speed centrifugation. Therefore, we have developed a simple and swift sample processing method named PURE. Thus far, it has been confirmed that PURE can be successfully applied to sputum, blood, serum, and swab samples. The mechanism of PURE is described below:

1. An aliquot of sample (blood, sputum, etc.) is added to the alkaline-based extraction solution and treated by heat to lyse the pathogens.
2. The sample solution is treated with adsorbent powder to remove inhibitory materials contained in samples and to neutralize the solution without any loss of target DNA.
3. After separating the solution from the powder by filtration, the obtained filtrate containing target DNA molecules can be used for reconstituting dried LAMP reagents, which are deposited to the lids of LAMP reaction tubes.

A)

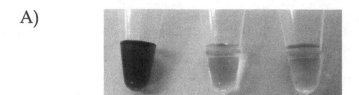

B)

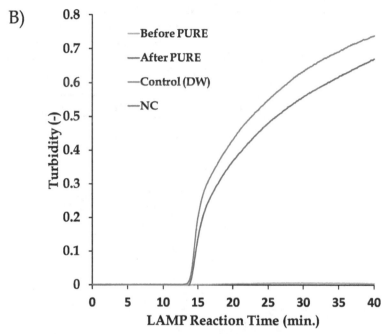

Fig. 3. Performance of the PURE–LAMP system applied for blood processing
A) Pictures of the blood sample solution (3.6% blood in an alkaline-based extraction solution) before and after PURE treatment. Left, Before PURE treatment; Centre, After PURE treatment; Right, distilled water (reference).
B) LAMP kinetics obtained by real-time turbidimetry for the 3 sample solutions with 1,000 copies of a template DNA spiked prior to PURE treatment.Green line, Before PURE treatment (directly added the solution to LAMP reaction); Red line, after PURE treatment; Blue line, control (distilled water); Purple line, negative control.

Figure 3 shows the performance of the PURE method applied for blood processing. An aliquot of blood was mixed with the extraction solution and heated at 70 °C for 5 minutes. Almost colorless solutions have been obtained by mixing the solution with the adsorbent powder (Fig. 3-A). The graph of real-time turbidimetry (Mori et al., 2004) in figure 3-B shows the LAMP kinetics for the 3 samples using 1,000 copies of a spiked template DNA. Untreated blood samples did not provide a positive reaction due to the inhibition from blood and extraction solution. However, PURE-treated blood samples showed almost the same kinetics as those of distilled water, indicating that PURE can remove inhibitory materials quite effectively from the blood samples without any loss of DNA.

Figure 4 shows the overall process of the PURE-LAMP assay system. First, an aliquot of sample is placed in a heating tube and heated at an optimized temperature (70–90 °C) to lyse the target pathogen. Then, the heating tube is attached to an adsorbent tube, and the treated solution is vigorously mixed with adsorbent powder. Next, the injection cap is inserted into the absorbent tube, which is then squeezed to elute the solution containing purified DNA. These processes can be performed in approximately 10 minutes or less for a particular sample. The LAMP reagents deposited in the lid of the tube are reconstituted by shaking the tube several times and then incubating it at around 65 °C for 30–40 minutes. Finally, the results of amplification are detected by simply observing the fluorescence using the LED lights provided in the incubator.

As mentioned above, we have successfully developed simple technologies for all the 3 steps required in molecular diagnostics, that is, the PURE method for sample preparation, the LAMP for amplification, and the calcein method for detection. Therefore, a combination of these technologies can be considered as a platform for a new molecular diagnostic tool with the desired simplicity.

3. Application of the newly developed platform for diagnosing tropical diseases

The developed platform has been applied to the following 3 tropical diseases to evaluate its performance as a practical diagnostic system.

3.1 Malaria and human African trypanosomiasis

Malaria is 1 of the 3 major infectious disease endemics in most tropical countries. More than 500 million people have been infected, and more than 1 million people die from malaria each year, mostly infants and pregnant women. Of the 4 malaria causing species, *Plasmodium falciparum* often causes severe, acute, and fatal malaria. In most developing countries, malaria is confirmed mainly by a blood smear test, although the sensitivity of the test is not sufficient to detect the parasites in patients with early-stage malaria.

Dried LAMP reagents using *P. falciparum* (Pf)-specific primers and pan genus (Pg) primers were developed in this study. The Pg LAMP primers were designed on the basis of the homogeneous sequence shared by all the 4 malaria species, thus providing the same primer specificity for all the 4 species. The Pf-specific LAMP primers were designed based on mutations between the Pf sequence and the other 3 sequences, making the primer specific only to *P. falciparum*. If both Pf and Pg LAMP assays give positive results, it can be interpreted that the patient is infected by *P. falciparum*. On the other hand, if only the Pg LAMP assay gives positive results, the patient can be diagnosed with malaria caused by 1 or more of the other 3 malarial parasites.

The sensitivity of PURE and malaria-LAMP have been evaluated by using of cultured *P. falciparum* parasites obtained from the American Type Culture Collection (ATCC). As shown in figure 5, both Pf and Pg malaria-LAMP assays can detect down to 1 parasite in 1 µl blood, processed by the PURE method. This sensitivity of 1 parasite/µl blood is much higher than that of smear microscopy test (~50 parasites/µl blood for routine tests in an endemic area (Moody, 2002)). It has been reported that the initial malarial symptoms appear after the accumulation of approximately 1,000 parasites/ml of blood (Andrews et al., 2005). Therefore, PURE-malaria-LAMP is sensitive enough to detect parasites in patients who present with the initial symptoms of malaria.

Human African trypanosomiasis (HAT) is one of the most neglected disease endemics in central African countries (Hotez, 2007). HAT is caused by an infection of protozoa

Trypanosoma brucei gambiense or *Trypanosoma brucei rhodesiense* transmitted by tse-tse flies. The symptoms of HAT occur in 2 phases: hemolymphatic phase, followed by the neurological phase. If left untreated, the hemolymphatic phase permits the parasites to invade the central nervous system of the patient, resulting in fatal neurological symptoms such as coma and eventually death. Because no vaccine or preventative drug for HAT is available, and therapeutic drugs for HAT patients in the neurological phase causes severe side effects, a simple and sensitive diagnostic method is in high demand.

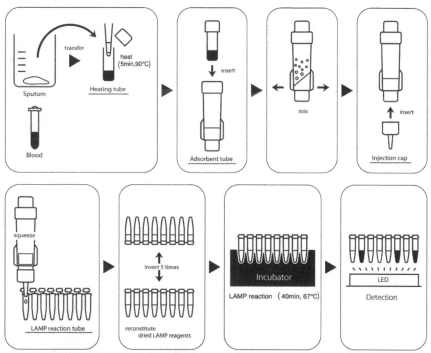

Fig. 4. Diagram of the procedures involved in the PURE–LAMP system

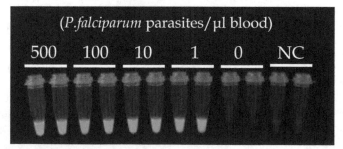

Fig. 5. Sensitivity of PURE-Malaria-LAMP
Thirty-five microliters of control blood spiked with cultured parasites (*P. falciparum*, from ATCC) was treated with PURE and tested by *P. falciparum*-specific and Pan-genus LAMP. Left and right tubes contain the same parasite numbers and are those of Pf-LAMP and Pg-LAMP, respectively.

To enhance sensitivity, the LAMP primers for HAT are designed on a multi-copy gene named RIME, which contains 80–250 copies in a parasite genome (Njiru et al., 2008). The efficacy of the PURE-HAT-LAMP assay was also evaluated by using uninfected control blood spike with cultured parasites. Positive results have been successfully obtained from samples with a parasite density of 100/ml, indicating that the overall analytical sensitivity of PURE-HAT-LAMP can be estimated to be approximately 100 parasites/ml blood. The sensitivities of the currently available smear microscopy tests have been reported to be between 100 and 10,000 parasites/ml blood (Chappuis., 2005). The sensitivity of PURE-HAT-LAMP has been found to be over 10 times higher than that of the simple Giemsa-stained smear microscopy test, which is one of the most common diagnostic tests in HAT endemic areas, and is almost comparable with that of the mini-anion-exchange centrifugation technique, which is quite tedious and time consuming.

3.2 Tuberculosis
Tuberculosis (TB) is one of the most threatening airborne diseases worldwide. One-third of the world's population is thought to be infected with *Mycobacterium tuberculosis* and new infections occur at a rate of about 1/second. Since the TB patients are concentrated in developing counties, including many tropical countries, TB is considered as a major poverty-related disease (Walker et al., 2003).

The sputum direct smear microscopy test is the only diagnostic method available for the detection of TB at peripheral laboratories in developing countries (Keeler et al., 2006). Because of the low sensitivity of the smear test, few patients with a low number of infected TB cells are often misdiagnosed as negative, thus preventing eradication of TB. In order to overcome this situation, we attempted to apply the novel platform PURE-LAMP system for the diagnosis of TB.

As summarized in Table 1, PURE-TB-LAMP provided positive results for both smear- and culture-positive sputum samples collected from patients suspected with TB. Furthermore,

Direct Smear	Culture(Ogawa)		PURE-TB-LAMP (Positive/Total)	% positive
Positive	Positive		34/34	100
Negative	Positive		15/25	60
	Colony Counts	100-200	7/7	100
		20-99	6/8	75
		1-19	2/10	20
Negative	Negative		9/91	9.9

Table 1. Summary of clinical performance of PURE-TB-LAMP
Sixty microliters of sputa obtained from patients suspected with TB in the Pham Ngoc Thach Hospital (PNTH; Vietnam) were analyzed by PURE-TB-LAMP. The performance of PURE-TB-LAMP was compared to those of the direct smear and culture method (Ogawa media) in terms of the positive ratios. Smear and culture tests for each sample were conducted according to the standardized protocols in PNTH.

the PURE-TB-LAMP assay can detect the pathogen with 60% accuracy in smear-negative but culture-positive samples, and with 75% or more accuracy if 20 colonies are detected by the culture test using Ogawa media. This data clearly shows that the PURE-TB-LAMP method is reliable enough to be applied to the targeted peripheral smear centers in developing countries as an alternative method for the direct smear test.

4. Conclusions

As mentioned above, PURE and LAMP system have been newly developed and successfully applied as a novel diagnostic platform for the detection of infectious diseases, which are wildly endemic in the developing world. This platform has the advantage of being simple enough to be applicable in resource-limited facilities and its performances is higher than those of the existing diagnostic methods routinely employed in rural laboratories of most of the developing countries. Recently, a novel idea for performing LAMP without electricity has been proposed (LaBarre et al., 2011). Combination of that technology with the platform mentioned in this chapter would make it possible to realize the use of molecular diagnostics in poorer settings or even in field conditions.

Since the geographical distribution of malaria, HAT, and TB overlap in many of tropical countries (Cook & Zumla, 2003), diagnostic tests for these diseases are often performed at the same rural laboratory in developing countries. The developed platform described in this study is a very useful tool in such laboratories because all the above mentioned diseases can be diagnosed using almost the same technique and the same simple incubator. This new technology can be beneficial as it reduces the initial costs associated with installing new equipments and preparing trained technicians for each target. This platform is potentially applicable to other pathogens, including those causing other neglected diseases such as leishmaniasis and Chagas' disease. The application of this platform could be extended to other diseases that threaten the heath and quality of life of patients in many tropical countries. This can also contribute to distribute them at more affordable rates because of the effect of mass production.

This platform can be considered as a gene point-of-care testing (g-POCT) device, which can also be used in developed countries. In fact, TB-LAMP has been approved as clinical in vitro diagnostics (IVD) in Japan and used along with PURE as a simple and fast screening test for patients suspected with TB. Since NALC-NaOH treatment for sputum is not necessary for PURE-TB-LAMP, turn-around-time of PURE-TB-LAMP is less than that of the decontaminated smear test, which is commonly adopted as the standard screening test for TB in most developed countries. Furthermore, LAMP reagents using similar concepts have been developed for the detection of the influenza virus (Nakauchi, 2011). We hope that the platform will contribute to the improvement of global health and benefit all those under the threat of infectious diseases.

5. Acknowledgments

We sincerely thank Dr. Satoshi Mitarai from the Research Institute of Tuberculosis in Japan, Dr. Noboru Inoue from Obihiro University of Agriculture and Veterinary Medicine in Japan, Dr. C.J. Sutherland and Dr. S.D. Polley from the London School of Hygiene and Tropical Medicine in the UK, and Dr. N.T. Lan from the Pham Ngoc Thach Hospital in Vietnam for their valuable help. This research was supported by the Foundation for Innovative New Diagnostics (FIND) in Switzerland.

6. References

Andrews L, Andersen RF, Webster D, Dunachie S, Walther RM, Bejon P, Hunt-Cooke A, Bergson G, Sanderson F, Hill AV, Gilbert SC. (Jul 2005). Quantitative real-time polymerase chain reaction for malaria diagnosis and its use in malaria vaccine clinical trials. *Am J Trop Med Hyg*. Vol.73, No.1, pp.191-8.

Aziah I, Ravichandran M, Ismail A. (Dec 2007). Amplification of ST50 gene using dry-reagent-based polymerase chain reaction for the detection of Salmonella typhi. *Diagn. Microbiol. Infect. Dis*. Vol.59, No.4, pp. 373-7.

Bendall K.E., Setzke E., Quandt A. (2002). Purification of Viral Nuculeic Acid, In: Nuculeic acids isolation methods, Bowien B. & Dürre P. (Eds.) pp.53-59, American Scientific Publishers, ISBN 1-58883-018-7 2002

Chappuis F, Loutan L, Simarro P, Lejon V, Büscher P. (Jan 2005). Options for field diagnosis of human african trypanosomiasis, *Clin. Microbiol. Rev*. Vol.18, No.1, pp. 133-46.

Cook G.C. & Zumla A. (Eds.) Manson's Tropical Diseases Twenty-first edition Elsevier Limited, ISBN 0-7020-2640-9

Goto M, Honda E, Ogura A, Nomoto A, Hanaki K. (Mar 2009). Colorimetric detection of loop-mediated isothermal amplification reaction by using hydroxy naphthol blue. *Biotechniques*. Vol.46, No.3, pp. 167-72.

Hotez PJ, Molyneux DH, Fenwick A, Kumaresan J, Sachs SE, Sachs JD, Savioli L. (Sep 2007)Control of neglected tropical diseases. *N.Engl. J. Med*. Vol.357, No.10, pp. 1018-27.

Iwamoto T, Sonobe T, Hayashi K. (Jun 2003). Loop-mediated isothermal amplification for direct detection of Mycobacterium tuberculosis complex, M. avium, and M. intracellulare in sputum samples., *J.Clin. Microbiol*. Vol. 41, No.6, pp. 2616-22

Jorgensen P, Chanthap L, Rebueno A, Tsuyuoka R, Bell D. (May 2006). Malaria rapid diagnostic tests in tropical climates: the need for a cool chain. *Am J Trop Med Hyg*. Vol.74, No.5, pp. 750-4.

Keeler E, Perkins MD, Small P, Hanson C, Reed S, Cunningham J, Aledort JE, Hillborne L, Rafael ME, Girosi F, Dye C. (Nov 2006). Reducing the global burden of tuberculosis: the contribution of improved diagnostics. *Nature*. 23;444 Suppl 1 pp. 49-57.

Kubo T, Agoh M, Mai le Q, Fukushima K, Nishimura H, Yamaguchi A, Hirano M, Yoshikawa A, Hasebe F, Kohno S, Morita K. (2010) Development of a reverse transcription-loop-mediated isothermal amplification assay for detection of pandemic (H1N1) 2009 virus as a novel molecular method for diagnosis of pandemic influenza in resource-limited settings. ., *J Clin Microbiol*. Vol.48, No. 3, pp. 728-35.

LaBarre P., Hawkins K.R., Gerlach J., Wilmoth J., Beddoe A., Singleton J., Boyle D., and Weigl B. (2011). A Simple, Inexpensive Device for Nucleic Acid Amplification without Electricity—Toward Instrument-Free Molecular Diagnostics in Low-Resource Settings, *PLoS One*. Vol. 6, No.5, e19738.

Moody A., (Jan 2002). Rapid Diagnostic Tests for Malaria Parasites, *Clinical Microbiology Reviews*. Vol.15, No.1, pp. 66-78

Mori Y, Hirano T, Notomi T. (Jan 2006). Sequence specific visual detection of LAMP reactions by addition of cationic polymers. *BMC Biotechnol*. Vol.10 6:3.

Mori Y., Kitao M., Tomita N., Notomi T., (2004). Real-time turbidimetry of LAMP reaction for quantifying template DNA, *J Biochem Biophys Methods*., Vol.59, No.2, pp. 145-57.

Mori Y. & Notomi T. (2009). Loop-mediated isothermal amplification (LAMP): a rapid. Accurate, and cost-effective diagnositic method for infectious diseases, *J.Infect Chemother.*, Vol.15, No.2, pp.62-69.

Nagamine K., Hase T, Notomi T. (Jun 2002).Accelerated reaction by loop-mediated isothermal amplification using loop primers. Mol Cell Probes. Vol.16, No.3, pp. 223-9.

Nakauchi M, Yoshikawa T, Nakai H, Sugata K, Yoshikawa A, Asano Y, Ihira M, Tashiro M, Kageyama T. (Jan 2011). Evaluation of reverse transcription loop-mediated isothermal amplification assays for rapid diagnosis of pandemic influenza A/H1N1 2009 virus. *J Med Virol.* Vol.83, No.1, pp. 10-5.

Notomi T Okayama H., Masubuchi H., Yonekawa T., Watanabe K., Amino N. & Hase T. (2000). Loop-mediated isothermal amplification of DNA, Nucleic Acids Res. Vol.28, No. 12, e63.

Njiru ZK, Mikosza AS, Matovu E, Enyaru JC, Ouma JO, Kibona SN, Thompson RC, Ndung'u JM. (Apr 2008). African trypanosomiasis: sensitive and rapid detection of the sub-genus Trypanozoon by loop-mediated isothermal amplification (LAMP) of parasite DNA. *Int J Parasitol.* Vol.38, No.5, pp. 589-99.

Parida M, Sannarangaiah S, Dash PK, Rao PV, Morita K. (Nov-Dec 2008). Loop mediated isothermal amplification (LAMP): a new generation of innovative gene amplification technique; perspectives in clinical diagnosis of infectious diseases. *Rev Med Virol.* Vol.18, No.6, pp. 407-21.

Polley SD, Mori Y, Watson J, Perkins MD, González IJ, Notomi T, Chiodini PL, Sutherland CJ. (Aug   2010). Mitochondrial DNA targets increase sensitivity of malaria detection using loop-mediated isothermal amplification. *J Clin Microbiol.* Vol.48, No.8., pp. 2866-7.

Rodrigues Ribeiro Teles FS, Pires de Távora Tavira LA, Pina da Fonseca LJ. (May-Jun 2010) Biosensors as rapid diagnostic tests for tropical diseases. *Crit Rev Clin Lab Sci.* Vol.47, No.3, pp. 139-69.

Tao ZY, Zhou HY, Xia H, Xu S, Zhu HW, Culleton RL, Han ET, Lu F, Fang Q, Gu YP, Liu YB, Zhu GD, Wang WM, Li JL, Cao J, Gao Q. (Jun 2011) Adaptation of a visualized loop-mediated isothermal amplification technique for field detection of Plasmodium vivax infection. *Parasit Vectors.* Vol.4, No.1, pp. 115.

Tomita N, Mori Y, Kanda H, Notomi T. (2008). Loop-mediated isothermal amplification (LAMP) of gene sequences and simple visual detection of products. *Nat Protoc.* Vol.3, No.5, pp. 877-82.

Walker D, Stevens W. (2003). The economics of TB control in developing countries. *Expert Opin Pharmacother.* Vol.4, No.3, pp. 359-68.

11

Neonatal Thermoneutrality in a Tropical Climate

Hippolite O. Amadi
Imperial College London
United Kingdom

1. Introduction

Sub-Saharan African countries are notably among the nations with high neonatal mortality (NNMR) and morbidity rates (WHO, 2009). A number of issues have been previously raised in the literature in attempt to define some of the factors that contribute to these such as level of illiteracy among mothers and short supply of healthcare workers (Amadi et al., 2007). However, little has been said of the impact of environmental temperature regulation on the wellness and survival of neonates in this region. The sub-Saharan Africa is well-known for its harsh climatic conditions of high sun intensity and ambient temperatures, often in excess of 35°C, coupled with societal condition of abject poverty. Nursing environment of the neonate, especially pre-terms, is a crucial factor for the maintenance of appropriate body temperature for the physiological stability of the newborn. Classical management of neonatal thermoneutrality in this region of Africa has been dominated by procedures that were handed down from industrialised societies; these being fundamentally compliant to the peculiar climatic factors and social advantages of the countries of origin.

In the last decade, there has been concerted effort to scientifically investigate factors that may be subtly contributing to high neonatal mortality and morbidity in this region. These include meteorological, socio-cultural and technological factors that define the macro- and micro-environments immediate to the neonate. This knowledge is fundamental for the tweaking or outright replacement of the present morbidity-high techniques. This chapter will attempt to explore these factors and their consequences, and discuss the present interventions and techniques that are coincidentally yielding improved outcome in some neonatal centres in the region. The ideas expressed in this chapter were drawn from on-the-spot clinical practice experiences in a decade-on collaborative project that has involved up to 21 neonatal referral Centres across the entire geographical region of the West African state of Nigeria (Figure 1). Recent publications show that this region of African is currently far behind the United Nation's Millennium Development Goal (MDG) target on the survival of infants, and neonatal mortality rate is steadily making this worse (Federal Ministry of Health [FMOH], 2011). Neonatal survival might not necessarily improve by the flooding of the region with 'foreign-culture-biased' sophisticated incubator systems that are not so easy to handle by the users despite the high pricing of these that limit their procurement by the poor countries. There is a perceived socio-cultural dimension of the work place attitude that militates against effective practice of neonatal thermoregulation. This needed to be properly addressed perhaps by the use of affordable and manageable appropriate incubation technology that the people can easily identify with.

Ineffective thermoregulation leads to other complications and patients' poor response to treatment. Neonatal physiological stability enhanced by adequate thermoneutral control and humidification is an essential factor that enables the neonate to respond well to treatment thereby enabling effective management of associated tropical diseases. An adequate and hygienic incubation technique, appropriately designed for the peculiar tropical settings, will minimise neonatal cross-infection and also reduce disease transmission by the often freely roaming insects in and out of the incubators. Adverse climatic conditions and observed procedural inadequacies of incubator application often lead to overheating, compelling attendants to open up the incubator portholes and windows thereby compromising the microenvironment. The present work seeks to extend the incubator application to create procedures that ensures the minimisation of such compromises.

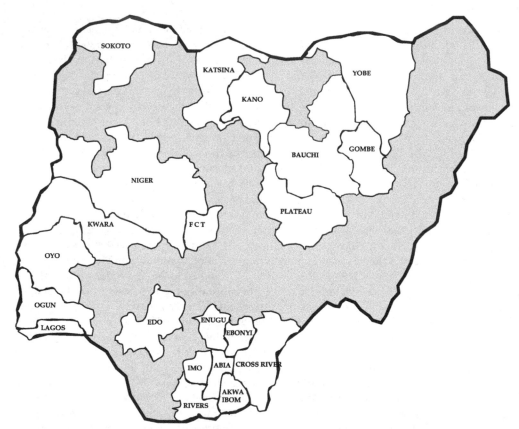

Fig. 1. Map of Nigeria showing all the states where the collaborating tertiary hospitals are located

In this chapter, four different environments that impact on the new-born baby would be examined. This knowledge is important to be able to effectively understand the thermal needs of the new-born during neonatal care, whether inside an incubator or an open cot. These are:

1. The prenatal environment or the mother's womb that provides for the nurturing of the foetus.
2. The micro-environment or the baby's compartment of an incubator or wrapping in an open cot.
3. The macro-environment or the outer room comprising the interior of the nursery building where the incubators and cots are situated for the nursing of the new-born.
4. The regional-environment or the outside surrounding of the nursery building directly being influenced by the regional climate.

2. Prenatal environment

The neonate's body system observes the law of "garbage in garbage out" in terms of what it does with the ambient temperature of its immediate environment. From clinical experience, it is very easy to observe that an extremely low birth weight neonate will quickly assume a body temperature equal to the ambient temperature of its immediate environment. This has been frequently observed at one of our collaborating neonatal centres in the very hot town of Nguru in Nigeria. In an overheated room, baby becomes hyperthermic and in a cold room, baby becomes hypothermic. Both extremes are devastating conditions, capable of claiming the baby's life and must be avoided. This is why the regulation of baby's environment must be done on patient-specific basis involving the exact extra warming or wrapping required to thermally stabilise such baby. Nature has made an adequate environmental provision for the prenatal period. Baby's immediate past housing, the womb, is a separately controlled environment independent of the foetus's body system and providing it with no worries for self-thermoneutral control. It is therefore essential to anticipate the possible fatal environmental shock that awaits a premature new-born as its organs are not yet functionally ready to completely support the baby outside the womb environment.

The body temperature of a healthy adult is physiologically stabilized about 37°C whether in a temperate climate of 1°C or tropical sub-Saharan African climate of 45°C. The adult expectant mother may be physiologically acclimatised to her 'freezing' or 'burning' weather respectively; however, the foetuses in both climates are accustomed to approximately the same thermal environment of the womb. Individual climatic adaptation for the baby only begins at birth. Therefore the design of a supportive environment for a premature baby must integrate the climatic peculiarities such foetus would be graduating into.

3. Neonatal micro-environment

It is an absolute necessity to provide an enabling environment immediately following premature birth. This calls for a sustainable artificial environment to allow the neonate enough time for its organs to fully mature to provide independent support to withstand the tougher climate of the outside world. This practice ameliorates the shock of a sudden change in environmental conditions that can become catastrophic for the premature new-born. What should such artificial environment possess then? A good design of controllable micro-environment for the baby might be achieved by applying constraints that are enriched with the good knowledge of the womb as well as the climatic and social factors of baby's place of birth. Incubator comes to mind in a clinical setting when neonatal microenvironment is mentioned. In a classical and basic sense, neonatal incubation might speak more of the provision of a controlled warming for the new-born. It is understandable that provision of uncompromised all-day warming is essential for the neonate in a temperate regional climate of average room temperature of less than 10°C, for example. The baby's inability to maintain its own homeostasis meant that the extra 27°C or more required to attain a body temperature of 37°C must be provided and sustained artificially. The definition for this separate microenvironment for the new-born must however begin to modify when the regional climate changes to another of room temperatures in excess of 40°C. Such elevated ambient temperature in poor hygienic settings as the tropical culture would normally encourage fast breeding of disease transmitting insects even around hidden corners of the incubator. Therefore, appropriate incubation technique capable of effective neonatal care must recognise and integrate the climatic characteristics of the culture the neonate is graduating into. Neonatal incubator care, as is presently practiced in the high ambient sub-Saharan Africa is deficient of this fundamental factor. The race to lower neonatal mortality rate in Tropical Africa might hence not necessarily be dependent on increase of drug donations or over flooding the health facilities with sophisticated incubators. The race might however be won by going back to the fundamentals of neonatal thermoneutral care that are compliant to the conditions of the region. This is a natural 'preventive technique' that would lead to the minimisation of disease occurrences. An effective and climate sensitive neonatal care would ensure a healthy start in life for the promising infant.

Classical incubation techniques in this tropical African climate might not have been fully successful because these were designs developed and originally practiced in climates and cultures that were completely different. This creates opportunities for deficient practices that expose the delicate neonates to unhygienic conditions, insects and infections that soon make them morbid and eventually claim their lives. An unstable thermoneutral environment does not provide the thermal stability the neonate's body system requires to effectively respond to treatment. In response to this, an on-going research adopting new practice procedures in collaboration with 15 different neonatal centres across the region was initiated to address various adverse incubation factors. This has so far proffered solutions that coincidentally improved survival rates in the centres (Amadi et al., 2010). The aim of this work was to present the various thoughts, considerations and incubator care approaches that might have improved neonatal defence against exposure to tropical epidemics that could easily claim their lives.

4. Effect of poverty and illiteracy

A well-looked after pregnancy and professionally efficient antenatal care are essential factors that could promise a healthy baby. These factors would characteristically help to avoid the complications of preterm birth. Poverty and illiteracy create a clear distinction in neonatal mortality rate between developed nations such as the United Kingdom and any sub-Saharan African country such as Nigeria. This is evident from literature reports on neonatal and perinatal mortality rates from these regions (FMOH, 2011; Centre for Maternal and Child Enquiry, 2010). Societal abject poverty and high degree of illiteracy are factors that do not allow the expectant mothers to nurture healthy foetuses or seek professional antenatal care when these are available. It is arguable that most mothers would be happy to observe any rules that would guarantee them a healthy baby. Maternal poverty and illiteracy are outside the scope of the present work; however it sounds reasonable to mention that tackling poverty in sub-Saharan Africa as part of an assembly of measures would go a long way in lowering NNMR of the region.

4.1 Incubator availability

The odd effect of poverty shows up again during the management of the premature baby in terms of inadequacy in the supply of equipment for neonatal nursing. There is endemic insufficiency of functional incubators for the teaming population of the neonates requiring incubator care in a typical referral centre among those involved in the present study. The situation in the region was such that it was common to have only one centre where neonatal special care might be obtained in a catchment population of over 5 million, covering over 30,000 km^2 of land area. Journeys could take as much as 3 hours to reach the centres and often involving very poor access roads. Such a centre would normally have an average of 35 neonates on admission at any time, yet working with no more than two functional incubators and grossly under-staffed with qualified nurses and doctors. Sadly, up to three babies from different mothers were at times crammed into the same incubator in one of those horrible thermoneutral malpractices to be treated in later sections of this chapter. Our strategic plan to lower neonatal loses due to complications of thermal instability had to be carefully designed to discourage such wrong applications. Ibe (1993) indicated a culture of high admission deliveries for very low birth weight babies within the study region. This is compounded by a high number of referral cases of distressed tiny babies, often stretching the facilities beyond capacity as observed in our study centres. This therefore suggests that a hospital with average on-admission of over 30 patients should operate with a minimum of 20 well-maintained functional incubators, up to 3 radiant warmers, up to 10 phototherapy machines, up to 30 units of cot/incubator installable apnoea monitoring systems and enough attending nurses to guarantee a patient-to-nurse ratio of 5 during every shift. The provision of twenty functional incubators in one hospital alone is almost impossible when the poverty factors of these tropical countries come into play. Hence, an extra ordinary approach to this seemingly impossible situation had to be sought for.

4.2 Budget re-equipping of functional incubator

An earlier study in the tropical region of Africa by Ogunlesi et al (2008) indicated that high point-of-admission hypothermia and general thermal instability contribute a great deal to the high NNMR, stressing the need of incubators in adequate number to re-equip the centres. Many centres were discovered to have several units of broken-down, old and obsolete incubators stacked in equipment stores; others littered the walk ways of the hospital complexes, breeding insects and rodents, promoting environmental pollution and unhygienic facility. Many of these were kept back in the neonatal wards and being used as 'cages' for these babies in such unhygienic manner that could enhance infections and disease transmission (Figure 2). The horrific dirty sights that were revealed upon removal of the mattress trays were enough to wonder why any baby survived at all from the cages. Careful inspections would reveal that many of these still had reusable canopies and trolleys. Proposals for the purchase of adequate number of functional incubators during joint-task meetings with hospital managements would not go well. Lack of adequate funding for the hospitals meant that it was nearly impossible for any of them to acquire enough systems at the local prevailing costs of incubators. These were to be supplied to hospitals at costs higher than €20,000 per unit of incubator. This meant, for a Unit requiring up to 20 incubators, a huge budget of over €400,000 for the purchase of incubators alone in a poorly funded hospital with many other departments to run. The local repair of the broken-down incubators was not a feasible option as the spare parts of few of the current models could not be acquired due to poor supply chain. None of the companies that produced these systems had any assembly plants or technical representatives to provide the needed technical support. Therefore sustainable solution was not envisaged through this approach. To acquire brand new systems, unlike the use of extended price-plan and after sale maintenance in developed countries, the hospitals in these poor nations would be required by the foreign companies to make outright payment of the full cost. High cost of logistics and unfavourable operating environments might have compelled these companies from any extended technical support to a country like Nigeria at the moment. They hence demanded full out right payment for the systems, leaving the country to bear the full liability of the carcasses when they broke down. An inventory carried out in a certain Teaching Hospital in Nigeria during this period revealed the presence of 45 carcasses of different models of dysfunctional baby incubators in their stores whilst they had no functional one to save tens of babies in its new-born Units.

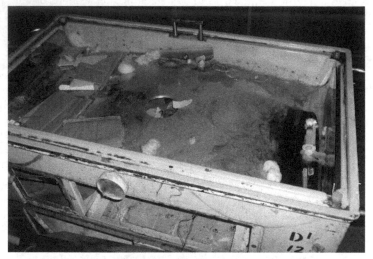

Fig. 2. An incubator carcass showing the inside immediately below matrass tray (removed); system was in use as is when retrieved

At this junction it was clear that the idea of a new approach to this was inevitable. The old carcasses of incubators that littered the hospitals were again considered and fresh investigations revealed the high availability of these across all the 5 collaborating tertiary (university teaching) hospitals at the time. A research was hence initiated to evaluate and design a process that might apply to re-introduce these obsolete systems to active services in a neonatal ward without necessarily taking recourse to original manufacturers or spare parts. This was to consider the maintainability of the resulting system, carefully selecting options that would ensure availability of spare parts and simplifying the technology to make it easy for the local technicians to handle. Typically available carcasses to apply in these hospitals were of all sorts of brands, age and models, the state of some could be best described as 'horrible' (Figure 3). Carcasses were also literally recovered from hospital dump sites where they were abandoned awaiting evacuation. However, these constituted the closest solutions to the problem required to be solved. The wide variability of these carcasses resulted in the constraint requiring that a workable design must be easily adaptable to any 'model' and 'make' of an item of incubator carcass.

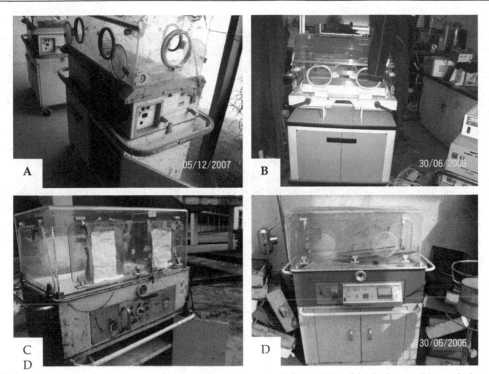

Fig. 3. Abandoned incubators for recycling, recovered from (A) rubbish dump (B) workshop (C) neonatal ward in use (D) scrap metal yard

5. Modelling Recycled Incubators

Recycled Incubator Technique (RIT) speaks of the successful application that most Nigerian tertiary hospitals have used to re-equip their Special Care Baby Units (SCBU) using their formally condemned or obsolete incubators. Many of these old systems were abandoned in the stores or used as ordinary cages (cots) in the Special Care Baby Units.

In the recycling technique that was designed in this study, the casings of the obsolete system were re-used but the functional assemblies of the power unit were completely re-engineered with customized generic digital components. RIT incubators currently make up 80% to 100% of the functional incubators in many Nigerian tertiary hospitals at the time of this report. These included University of Benin Teaching Hospital (UBTH) Benin-City, Lagos University Teachning Hospital (LUTH) Lagos, Jos University Teachnig Hospital (JUTH) Jos, Ebonyi State University Teaching Hospital (EBSUTH) Abakaliki, Aminu Kano Teachnig Hospital (AKTH) Kano, Federal Medical Centres (FMCs) at Nguru, Gombe, Owerri, EbuteMetta and Abeokuta. Others were University of Nigeria Teaching Hospital (UNTH) Enugu, University of Calabar Teaching Hospital (UCTH) Calabar, University of Ilorin Teaching Hospital (UITH) Ilorin and University of Abuja Teaching Hospital (UATH) Gwagwalada. An RIT system comparatively saves up to 75% of the cost of procuring and maintaining a modern state-of-the-art incubator whilst being functionally akin to these (Amadi et al, 2007). RIT has presently made it possible for some of these hospitals to currently maintain up to 25 functional incubators whereas they could not simultaneously own up to 3 or none at all in the recent past. This has therefore been described by a Nigerian healthcare organisation as a significant contribution to national development in the Nigerian healthcare system (Committee of Chief Executives of Federal Tertiary Health Institution [CCEFTHI], 2007).

5.1 Original concept
The initial hypothesis proposed that the application of generic assemblies in the rebuilding of the functional mechanisms and electronics of an incubator would drastically reduce the unit cost of incubation in low income countries. To verify and implement this, modern manufacturing techniques based on standard generic assemblies was exploited in a careful design of interfaces for the linking of the generic assemblies. Using the internet market, individual mechanical, electrical and electronic assemblies that could apply to design the functional mechanism of an incubator were cost-competitively selected. These were assembled by design to yield desired outputs necessary for effective maintenance of the unique standard conditions required in an incubator's micro-environment.

5.2 Casing and trolley
System functionality was the primary focus of the RIT, however the overall peripheral finishing must be appealing necessitating a careful investigation of the abilities of self-employed local artesans. It was discovered that individual fabricators, welders and car painters around major cities in Nigeria were good enough in their arts such that with very close supervision these could do excellent jobs. Therefore the best of these artisans were identified and separately guided to renovate the old incubator casings and to finish these with the best possible standards.

5.3 Canopy and plastic components
There were identified artisans that worked on Perspex materials in the small and big cities. Some of these demonstrated good skills in the methods they used in their jobs. Various plastic components of different models of incubator amongst the carcasses were re-designed to be produced as spares for the replacement of the originals; the new designs being such as would be easy to fit into the crafting techniques of the local artesans. Most of the new designs therefore resulted in different shapes from those of the original incubator manufacturers. The changes in the RIT designs for these plastics/Perspex parts were necessary in order to simplify their production as required to ensure good finishing by a closely supervised artisan. The incubator hoods were assessed. Old age and handling could make some of these to become opaque after technical cleaning and must not be reused if not completely clear and transparent. Effort was hence made to reproduce the discarded hoods with locally available Perspex materials by applying simple procedures of working and reshaping of the materials.

5.4 Power unit modules
This is a detachable unit that houses the operational control elements in most incubator designs. A repairer intending to fix a broken-down incubator would normally detach and take this unit away in attempt to diagnose the source of a wrong system signal.

Unfortunately, many of these that were taken away from some of the hospitals by prospective repairers were returned without success as the spare parts were no longer available. Some repairers lost or did not even bother to return the removed power-units after their unsuccessful attempts. In RIT, the casing of the power module was normally reused. However, when these could not be traced to where they were sent to or by whoever removed them, a new simplified casing was designed and locally produced. In some cases, the high aesthetic finishing of the incubator was not altered by this major reconstruction. The Airshields model C100 systems at the Ebonyi State University Teaching Hospital (EBSUTH) Abakaliki and one of the C200 models at University of Benin Teaching Hospital (UBTH) were examples of incubators that were recycled with re-engineered power module casings (Figure 4).

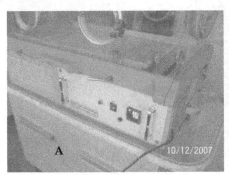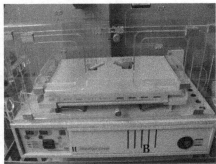

Fig. 4. Recycled incubators, originally carcasses of (A) Airshields model C200 (B) ISIS Mediprema system

5.5 Operating system
Designing and developing a new assembly of an operating system to power the incubator was the most challenging step in the RIT procedure. The chain of electronic and digital communications that powered the intelligence system was generally achieved by interconnectivity of distinct units of circuitry. These were called assemblies and were generic constructs by different companies but selected and arranged by design in RIT systems (Figure 5). All used circuitry could be sourced for internationally through the internet. Specifications of input requirements and expected outputs of such units of assemblies enabled effective integration of these to achieve the ultimate incubator output during the design stage. Ability to design a functional system with this method required a good understanding of how the incubator worked and the different functions of the assemblies that powered it. A good knowledge of human anatomy and neonatal physiology were essentially applied to relate to the outputs of these assemblies to ensure the clinical suitability of the resulting system. These different assemblies or components were then purchased from their individual companies or marketers, appropriately reconfigured to design specifications and mounted in the power module casing. The various outputs, signals and actuations specified in the design were compatible with the applied transduction elements in the incubator; else design adjustments or matching transducers were sought for and applied.

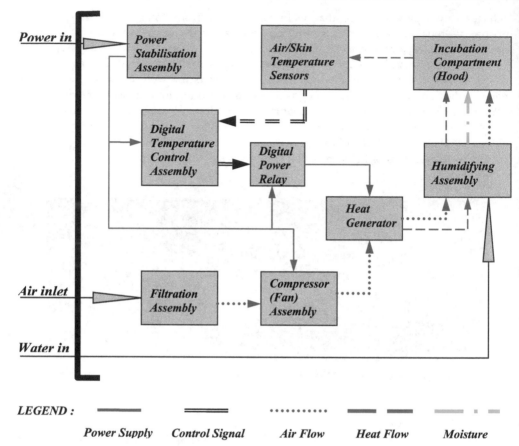

Fig. 5. RIT Assembly Block Diagram (Amadi et al, 2007)

6. Recycling own old incubators

The successful clinical trials of the initial RIT systems paved the way to the present in-depth study on neonatal thermoneutral control in this African tropical climate. The cost of producing an RIT system from a hospital's fleet of carcasses was demonstrated to be less than 20% of the cost of purchasing one state-of-the-art (STA) incubator (Amadi et al., 2007). This made the idea of incubator re-equipping of the SCBUs an attractive project to administrators of many of the tertiary hospitals that participated in the study. More hospital centres were later attracted to participate in Nigeria when the government approved the supply of STA Draeger Caleo system at a unit cost equivalent to the cost of recycling 7.5 old incubators. It was important to strategically tackle the provision of adequate number of functional micro-environments (housing) for the teaming population of the neonates within the limits of the available funding. It was well-understood that the STA systems have got the excellent finishing of modern technology and sophistication, however, it was necessary to consider the number of babies the same amount of money could house per unit time. RIT approach was hence the easy way of populating the SCBUs with many functional incubators using the available meagre funding. This would hence create the platform to properly study thermoneutral application in a tropical busy centre. In order to keep the project focused and on course, some of the collaborating hospitals Managements were advised to adopt a 'slow but steady batch-by-batch' recycling approach. This approach allowed a hospital to put a time frame vision for the completion of the recycling of all available carcasses of incubators. The Lagos University Teaching Hospital, for example, had no functional incubators at the start of the project. Ten incubators were initially recycled; there after the Hospital Management recycled 5 more each year to achieve a fleet of 25 functional incubators in three years. This boosted patient flow and staff enthusiasm for work thereby enabling better investigations of the objects of this study in the Centre (Amadi et al., 2010).

The good dedication of most of the collaborators soon led to the successful recycling of all available old incubators in most of the participating hospitals. However, the drive to provide adequate number for the SCBUs meant that some of the hospitals had to take another step of procuring more incubators from the market. The confidence already reposed on RIT made it possible for the Hospitals Managements to use available funds to purchase affordable systems they could easily re-power with RIT component when these failed. This hence secured a sustainable fleet of functional incubators required for the study in each of the participating Centres. The Centres were also encouraged and assisted to add one or more transport incubators in the fleet. This helped to reduce the distress some of the neonates suffered during intra-hospital transports using inappropriate and crude techniques.

6.1 Incubator routine maintenance and functionality auditing

The high neonatal admission delivery in these hospitals coupled with high influx of referrals resulted in extensive demands on the incubators. Many of these functioned continuously for weeks and months without break except when they were to be cleaned for another waiting baby. There was then need to initiate another supportive programme to guarantee sustainability of the functional status of the incubators and freedom from frequent unexpected system failures. This was ensured by the introduction, in each Centre, of a routine maintenance culture. By this the Hospital Managements allowed all the RIT systems to undergo professional functionality auditing and thorough system servicing by qualified RIT in-country technicians once in every 6 months. Some employees of the hospital's engineering department were deployed to be trained to assist in the technical upkeep of the recycled systems. This programme ensured the replacement of any damaged or damaging part of the incubator before this could lead to the system being run to a stop.

7. Paediatrics incubation technique course

It was discovered that generations of medical students and staff had come and passed on from the Units without ever practicing with a really functional incubator. This created generations of staff who knew no better than how to crudely improvise cages to do the work of an incubator. This hence meant an absolute lack of the fundamental knowledge of how to operate and nurse babies in proper incubators. There was initial 'general' staff training on how to operate the newly recycled systems. This basically familiarised the systems to the nurses, clinical staff and the engineering technicians, demonstrating the various assemblies of the machine and how it worked. The course was basic enough to introduce the system with the assumption that the attending staffs were already trained in various aspects of new-born management including incubator care. Over the succeeding months and across the peculiarities of the various participating hospitals in the region, there was continuous monitoring of how the nursing and clinical staff (care providers) attended to the patients with the incubators. Practice errors were thus identified; building up what was later to form the contents of a proper course work that would treat the fundamentals of incubator care in the tropical climate. This was to collate environmental, socio-cultural, human and technical factors as observed to design an elective course to demonstrate a customised approach to neonatal incubation within the climatic setting. This was to demonstrate to the attending care-providers how various wrong practices could have contributed to the mortalities in their Units. The second aspect of the course concentrated on educating participants on the 'dynamics of neonatal thermoneutral control' based on the best practice approach for achieving a steady body temperature for babies in incubators in the tropical climate. This two-graded elective course coined 'Paediatrics Incubation Techniques' thus had level 1 as 'fundamentals of neonatal incubator care' and level 2 as 'dynamics of neonatal thermoneutral control'. The general aim of level 1 was to apply theories and on-the-spot practical demonstrations to explain the basic physics of incubation and how the incubator achieved this. This also demonstrated how familiar wrong practices could have prevented the incubator from properly achieving its aims thereby delimiting the overall neonatal care quality. Level 2 was a short course that taught participants how to interactively set and re-set the incubator set-point to avoid the common confusions encountered when using the incubator to thermally stabilise the baby. The contents of these courses are briefly set out below.

7.1 Fundamentals of neonatal incubator care

The course was started with an introductory segment that was aimed at making participants to understand the general make-up of the incubator. This presented its features and mode of operation in a way as to simplify any complexities that would make care-providers see this as a mystery machine. This emphasised that Newborn babies were precious and generally delicate while the premature, among them, were much more delicate to nurse, especially during the first few days of their arrival. The premature baby, during the first few days of its arrival, needed above every other thing, controlled and regulated warmth that could provide it with a comfortable environment in its struggle for survival. The Incubator, in doing this job, becomes the obvious best friend of the premature baby during this period. A mishandling of the Incubator would mean everything DANGER to the precious premature baby inside it. Therefore a carefree attitude towards an incubator on duty could expose the child to suffocation, electric shock and many other dangers that could claim its life. Hence it was necessary that every nurse and clinician was adequately informed and trained before he/she could effectively nurse a baby with it. This emphasized that the incubator was precious and delicate just like its best friend and hence must be handled with care.

The course module explained some differences in designs of infant incubators, describing these as diverse and versatile, pointing out probable constraints necessitating the design variations. Although there is a generally acceptable basic programme of operation of an incubator, different manufacturers enhanced their designs over others with automation technology that improved their values. Modern designs incorporate microprocessors that aid automatic operation of the machine, enabling it to do much more than what older analogue and hybrid systems could do. The microprocessors fostered advanced artificial intelligent systems that regulated the humidity of the incubation chamber or neonate's compartment. Some apply affixed probes to independently monitor baby's temperature, breathing, heartbeat rates and weight-gains.

The module explained why some infant incubators were designed as "Transporters" or "Rescue" Units; discussing the kinds of "Power Sources" that keep the system functional whilst on transit. The power source could be assemblies incorporating a lead-acid accumulator (car battery) or rechargeable uninterrupted power supply (UPS) units. Transporter designs are used for ambulatory services, i.e. to move premature babies, for example, from the labour room to the neonatal intensive care unit. During such transport operation, the machine power source would be switched to battery or UPS. In cases where the baby arrives in a distant hospital or maternity, the transport incubator could be inter-phased with the car or ambulance electrical systems for operation throughout the drive or flight. More sophisticated transport incubators are designed with integral neonatal ventilators for life support and to minimize the possibilities of successful apnoea attack. Transporter units are designed to also make use of the conventional electric mains supply during normal operation in the ward. Diagrams and photos of different models of transport incubators were used to buttress on the diversity of transporter designs where none was physically available in the hospital.

The ability of the incubator to make artificial (programmed) decisions was explained. This facility is installed in incubators at different capacity levels depending on the taste and design constraints of the manufacturer. The intelligence is mostly installed take care of

a.   Incubator over-heating through 'air' temperature sensors or baby over-heat through 'skin' probes on baby.

b.   Electric Current leakages which can cause electric shock and hence harmful to both the attendance and the premature baby inside it.

c.   Humidity control for the comfort of the baby. Most of the earlier designs incorporated manually operated humidity controls.

Other primary allowable design capabilities, either automatically operated through its artificial intelligence or manually were explianed. These included Weighing features for checking baby's weight gains; Oxygen supplies through inbuilt oxygen concentrators or direct feed through independent oxygen cylinders or supply plants. The need and necessity for incorporation of cooling facility in tropical incubator designs to aid heat extraction for climatically overheated incubators was also explained.

Participants were also taken aback in history to trace the origin of modern neonatal incubation. This segment of the course endeavoured to show the progress in the development of the ideas and technologies that led to the design and production of the modern systems that could be seen today. The contributions of early players were discussed, including: the early Egyptian applications, the 1588 Giovanni Battista della Porta's idea, the 1609 Cornelius Drabbel's 'Athenor incubator' with thermostat, the 1770 John Champion's London design and patent of 1846. Other pioneering works examined were those of 1837 work of Dr Crede of Leipzig, Odile Martin's 'Couveuse' at Paris Maternity Hospital and the remarkable 1896 Earl's Court exhibition in London [Drebbel, 2011; Neonatalogy on the web, 1897].

The course isolated different basic assembly modules of an infant incubator and practically demonstrated these features to intimate students on the operational links of these to achieve regulated warmth for the baby. This includes: (a) Power source/input assembly (b) Electromechanical/Electronic compartment (c) Compressor/fan assembly (d) Thermal generation assembly (e) Humidity assembly (f) Incubation chamber/Neonate's compartment (g) Thermostatic assembly and (h) External communication assembly. Cartoon illustrations were applied in some instances to ensure fair understanding of the ideas behind these various assemblies (Figure 6).

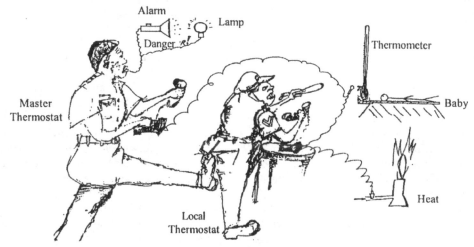

Fig. 6. Cartooned illustration of thermostatic operation

[This assembly is the thermal policeman of the incubator. It controls and gives the thermal generators instructions on when to supply heat and when to stop. It always checks up the temperature of the incubation chamber and compares it with the operator's input (set point). The thermostat's 'ON and OFF' or 'REDUCE and INCREASE' commands to the thermal generators help it to keep a check and guard against an under- or over -shoot of incubation temperature. It does this by what is known as "feedback control mechanism"]

7.1.1 Operational safety
This was a special segment of the course taught in relation to the neonate, the care-provider, the immediate nursery ward and the incubator itself. Necessary steps for the care of incubator were examined so that participants would appreciate the conducts that were required for their systems to remain functional and hygienic. Some of these were:
a. Preventive Maintenance Culture (PMC): This was an important routine that every newborn intensive care manager was encouraged to imbibe. The PMC is a practice of keeping the incubators and all other neonatal equipment in the neonatal intensive unit under a regular and routine technical check by qualified service personnel to ensure safety and avoid frequent breakdowns. Such breakdowns can occur at odd times especially when the services of the machine are most needed by a neonate. The PMC helps to put the systems in regular six or four monthly technical check-ups and performance auditing.
b. Cleaning: There was need for a regular cleaning and dusting of the machine outer casing everyday so long as the machine was in use. A thorough 'in and out' cleaning is very important before the machine is put into use after a long time of being parked. Various tested locally available disinfectants were recommended for use during such cleaning exercise. The cleaning of the incubators was discouraged from being grouped among the relegated menial jobs given to recruited 'ordinary' people to do. These often

low-paid casual workers were recruited to mop floors, clean windows and dust chairs. These also went ahead to handle the incubators, often with neonates inside, the same way as they cleaned chairs using same filthy and smelly rags. What a perfect way of introducing bugs that reduce neonatal survival and also cause damages to the incubator! The course stressed the need for hygiene around the neonates and the incubators and to keep off such infection vendors as outside visitors, improperly masked staff and mothers. Participants were encouraged to use their improved understanding of the neonatal microenvironment during the course to ensure effective cleaning standards that would be professionally acceptable.

c.   Mains Input: There was always insufficient power sockets on the walls of nursery wards to take up all electrical appliances required to be on at the same time. This was an observed failure common to all participating neonatal centers without an exception. This deficiency in the nursery electrification often causes care-providers to multiply power ports by the use of 'cabled extension'. Unfortunately, this indiscriminately run all over the place, staying in the way for movement and potentially posing the hazard of a staff tripping over them. This might result in injury to the staff or the baby such may possibly be carrying. The use of extensions causes care-providers to innocently overload these cables and the host power sockets causing electrical sparks and shocks, endangering lives and damaging equipment. This was therefore labeled a hazardous and unprofessional practice that must be discouraged. New wiring designs were proposed and implemented in each Centre to correct this deficiency.

d.   Humidity Reservoir: The care of the humidity reservoir was a segment that highlighted on the effective management of the incubator humidifiers. This explained how the reservoir might be kept from becoming nursery for infection-causing micro plants and organisms. Hence, humidifier tank must be drained of water whenever the machine was discharged of a neonate and kept dry if not in use. The tank should however be refilled with distilled water whenever the machine was to be used again. Water could be boiled and stored in a clean plastic container for use as an alternative to the use of distilled water if unavailable.

e.   Thermometer: The operator must closely monitor the temperature of the incubator with the thermometer provided to probe the microenvironment. This helps to notice when the temperature might be indicative of unfavorable condition inside. This is important especially for cases when there is a thermostatic assembly failure.

f.   Voltage Stabilizer: Use of single incubator-specific automatic voltage regulator (AVR) sets was introduced and encouraged to be applied. Erratic, poor quality and incessant power failures in these tropical countries often exposed the incubators to power surges and under voltage supplies that crippled their effective function (Figure 7). The functional inadequacies of this phenomenon were demonstrated diagrammatically to enable self-appreciation of the problem by the trainees so as to have personal drives to protect the systems during use.

g.   Earthed Lines: Trainees were encouraged to carefully inspect incubators being delivered for use before acceptance. It was important to reject incubators with obvious electrical hazards such as un-fused systems and the absence of the 'earthing line' pin (E) on the plug head, whether the system was a new product from a supplier or repaired system from the maintenance workshop. Cartooned illustrations were used to demonstrate how these related to the general building earthing and how these served as safety devices to protect baby and care-providers from 'static' and 'mains' electric shocks (Figure 8).

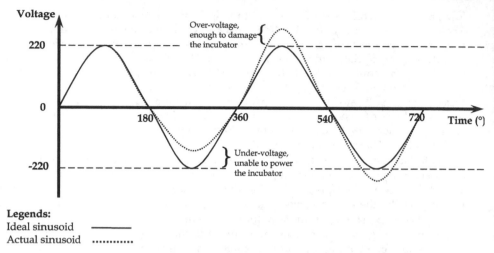

Legends:
Ideal sinusoid ———
Actual sinusoid ....

Fig. 7. Exaggerated sinusoids illustrating unsteady power supply

[There may be need for a voltage stabilizer set to run an incubator in these countries, especially for modern microprocessor based systems that might not operate with deficient power supplies. However, it must be noted that at adverse, erratic power supplies as has been witnessed, the stabilizer also stood in danger of being blown up together with the incubator it was supposed to be protecting. At this condition, if need be, it was necessary to power down the incubator.]

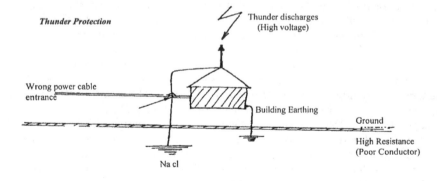

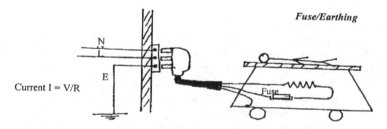

Fig. 8. Cartooned illustration of earthing line

[There must be a regular check of the effectiveness of the electrical earth conductor of the building that is housing the incubators. Improper 'earth' conduction or failure of the electrical earth line is an electrical hazard and can cause such accidents as electric shock to the baby or attending clinician. Poorly installed earth conductor such as shown in the diagram can cause interference of thunder discharges with the power supply to the machines. This can lead to damages to the incubators and other systems. Inexperienced contractors as has been noted can wrongly pass the copper conductor of thunder discharges directly over an electric cable that supplies the building. The interference that resulted from this in one occasion destroyed all connected appliances in the nursery.]

h. Socket Pin: Burnt wall sockets and plug head were observed being used to power incubators and appliances in the nursery irrespective of their conditions. The dangers of this practice were communicated and the continuous use of incubators with broken or partially burnt plug heads was discouraged. Hence, every broken power plug, burnt socket or wrong fuse must be changed before these were used to power the incubators. Figure 9 shows a couple of dangerous plug head/socket applications captured during usage.

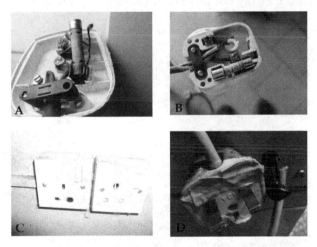

Fig. 9. Unsafe socket and plug heads (A) plug head with hair wire instead of properly rated fuse (B,D) broken plug head with missing earth-pins (C) burnt socket

i. Operator: Unit Heads were encouraged to ensure that untrained operators or nurses should not be allowed to man the machines until these were properly lectured on how to use them to provider effective care for the neonate. This pointed out the dangers of wrongly operating an incubator and how this might turn around to destroy the baby rather than saving it.

7.1.2 Incubator overheat

It was a common event across all centres to observe practices that led to an incubator overheating beyond their set point values. Such situations often resulted in neonatal hyperthermia for the babies inside the incubators. It was therefore necessary to carefully study how the identified conditions and practices resulted in the malfunctioning of the incubators. A segment of the course module was dedicated to this, emphasising possible remedies as peculiarly applied to each Centre. The identified causes were of two types, namely externally induced warming and locally induced warming. External warming of the incubators happened as a result of wrong positioning of the system within the nursery building or close to other heat generating gadgets in the same rooms. The consequence of external sources of incubator warming is not necessarily a new discovery as this has already been commented in the literature (Lyon, 2004). However there was no practical evidence of a working knowledge of this in any of the Centres. Related errors were therefore identified, studied and included in the course module to educate users on how their habits were contributing to the situation. Few of these are briefly explained below.

a.   Incubator access doors: Wrong usage of the incubator access doors and portholes was the primary cause of locally induced extra warming of the incubator. Attendants were often observed to carry out long procedures on the neonate right inside the incubators with all portholes or access doors left wide open whilst the incubator was still on (Figure 10). Such procedure might start at a time when incubator had already attained and maintained the set-point value. Opening of the portholes for a long period of time compromises the integrity of the microenvironment by a sudden drop in temperature within the chamber. This happened as a result of the nursery cooler air that uncontrollably rushed into the incubator chambers.

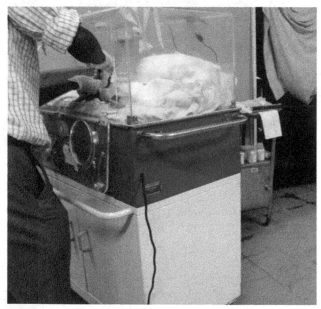

Fig. 10. A long clinical procedure being carried out inside a functioning incubator

The incubator air probe senses the drop in the chamber temperature and sends signals to the controller. This makes the thermal generators to increase heat output in attempt to counter the losses through the open portholes. This condition could cause the thermal generators to maintain an unnecessary 100% heat output for the period of the procedure without this being noticed because the extra heat was being fed to the wider nursery. However, soon after the procedure has been completed and the portholes and access doors closed, the extra heat already generated within the thermal compartment is then concentrated in the recovered microenvironment overshooting the set-point value. The incubator intelligence would sense this and automatically withdraw heat generation. However it would take a long time for the accumulated chamber temperature to fall, within which this effect could instigate neonatal hyperthermia. Following from other studies, the literature has commented that the use of open bed is more convenient than the closed incubator during special procedures such as endotracheal intubation or arterial catheterisation (Tunell, 2004). Procedures requiring long period of time was advised to rather be carried out on a resuscitaire or 'work-bench' under a radiant warmer as this also allows the clinician enough space to work. Alternatively, the incubator should be switched off if such procedures must necessarily be carried out inside the incubator. This overheating effect was also practically demonstrated during normal working periods when such errors occurred and this helped to accelerate a change in this attitude of workers within the Centres. This practice was also identified to be unhygienic as many of the incubators were observed to contain various leftover items of work materials such as syringes, needles, wrist bands, cotton wool, plaster, sample bottles etc (Figure 11). A currency note and caps of water bottles were also items recovered right inside the incubators in some cases.

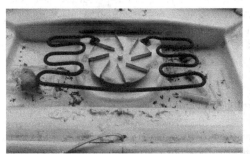
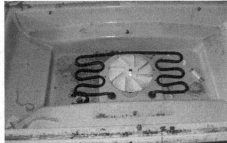
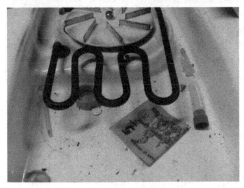

Fig. 11. Items of clinical and other materials trapped inside humidifier/heater chambers of three different incubators on active service.

b. Radiant warmer: Literature has previously pointed out external heat sources that could contribute to incubator overheat (Lyon, 2004). All through the observatory period of the present work, Centres never paid attention to incubator positioning relative to open radiant warmers. This hence contributed a great deal to the re-occurring cases of incubator overheat and neonatal hyperthermia for systems located very close to warmers. Causes to this were mistaken by attendants to be local to the incubators until these were practically demonstrated during the series of trainings to show how the incubators displayed 0% local heat output whilst the chamber temperature was steadily rising. The practice of incubator positioning in these Centres were hence modified, avoiding incubators to be located next or very close to the location of open radiant warmers.

c.   Phototherapy lamps: Neonatal jaundice is a widespread disease simultaneously treated whilst baby is being incubated. Therefore it was common to observe various kinds of phototherapy machines set over incubator canopies. Many of these often locally-produced systems operated on conventional household fluorescent lighting tubes. These deliver very high intensity of heat across the canopy to the baby, uncontrollably overwarming the microenvironment. The operating heights of these systems were often not adjustable or professionally fixed to avoid the consequent induction of incubator overheat and neonatal hyperthermia. It was hence demonstrated that the use of scientifically recommended phototherapy light tubes would ensure effective outcome without compromising baby's thermal stability. Constructions to adjust the operating heights of the local systems were recommended and carried out, especially when lack of spare parts or poor financing was the cause of resorting to the make-shift systems.

d.   Nursery windows: There seemed to be no guiding rule for positioning an incubator in the nursery as some of these were placed directly behind windows. High heat intensity of sunlight gained easy direct access into the nursery through the glassy windows. This takes over the warming of the microenvironment through the transparent canopy. This uncontrollable external heating was often the cause of incubator overheats and hyperthermia during the day times. Incubators were therefore discouraged from being placed against glassy windows as much as possible within the nursery. Alternatively, appropriate window blinds that were able to minimise the solar radiation were fixed; these could be chosen to be drawn when necessary.

e.   Nursery walls: Incubators were recommended to be placed no less than 45 centimetres from the nursery walls. This minimised the adverse effect of heat radiation from the overheated walls by the sun. The structural building pattern for new-born wards did not have any special consideration to minimise radiant heat storage. The observed poor designs easily made the walls work like a capacitor, being recharged by the sun from the outside during the day's heat. This retained the heat which was later discharged into the nursery, uncontrollably warming the incubators and babies in cots. This 'capacitance effect' was identified to be responsible for the common cases of periodic feverish attack on most babies in the ward. Though not yet reported in any medical literature, this experience is prevalent in all the Centres that participated in this study. This was observed to begin in many of the Centres at different times during the 'pm' periods of the day. This uncontrollable 'evening fever syndrome' would often confuse care-providers as they struggled to narrow the feverish event to any particular pathological or clinical cause. Most Centres were also observed to resort to using water to sponge babies to lower their temperatures. Others opened all incubator portholes and doors in attempt to lower temperatures thereby exposing neonates to the open environment and all kinds of air-borne infection vendors.

7.1.3 Further common errors

There were other commonly identified errors that might have contributed negative impact on the general wellness of the neonates, impoverishing practice outcomes. These were studied as applied to the local setting, trying out and proffering some coincidental effective solutions. Some of these were:

a. Humidification: Adequate humidification of the microenvironment has been said to enhance effective neonatal incubation (Silverman et al., 1958, 1963). Humidifier assembly is therefore a basic feature of a standard infant incubator. In most incubator designs this is located beneath the mattress tray at the covered lower aspect of the machine. Humidifier fill-ports from which this could be refilled or drained of water are usually visibly located in front or at the sides of the incubator for easy access. The often harsh climatic weather brings about a very low atmospheric Relative Humidity (RH), as low as 20% in the northern parts of Nigeria. It could therefore be a serious clinical challenge to keep baby adequately hydrated during resuscitation and neonatal nursing if this facility was not properly applied. The practice of running an incubator with dry humidifiers whilst baby was inside was a common failure observed in all the Centres at the beginning of this project. Quick staff interviews revealed that some attendants were not aware of any humidification facilities in incubator designs. Many of those aware of this confessed never bothered or remembered to add water to operate this. Many practical incidents occurred in Centres that perfectly assisted as good traditional events to convey the reasons behind these inevitable scientific procedures.

On one occasion during a whole day consultation in one of the collaborating centres, a certain incubator was running at a set point of 35.5°C. It was on a sunny dry 'harmattan' period, described as a West African season of hot, dry and dusty trade wind that normally blows from the Sahara during the month of November, carrying large amounts of dusts out over the Atlantic Ocean (Wikipedia, 2011; Britannica Online, 2011). The afternoon of the said day was about 35.2°C outside air temperature, nursery room temperature and RH of 34°C and 22% respectively. About half an hour later the same incubator with the same 5-day old baby was observed to have been reset to 37°C. The set-point of this was again, another 1hour 45 minutes later seen to have been increased to 40°C. The system was a 'dial-knob control', mercury meniscus-guide thermometer, Narco Isolette Airshields incubator model C86 at the SCBU of UPTH Port-Harcourt. Upon the observer's request, baby's skin temperature at that instant was measured to be an extreme hypothermic 33.2°C. The baby was said to have been on a steady temperature decline over several hours and throughout the period the incubator set-point was being raised. There was the presence of obvious clinical confusion as the attending clinician seemed to have eliminated some possible reasons for this situation and expressed fears of losing the baby. This true situation recalled similar events that had been observed in other Centres across the country. The incubator humidifier was at this point checked and discovered to be completely dry. As this called for emergency, available 'clean' water was called for and introduced, incubator set-point arbitrarily lowered to 37°C and humidification set at 'maximum' mark. This was also advised for the rest of the incubators in the ward as these were also being operated without functioning humidifier. To the amazement of the clinicians and nurses on duty who got involved in the frenzied situation, baby's condition dramatically reversed. Baby started to improve, gaining skin temperature after only 10 minutes and reaching 36.2°C in 35 minutes. This obvious wrong practice culture at UPTH at the time was to change forever as the science behind the drama of this event was explained to the wider audience of the Unit's care-providers.

Etiology: The science of molecular equilibrium in an open environment expects molecular migration from an area of higher concentration to a lower one. This general law was also expected of a microenvironment with very low RH as in this real life example. As baby was incubated 'naked', i.e. without clothes or wrapping, the microenvironment was a continuum with the porous-skinned neonate. This meant that baby, having more water than the immediate surroundings, was dehydrating by losing water to a thirsty atmosphere as the microenvironment sought to reach its saturation. Unfortunately, this instigated another general law of basic physics that 'evaporation causes cooling' and manifested in the dropping of baby's skin temperature. The subsequent practice response of the increased incubator heating made things worse because the microenvironment became dryer and hungrier for more water thereby exacerbating the baby's condition. Hence, this practice was never going to improve baby's condition under the present circumstances. Introduction of water in the humidifier chambers quickly saturated the microenvironment's atmosphere, reversing the concentration gradient of water molecules in the continuum in favour of the baby. As baby gained moisture and headed for saturation, evaporation immediately seized and neonatal cooling stopped. Hence, baby began to regain thermal stability as it retained the moderately supplied warming. It was possible for other neonatal complications to result in baby's loss of temperature as this; however, practice experience in this climatic region showed that elimination of possible causes should start with a check on humidification.

A near opposite of this occurred during heavy torrential rainy season that was also common to this climate, around the months of June. This would leave pockets of surface puddles scattered all over the area due to poor drainage systems. The atmospheric humidity of nearby neonatal nurseries had been measured to reach full saturation affecting the functioning of certain models of incubator such as the Vickers models 59, 79 and 77. The humidity control mechanism of such systems did not allow full stoppage of moisture supply to the microenvironment, especially when the humidifier contained maximum water. The reluctance of the wider nursery atmosphere to accept escaping moisture from the incubator soon led to saturation and condensation within the inside walls of the canopy. The resulting misty covering, often referred to as 'steaming' by the care-providers, blinds the see-through canopy, confusing the less experienced workers. The direct effect of such over-humidification on the wellness of the neonate had not been fully studied within the present project, however, literature points to a possible neonatal discomfort and a poor overall outcome (de Carvalho et al., 2011). A coincidental practice remedy to this was to fully minimise the setting of the humidity control followed by a possible drastic reduction of the humidifier water level.

b.   Incubator overcrowding: This term refers to the wrong practice of putting more than one baby into a single functioning incubator, a common method initially observed in all the collaborating SCBUs (Figure 12). There are a lot of imaginable consequences of this practice on the general outcome.

i.   This can easily lead to neonatal cross infection among the inmate babies and can potentially cause the loss of all of them to the same infection outbreak.

ii.   This makes it absolutely difficult to regulate the incubator to suit all babies at the same time. Neonatal thermoneutrality is supposed to be a patient-specific application because thermal responses to the same environment can rapidly differ among neonates. This practice hence has the potential of saving one baby whilst adversely chocking the rest to death. Therefore this must be avoided where possible, even for a possible lower-risk carrying cohorts of a multiple-birth.

iii. There is a potential risk of mistaken administration of the wrong medication to the wrong patient by the often over worked nurses on duty.

iv. This increases the dangers of possible fall through less secured incubator portholes as reported by Health Devices (2010).

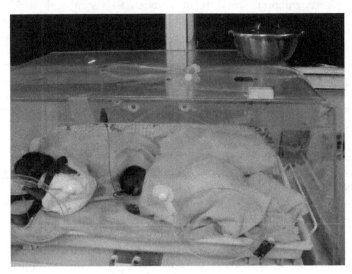

Fig. 12. Two babies sharing a single incubator.

This wrong approach was reported to be due to inadequacy of functional systems to independently support all needy babies, mostly blamed on poverty and poor funding. The seemingly moral reason of giving equal share to all needy babies as argued by some care-providers must be seriously weighed against the above consequences and for the sake of clinical hygiene.

7.2 Dynamics of neonatal thermoneutral control

This was the level 2 aspect of the 'Paediatrics Incubation Technique' course. The content of this aspect was drawn from lots of observed unscientific manner the incubators were operated during neonatal nursing. There was absolute lack of knowledge or any algorithm on how to re-regulate the incubator set-points based on the state of the neonate to achieve a physiological thermal equilibrium for the baby. Modern incubation techniques rely on algorithms that have been discussed in the literature stemming from the knowledge of 'central or core temperature' (t_c) and 'peripheral temperature' (t_p) of the neonate (Lyon and Oxyley, 2001). This technique requires the probing of the baby's skin temperature at two separate spots, notably the t_c from baby's back, in-between the scapulae and the t_p from the sole of baby's feet. This technique primarily measures a differential blood temperature (t_d) based on blood stream closest to the cardiac exit (chest level) and farthest travelled stream (foot level); $t_d = f(t_c, t_p)$. Instantaneous values of t_c and t_p are applied to proposed equations and situations to obtain the appropriate marginal values for upward or downward resetting of the set-point (Lyon and Oxyley, 2001). The proposed equations and resetting algorithms are theoretically sensible and supposed to be practically helpful for application in any setting of clinical practice. However, there were observed difficulties in its clinical usage in the present situation as most of the clinicians and nurses would require a standby calculator to work out the values of t_d each time the incubator was to be reset. This soon became more frequent than to be tolerated by the often too busy few staff on shift. This difficulty was made worse by the high volume of neonates that were usually on admission during the shifts. In probable recognition of this difficulty, modern STA incubators such as the Draeger Caleo system are designed with a similar algorithm inbuilt in them. Therefore it is possible to permanently affix the temperature probes on the designated portions of baby's skin for the incubator to automatically and appropriately reset the incubator when baby's condition changed. Unfortunately, over 97% of the incubators in use in the studied tropical region were of older generation of incubator systems, requiring manual application of this modern algorithm by the attendants. On-the-spot monitoring and study of how attendants operated the few STA systems was carried out. The findings however raised new concerns for the consequences of inaccurate application of the temperature probes.

7.2.1 Dangers of 'skin mode' control
The presence of some skin-mode servo-controlled modern incubators and open warmers should have been a welcomed advantage for the few Centres that had them. However, a sound knowledge of the working principles of such advanced systems was extremely crucial for their services to produce effective automatic neonatal thermoneutral control. Unfortunately, our initial practice observations in these Centres showed insufficient understanding of these as has been expressed in the literature (Perlstein et al., 1997; Dollberg et al., 1993; De La Fuente et al., 2006). Users knew little about the possibilities of true skin temperature attenuation as the thermistor probes placement was always improperly done. These reported their previous experience and fears when baby's temperatures were noticed to soar whilst incubator displayed a desired 36.5°C. These could not effectively interpret the reason and hence resorted to manual control via 'air' mode. It was reported that some instances produced serious consequences of neonatal hyperthermia before baby's ordeal could be discovered. Tunell (2004) pointed out the complexities of the 'servo control' technique and suggested the use of manual regulation during the first days after birth. The important steps and assiduous care required to ensure that such automatic machines did not pose any threat to the life of the babies might have been stressed in the working manuals or by a trained company representative. However lack of the presence of quality professionals from these companies does not allow this. Users are often left at the mercy of common market traders, with no professional understanding, who act as middlemen or vendors for the big companies in the developed countries.

7.2.2 Handy approach
Sophistications and cutting-edge technologies are good, especially in developed countries where expectations compare to the scientifically advanced culture. However, as relates to West Africans with a different culture of poverty, illiteracy and underdevelopment, how do we communicate this sophistication in a sustainable manner? The primary goal of any standard was to save the highest possible number of needy neonates within the limits of poor funding and manpower. A culturally compatible approach would therefore be (1) clinically functional (2) relatively non capital intensive (3) highly simplified, locally-sustainable technology; operational techniques must be (1) easy-to-remember (2) simple for quick mental evaluation of control parameters (3) based on simple but functional

algorithms. These factors guided the development of the 'handy' approach currently being used in all the collaborating Centres. This was a simplified operational algorithm for achieving thermal stability in neonates. A recent follow-up study reported that over 80% of applying nurses believed that the usage of the technique was a boost to their practice enthusiasm [Amadi et al., 2010].

Principles: The handy approach might not be the best technique ever used but this was definitely better than the unscientific 'trial and error' methods observed at the inception of this project. This was developed by a long study that paid very close attention to the worst case scenarios such as the weakness of an 'extreme preterm baby' in an 'extremely harsh weather' of Nguru town, Nigeria. Nguru is a north-eastern ancient city of Nigeria notable with up to 47°C ambient temperatures during certain periods of the year. One of Nigeria's Federal Medical Centres (FMCnguru) was located in this grossly under-developed town. During the periods of these experiments approved by the FMCnguru's ethical committee, informed consents were obtained from mothers that were happy to permit the extended neonatal observations required for the study. The allowable standards for neonatal body temperature in most Nigerian neonatal centres including FMCnguru was a lower-upper limits of 36.5°C-37.4°C, measured from the axilla. Baby's thermal reaction to prevailing room temperatures were noted and compared to how volunteer healthy adults responded to the same harsh weather. Baby's skin temperatures behaved differently with those of the adults as these were observed to be always equal to the room temperature even when this increased to 43°C or decreased to 34°C whilst the adults maintained a constant range of 36.2°C-37°C all the times. This pattern was not exactly the same with higher birth weight and older postnatal age babies. Although such babies were all the same observed to be hyper- or hypothermic during these periods, their body temperatures were slightly lower or higher than room temperatures respectively. The local responsorial procedure at FMCnguru during high ambient heats was to sponge babies with water to minimise hyperthermia. Based on these findings, it was assumed that the neonate was very likely going to become hypothermic or hyperthermic depending on the relative overheating or under-heating of its host incubator. A neonate's thermal equilibrium set-point was therefore defined as the incubator air-mode set point that thermally stabilised a neonate to a body temperature of 36.5°C-37.4°C; incubator being appropriately humidified. The mid-point of this range was set at 36.9°C and used as a target for neonatal stabilisation. Therefore a general guiding principle for restabilising a deviating neonate was to increase or decrease incubator set-point value by an amount equal to baby's deviation from 36.9°C. This also demanded a compulsory recheck of baby's situation at intervals of no more than 30 minutes until baby re-stabilised. This was to allow enough time for the incubator to achieve the new set-point and for the baby to fully respond to the new changes, incorporating a possible neonatal cyclic temperature changes described by De La Fuente et al (2006). A disease process such as infection would be suspected and investigation initiated if baby's situation failed to respond positively to these changes after the 2nd cycle. It must however be first established that hyperthermia was not due to any domineering external warming of the incubator as described in section 7.1.2 of this chapter.

In quick easy-to-remember steps, the handy approach sets a good stage for the admission and systematic management of a neonate in an incubator thus:

a.   Feeder Unit alerts SCBU: At the inception of this project the SCBU of most centres had poor or no existent system of pre-admission communication with feeder departments such as the labour-ward/theatre for the in-born babies and any available reception unit for referral neonates. Therefore there was always a routine of frenzy and chaotic emergencies at the sudden appearance of an unexpected baby with a group of panicking adults. The confusion often created distracted the normal work flow of attendance on the nursery inmates. A standard of 'feeder unit alert' was hence established mandating a pre-admission alert with expected arrival time (EAT). A fair knowledge of the EAT for a prospective inmate allowed the SCBU management to make adequate preparations and properly assign respective duties to the attending staff in good time for the arriving baby.

b.   Designation and readiness of the expected incubator: Following feeder unit alert, preparations and provisional designation of duties would start. The expectant incubator was the incubator chosen to host the expected baby upon arrival and after all the admission protocols and possible initial clinical routines has been completed on a resuscitation table. The steps for preparing the expectant incubator was: (1) Cleaning with a standardised disinfectant solution of a combination of antiseptic fluids and water, normally referred to as 'carbolisation'. The hood and matrass tray with all the interior of the canopy were thoroughly disinfected during this procedure. (2) Fresh cover spread was laid on the matrass and access portholes requiring replaceable covers were covered with fresh sterile blinds. (3) The humidifier that should have been completely drained of water after the last use was then re-filled with the appropriate incubation water. This was distilled water or in the alternative 'boiled and cooled' water. Reservation of the alternative incubator water was practiced provided this was done in a plastic container as the use of metal containers could generate rust and contaminate the water. (4) The incubator was then switched on. (5) Oxygen in-line supply was connected and tested for function. The supply was then turned off and kept on standby. (6) A provisional set-point for the incubator was fixed at the lower limit of the neonatal clinical range, i.e. 36.5°C. It was necessary to keep the provisional set-point closer to normal body temperature as the baby's point-of-admission temperature was yet unknown, whether this was going to be within acceptable range or not. (7) The incubator was then allowed to run to achieve this set point in good time before baby's EAT.

c.   Admission, resuscitation and stabilisation: Upon baby's arrival, all the normal protocols were carried out by the admitting clinician and baby handed over for neonatal nursing.

d.   Start of incubation: Initial thermal stabilisation started as soon as baby was introduced into the incubator. Baby's entrance temperature was checked and noted. Attendants would ensure that baby was securely place on the matrass and all the access doors and porthole covers were securely latched. Opening of all canopy access windows to work on the baby were kept at minimum. Baby's temperature was re-checked no later than 30 minutes after incubation began to confirm a possible re-adjustment of the incubator set-point, to search for the thermal equilibrium set-point.

e.   Subsequent thermal re-stabilisation: This followed the procedure described earlier in this section to find a new equilibrium set-point whenever baby's temperature deviated from the allowable range. Figure (13) shows the guiding flowchart for this dynamics.

8. Externally influenced deficiencies

Gradual elimination of the various identified and rectified SCBU errors has steadily improved practice in the collaborating hospitals. However, there are other highly influential

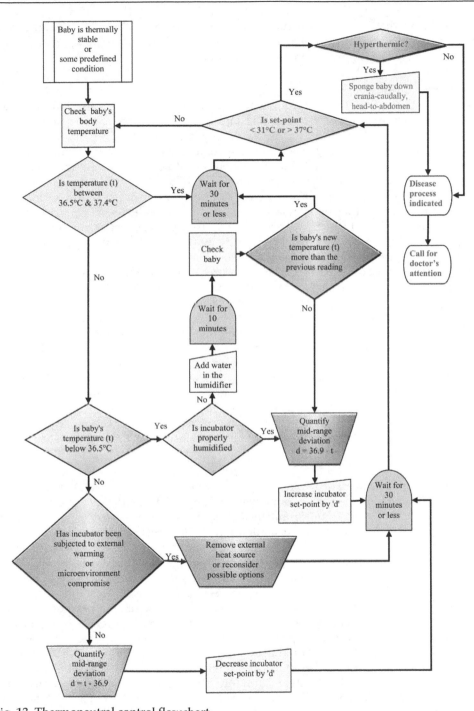

Fig. 13. Thermoneutral control flowchart

external factors that are possibly contributing to lower practice outcome. This category of problems might be beyond the ability of immediate SCBU to correct, hence required the cooperation of the higher institutional management to resolve.

8.1 Epileptic power supply

Inside a functioning incubator and yet wrapped! One would expect that a well-documented and known practice of nursing neonates naked inside a functional incubator would not need to be overemphasised anywhere in the world (Lyon, 2004). However this was initially observed to be one of the wrong incubator applications in the collaborating Centres. Some of the users showed evidence of this knowledge but could not stop because they needed to protect baby from cold stress that sets in upon power failure. However, there were no clear reasons given for this practice during the periods when the system functioned. Uninformed and indiscriminate electric power outages that last for several hours are common to West African countries. Unfortunately, very sensitive units as the SCBU of hospitals suffer from this problem at which point the incubator suddenly fails exposing baby to danger of cold stress and hypothermia. The use of 'standby' generators is widespread but this still does not effectively cover up this deficiency in most Centres. There were also reports of incubator damages due to power surges from malfunctioning generators. Full-sine-wave power inverting technology was therefore considered an option to investigate. A full-sine-wave power inverter system with a cascade of sealed batteries function to convert the DC power of the batteries to AC power required to operate the incubators upon conventional mains power failure. This operates with an automatic power change over system that allows it to stay 'on' to recharge the batteries when mains AC supply is available and switches incubators to draw inverted battery power when mains supply fails. A 5KVA system installed with up to 8 pieces of '12 volts 200 amp-hour' batteries was found to be able to continuously support up to 11 incubators simultaneously for up to 10 hours. This was enough to provide uninterrupted power supply to the most critical neonates in the few Units that could afford to implement this, hence minimising the effect of operating power deficiencies.

8.2 Inadequate nursing staff

The sudden increase in the number of patients seeking to be admitted for neonatal care as reported by Amadi et al (2010) meant that more hands were needed to cope with the present volume of work in each participating SCBU. The Units were hence faced with the lack of adequate manpower and challenges to retain the already experienced ones on employment. External issues of government policies on employment and local administration of the Nursing Department in these hospitals were contributing factors to the challenges. The direct effect of this to the present project was the resulting inability to effectively offer adequate care using all the developed techniques and procedures in this project. Some of these challenges as enumerated below are currently being tackled through engaging the various hospital managements to demonstrate the importance of discriminate staffing of the new-born Units.

1.   Maintaining a sizable number of SCBU nursing staff as compared to adult or young-adult wards. Most of the SCBUs are currently having up to 40 inmates on admission at the same time with as few as 3 nursing staff to look after them during some rota shifts. Our current study shows that the quality of attention offered to these babies becomes

clinically unacceptable at more than a patient-to-nurse ratio of 5. This mark is frequently being exceeded, hence calling for urgent review on nurses' deployment to the Units. This has also led to some preventable loses to apnoea as many attacks were not detected early enough to commence resuscitation. It therefore became important to propose and implement the provision of integral digital apnoea monitors on all incubators and cots. These raised audible alarms during attacks, enabling the few nurses on duty to be aware of the points of emergency even whilst they were busy with other babies.

2. Frequent shovelling of experienced nurses has militated against more excellent results from the Centres. It was a common routine in 80% (12/15) of the hospitals to re-shovel senior nurses among all the departments including the neonatal wards. This was entirely governed by the Nursing Department as a measure to allow nurses acquire experiences of how things worked in various departmental wards and happened as frequent as every two years or less. There might be good intentions for this; however, our findings from the present study showed that this was producing a serious counterproductive effect on the SCBU target. Nurses needed to stay in the Units for up to 18 months to fully understudy the new systems and procedures being implemented to positively alter the neonatal mortality as these ideas were completely new to most of them. During this period they would have attended the level 1 and perhaps level 2 of the Paediatric Incubation Technique courses. This has hence frequently created occasions when all three or four nurses on duty were completely untrained newcomers to the new procedures, hence slowing down the progress of the Unit. Minimizing the unequal shovelling of well-experienced and trained neonatal care-givers with inexperienced ones has therefore become a major issue to settle in all the hospitals. A proposal was drawn and negotiated with the various Nursing Administrative Departments of the hospitals to implement a 'neonatal 70-30' agenda whereby their normal shovelling exercise must ensure that 70% of SCBU qualified nurses were specialised or have at least 15 months experience and certified on the course levels 1 and 2. This excluded the numerous yet-to-qualify and short-staying nursing students that must work under full supervision of at least one experienced nurse on duty. This is presently working well and yielding good results in 6 of our 15 collaborating centres. Quantified in terms of incubation hours denied due to system breakdown, and comparing one calendar quarter before and after full implementation of the agenda, this has on the average saved 81% (10,886.4 hours) of the total incubation time lost to system breakdown before implementation. It is evident from these 6 Centres that frequency of system breakdown due to mishandling has dropped, thereby reducing maintenance costs and providing for more babies to save.

3. Compulsory theoretical course (requiring a pass in an end of course test) was initiated and currently being implemented by some of the Nursing Administrative Departments as a prerequisite for posting a new nurse to the SCBU. In the new guideline, resident doctors that were specialising on new-born care were advised to complete the 2 levels of the elective course.

9. Conquering the climate

The conclusions being drawn from the entire project suggest that culture and climate were major forces to conquer in order to realise the MDG target on neonatal mortality. Our ongoing studies at the University of Ilorin Teaching Hospital and the Federal Medical Nguru have identified a number of parameters that could be altered to reduce the negative impact of climate on new-born morbidity. We studied all the nursery buildings at our disposal, these being all distinctively different from each other in design, structure and relative location. The impact of high sunlight intensity as a source of uncontrollable external warming of the incubator was used to identify the parameters that were aiding or preventing the harsh climate. Incubators functioned well, adequately maintaining their set points, when these had absolute control of the warming of their microenvironments. This occurred during cooler periods of the day or the night when the nursery ambient temperature dropped well below 30°C. However this often changed during the day when the macro-environment of the inside of the nursery became excessively hot due to radiation from the sun. We therefore hypothesised that minimising the outside influence of climatic heat on the nursery would enhance effective thermoneutral control and achieve better success rates. It is understood that the use of air-conditioners could artificially cool the nursery wards to counter room warming during the day. This was tried but not considered a sustainable solution as the high frequency of breakdowns without immediate repair or replacement often sent the Unit back to the same ugly situation. Again, this was also noticed to present threats of hypothermia on the other full-term babies in cots as these shared the open nurseries with the incubator babies. It therefore became necessary to find enabling parameters that could be altered to attain the best naturally cooled condition in the nursery. Parameters were preliminarily identified by comparing nursery warming in any two Centres that have direct opposite circumstance. Parameters currently being studied in details were:

1. Siting of the nursery building within hospital complex. Nurseries that were cited as the eastern-most building among the rest in the hospital complex and without any other immediate building east to this seemed to be hotter than those elsewhere cited.
2. Locating nursery within building structure. Nursery apartments that were located on the topmost floor of a multi-storey building seemed hotter than those located on the ground floor.
3. Structural design of nursery outside wall. Nursery designs that provided the main ward at the middle of other flanking rooms, stores or side labs seemed cooler than designs where the wall of the main ward was directly next to the outside. This suggests that some kind of wall lagging designs might provide the needed natural cooling for the macro-environment.
4. Floor to roof height of nursery. Nurseries with higher roofs from the floor level seemed cooler than the shorter ones.
5. Nursery floor level, nursery window height and nursery window blinding material were also identified to seem to create some differences and hence also being studied.

10. Conclusion

This project has been an individual coordinating effort in a drive to lower neonatal mortality rate, restore nursing enthusiasm and patient- carer's confidence in the tropical region of West African state of Nigeria. The project originally set out to find alternative solution to the provision of functional incubators to re-equip the referral hospitals in the country. This began in each of the participated hospital at a time when most of these had no functional incubator. The development and application of the idea of Recycled Incubator Technique (RIT) helped to realise the initial objective as this has made it possible for some of the hospitals to move from a condition of having no functional incubator to having 15 or more within a short period of time. However, the restoration of proper usage of the incubator to nurse babies exposed the knowledge deficiency of care-providers in incubator application. It was evident that immediate cultural setting and the quality of care with the provided incubator were capable of promoting the spread of diseases among the neonates. Hence, this project extended to the study and proposition of corrective procedures that were easily applicable to the people.

The implementation of the various ideas developed in this study has brought cultural dimension to tweak already established practice facts. This was another way of using the local language to communicate the medicine of neonatal thermocontrol in this tropical region. The methods were easily acceptable and adaptable and seemed to have led to improved outcome among all participating Centres.

Overall, the entire project has achieved significant success across the landscape of Nigeria among all the applying hospitals as published by Amadi et al., 2010. This study was unable to explicitly isolate successes due to the provision of incubators as an initial project and the duo of training courses and modified thermoneutral algorithm as an extended application. These were applied simultaneously. It is commonly acknowledged among hospital administrators in Nigeria that the advent of RIT and the subsequent thermocontrol procedures represented a significant contribution to Nigeria's improving neonatal healthcare delivery (CCEFTHI, 2007). Further investigations are still continuing on how the climate is impacting and militating against overall outcome. We hope to fully define this and proffer solutions on how to ameliorate this and boost survival rate in the region.

11. Acknowledgement

The support of all the Chief Medical Directors of the hospitals that have so far collaborated is hereby acknowledged. Some of these were outstanding in their cooperation at various segments of this project. These were Akin Osibogun, Bello Kawuwa, Uriah Etawo, Dan Iya, Sulyman Kuranga, Abulhameed Dutse and Eugene Okpere. Other individuals whose supportive roles are worthy of mention are Jonathan Azubuike, Olugbenga Mokuolu and Peter Onyeri.

12. References

Amadi, H.O.; Azubuike, J.C.; Etawo, U.S.; Offiong, U.R.; Ezeaka, C.; Eyinade, O.; Adimora, G.N.; Osibogun, A.A.; Ibeziako, N.; Iroha, E.O.; Dutse, A.I.; Chukwu, C.O.; Okpere, E.E.; Kawuwa, M.B.; El-Nafaty, A.U.; Kuranga, S.A. & Mokuolu, O.A. (2010). The impact of recycled neonatal incubators in Nigeria: a 6-year follow-up study. *Int J Paeditr.* Vol.2010, Article ID 269293, 7 pages doi:10.1155/2010/269293

Amadi, H.O.; Mokuolu, O.; Adimora, G.N.; Pam, S.D.; Etawo, U.S.; Ohadugha, C.O. & Adesiyun, O.O. (2007). Digitally recycled incubators: better economic alternatives to modern systems in low-income countries. *Annals Tropical Paeditr*, Vol.27, No.3, (September 2007), pp. 207-214, ISSN 0272-4936

CCEFTHI. (July 2007). Communiqué issued at the end of the 58th quarterly meeting of the Committee of Chief Executives of Federal Tertiary Hospitals, University of Benin Teaching Hospital Nigeria, 16.02.2010, Availbale from ccefth.org/document/communique_53rd_meeting.pdf

Centre for Maternal And Child Enquiry. (2010). Overview of perinatal and neonatal mortality in the UK. In: *Perinatal mortality 2008: United Kingdom,* J. Dorling (Ed.), 9-15, CMACE, ISBN 978-0-9558055-3-0, London, United Kingdom de Carvalho, M.; Torrao, C.T. & Moreira, M.E. (2011). Mist and water condensation inside incubators reduce the efficacy of phototherapy. *Arch Dis Child Fetal Neonatal Ed*, Vol.96, No.2, (March 2011), pp.F138-F140

De La Fuente, L.; Campbell, D.E.; Rios, A.; Grieg, A.; Graff, M. & Brion, L.P. (2006). Frequency analysis of air and skin temperature in neonates in servo-controlled incubators. *Journal of Perinatology*, Vol.26, No.5, (May 2006), pp. 301-305

Dollberg, S.; Xi, Y. & Donnelly, M.M. (1993). A non-invasive transcutaneous alternative to rectal thermometry for continuous measurement of core temperature in the piglet. *Pediatr Res*, Vol.34, pp. 512

Drebbel. (June 2011). Incubator, In: *Cornelis Drebbel's inventions and instruments: references and descriptions*, pp. 3, 18.06.2011, Available from http://www.drebbel.net/Drebbels%20Instrumenten.pdf

Encyclopedia Brittanica. (June 2011). Harmattan wind. In: *Brittanica Online Encyclopedia*, 18.06.2011, Available from http://www.britannica.com/EBchecked/topic/255457/harmattan

Federal Ministry of Health. (2011). Saving newborn lives in Nigeria: Newborn health in the context of the Integrated Maternal, Newborn and Child Health Strategy. *Federal Ministry of Health Abuja, Save the Children, Jhpiego*, 2nd edition, 24.06.2011, Available from http://resourcecentre.savethechildren.se/content/library/documents/nigeria-newborn-health-report-context-integrated-maternal-newborn-and-chilHealth Devices. (2010). Hazard report-Infants may fall through insecure ports on incubators. *Health devices*, Vol.39, No.1, pp. 25-26

Ibe, B.C. (1993). Low Birth Weight and Structural Adjustment Programme in Nigeria. *Journal of Tropical Paediatrics*, Vol. 39, pp. 312-313

Lyon, A. (2004). Applied physiology: temperature control in the new born infant. *Current Paediatr*, Vol.14, pp. 137- 144

Lyon, A.J. & Oxley, C. (2001). Heat Balance, a computer program to determine optimum incubator air temperature and humidity: a comparison against nurse settings for infants less than 29 weeks gestation. *Early Hum Dev*, Vol.62, pp. 33-41

Neonatology on the web. (1897). The use of incubator for infants. *The Lancet*, pp. 1490-1491, Available from http://www.neonatology.org/classics/lancet.incubators.html

Ogunlesi, T.A.; Dedeke, O.I.; Adekanmbi, F.A.; Fetuga, B.M. & Okeniyi, A.J. (2008). Neonatal resuscitation - knowledge and practice of nurses in western Nigeria. *South African Journal of Child Health*, Vol.2, pp. 23-25

Perlstein, P.H. (1997). Physical environment. In: *Neonatal-Perinatal Medicine: Diseases of the Fetus and the Infant*, A. Fanaroff & R. Martin, (Eds.), 481-501, Mosby, Philadelphia, PA

Silverman, W.A.; Agate, F.J. & Fertig, J.W. (1963). A sequential trial of the nonthermal effect of atmospheric humidity on survival of human infants of low birth weight. *Pediatr*, Vol.31, pp. 710-724

Silverman, W.A.; Fertig, J.W. & Berger, A.P. (1958). The influence of the thermal environment upon survival of newly born preterm infants. *Pediatr*, Vol.22, pp. 876-885

Tunell, R. (2004). Prevention of neonatal cold injury in preterm infants. *Acta Paediatr*, Vol.93, pp. 308-310, ISSN 0803-5253

WHO African Region. (September 2009). Child and adolescent health. *World Health Organisation*, 07.09.2009, Availabe from http://www.who.int/countries/nga/areas/cah/en/index.html

Wikipedia. (June 2011). Harmattan. In: *Wikipedia, the free encyclopedia*, 18.06.2011, Available from http://en.wikipedia.org/wiki/Harmattan

12

Sexually Transmitted Infections in the Tropics

John C. Meade and Denise C. Cornelius

University of Mississippi Medical Center, Department of Microbiology, Jackson, MS
USA

1. Introduction

The burden of sexually transmitted infections (STIs) on the health and well-being of the population in the developing world is considerable. The World Health Organization (WHO) estimates that there are 340 million new cases of curable STIs in the world each year; 174 million new cases of trichomoniasis, 92 million new cases of *Chlamydia* infection, 62 million cases of gonorrhea, and 12 million new cases of syphilis (Table 1). Approximately three quarters of these infections are in countries encompassing tropical regions of the world in Latin America, sub-Saharan Africa, and South and Southeast Asia. The prevalence of viral STIs is even higher; infection with Herpes simplex virus-2 (HSV-2) is the most common STI worldwide and as many as 50% of sexually active individuals will be infected with human papillomavirus (HPV) during their life. The prevalence of STIs is considerably greater than many classical tropical diseases and it is unfortunate that they do not receive more attention and resources from international programs and donor groups. The public health impact of these diseases extends well beyond the immediate effects and morbidities of infection. STIs have been implicated in facilitating acquisition and transmission of HIV, in pregnancy complications such as pre-term births, low birth weight infants, stillbirth, neonatal death and blindness, in the inducement of cervical and prostate cancers, and in increased risk of pelvic inflammatory disease and infertility. Failure to diagnose and treat STIs at an early stage thus increases the already substantial burden these conditions impose on the populations of developing countries. Although effective diagnostic tests and treatments are available for these STIs, they are often unavailable or inaccessible in resource-limited tropical settings. As a consequence, syndromic management of STIs remains the option of choice for individual case management. The inadequate public health response coupled to ongoing socioeconomic and demographic trends have led to an epidemic of STIs in many countries in the developing world. The development of antimicrobial resistance is an on-going problem and new agents are often much more expensive, increasing the burden of control. The economic costs of these diseases and their infection sequelae place a considerable burden on national health budgets and household income. In developing countries, STIs are among the top five reasons for which adults seek medical care. Due to the prevalence and public health implications of STIs in the tropics a discussion of STIs should be included in any compilation of tropical medicine.

This chapter will cover sexually transmitted infections caused by *Trichomonas vaginalis* (trichomoniasis), *Chlamydia trachomatis* (chlamydia and lymphogranuloma venereum), *Neisseria gonorrhoeae* (gonorrhea), *Treponema pallidum* (syphilis), *Haemophilus ducreyi* (chancroid), *Calymmatobacterium granulomatis* (granuloma inguinale or donovanosis), and the viral STIs, herpes simplex virus and human papilloma virus. Each of these STIs spreads via vaginal, anal, and oral sex, as well as by inoculation of material from infected sores in some cases. All share many common risk factors and higher rates of infection are seen in marginalized populations; persons of low socioeconomic status, commercial sex workers, alcohol abusers, illicit drug users, men who have sex with men, prison populations, uncircumcised men, and those with multiple sex partners or who have partners with multiple sex partners. This chapter will cover both syndromic management of STIs as practiced in most areas of the tropical world (WHO 2003, 2005, 2007b) as well as individual descriptions of these diseases, their clinical presentation, diagnosis, and treatment. The treatment regimens presented are those recommended by the Centers for Disease Control and Prevention (CDC, 2010) and the World Health Organization (WHO, 2005).

	Latin America & the Caribbean	Sub-Saharan Africa	North Africa & Middle East	Southeast & South Asia	World Total
Trichomoniasis	18.5	32	5	76.5	174
Chlamydia	9.5	16	3	43	92
Gonorrhea	7.5	17	1.5	27	62
Syphilis	3	4	0.37	4	12
Total STIs	38.5	69	10	151	340
HIV/AIDS	1.4	22.5	0.46	4.1	33.3

Table 1. World Health Organization estimates of new cases of curable sexually transmitted infections and HIV, in millions (WHO, 2001; UNAIDS, 2010).

2. STIs and HIV

It is estimated that there are 34 million cases of HIV in the world with 68% or 22.5 million cases occurring in sub-Saharan Africa, where the prevalence is highest, and 4.1 million in South and Southeast Asia. The emergence of the HIV epidemic has complicated the control of STIs as HIV induced immunosuppression leads many patients to respond poorly to STI treatment regimens, requiring higher drug dosages and longer treatment schedules to affect cure. Sexually transmitted infections (STIs) also facilitate the transmission of other STIs, including human immunodeficiency virus (HIV). Several observational studies have been conducted that conclude there to be a strong association between STI and increased risk of HIV acquisition. An individual with a co-existing STI has a 2-5 fold greater risk of acquiring and transmitting HIV. Increased risk of HIV transmission has mostly been attributed to ulcerative STIs, mainly HSV-1 and 2, but also syphilis, chancroid, lymphogranuloma venereum, and granuloma inguinale. For instance the population attributable risk percent of HIV acquisition for HSV-1 and 2 varies from 15-30% in Africa. However, studies also show that non-ulcerative STIs, gonorrhea, *Chlamydia*, and trichomoniasis increase the risk of HIV transmission and acquisition as well. Studies that have examined non-ulcerative STIs and risk of HIV seroconversion have found an odds ratio of 1.8-4.8 for gonorrhea, 1.8-3.6 for chlamydia, and 1.9 for trichomoniasis. Therefore, early diagnosis and treatment of treatable

STIs could significantly impact the incidence of HIV transmission and acquisition. The number of individuals co-infected with HIV and an STI are high. Studies show increases in treatment failure of treatable STIs in HIV-positive patients. Studies in several countries show high treatment failure of syphilis in HIV-positive patients and in a trichomoniasis study, 18% of HIV-positive women were *T. vaginalis* positive 1 month after treatment. It is therefore possible that more aggressive treatment of non-ulcerative STIs may be necessary to cure an infection in HIV-positive individuals. STI treatment has been shown to significantly reduce HIV-shedding in both men and women. Follow-up for test of cure is also necessary due to the higher risk of treatment failure due to co-infection.

3. Syndromic management

The diagnosis and management of STIs in the tropics has a dual nature. Sophisticated testing equipment and facilities comparable to those available in developed nations can often be found in large urban centers and popular resort destinations in developing countries. However, in many parts of the developing world, the absence of etiologic diagnostic capacity due to constraints imposed by cost, lack of equipment or trained personnel, and time management has forced health care providers to rely on a syndrome-based approach to STI management. This approach employs clinical algorithms based on an STI syndrome to determine antimicrobial therapy. The following sections discuss management of the most common clinical syndromes encountered in STIs. Sexual partners of the index patient should also be examined for STIs and promptly treated for the same condition as treatment failures are common when partners are not treated. Often, treatment regimens to cover multiple infectious agents are recommended due to the difficulty in distinguishing between the overlapping clinical presentations of different STIs, the high prevalence of mixed infections in many areas, and to ensure adequate therapy in the case of loss to follow-up. Syndromic management enables many STIs to be treated and resolved at local clinics which may lack all but the most rudimentary laboratory capabilities. However, patients that do not respond to therapy or those that show systemic signs indicative of other disease conditions warrant referral to a clinic with more comprehensive facilities.

3.1 Urethral discharge in men

Neisseria gonorrhoeae and *Chlamydia trachomatis* are the major STI pathogens causing urethral discharge. In the syndromic management scheme, treatment of men with urethral discharge should cover both of these organisms. Treatment regimens may be found in the specific sections describing these STIs. Single-dose therapies are preferred. Whenever possible microscopic examination of the urethral smear should be performed; the appearance of more than 5 polymorphonuclear leukocytes per high power field (x1000) is indicative of urethritis. A Gram stain could also demonstrate the presence of gonococci and permit specific treatment. Patients should return in 7 days if symptoms persist. Treatment failure may be due to drug resistance necessitating use of one of the alternative drugs for these STI agents. Patients indicating poor compliance with therapy or the possibility of re-infection can be re-treated with the same drug regimen. *Trichomonas vaginalis* can also be a cause of urethritis in men. In areas of high local *T. vaginalis* prevalence, treatment for this organism should also be given at this time. If symptoms still persist, the patient should be referred to a facility possessing the resources for a more extensive workup.

3.2 Genital ulcers

Five STIs typically produce genital ulcers; herpes, syphilis, chancroid, lymphogranuloma venereum (LGV), and granuloma inguinale or donovanosis (Table 2). Physical examination should focus on the characteristics of the lesion(s): single or multiple, painless or painful, indurated or soft, irregular or regular borders, and how they began, as a papule or a vesicle. The examination should also determine the time since exposure, the presence or absence of lymphadenopathy, and the presence of systemic symptoms which may indicate another etiology. Syphilis ulcers are painless, indurated, sharply demarcated with a red, smooth base. When present, inguinal adenopathy is firm, rubbery, nontender and usually bilateral. Herpes ulcers begin as multiple grouped vesicles on a red base which forms shallow ulcers that may coalesce. Herpes inguinal adenopathy is bilateral, firm, and tender when present. Chancroid ulcers are shallow and often multiple with irregular shape, sharply demarcated borders, and undermined edges. Chancroid inguinal adenopathy is typically unilateral, fixed, and tender, with overlying erythema and may supperate. Granuloma inguinale ulcers are shallow sharply demarcated lesions with a beefy red friable base and usually without inguinal adenopathy. LGV ulcers are usually a single lesion, transient, and frequently not noticed. Inguinal adenopathy in LGV is usually unilateral, firm, tender, fixed, and may supperate or form fistulas. When genital ulcers present as vesicles only, syndromic management recommends treatment for both herpes infection and for syphilis if the patient has a positive RPR syphilis test, or has not received recent syphilis treatment. Patients with ulcers and no vesicles should be treated for syphilis plus either chancroid, granuloma inguinale, or lymphogranuloma venereum dependent on clinical presentation and local prevalence of these agents. In areas where herpes prevalence exceeds 30%, patients with ulcers should also be treated for herpes. Patients whose ulcers do not respond to both initial treatment and follow-up therapy should be referred for more extensive diagnostic testing.

Disease	Lesions	Lymphadenopathy	Systemic symptoms
Herpes	Small, painful, pruritic vesicles lesions shallow, usually multiple, grouped, and may coalesce	Tender, firm, bilateral nonsupperative inguinal adenopathy	Yes, primary infection
Primary Syphilis	Painless, indurated, round red smooth base, usually single, sharply demarcated	Nontender, firm, rubbery, nonsupperative, bilateral	None in primary stage Yes in secondary/tertiary
Chancroid	Tender, erythematous papules ulcers painful, purulent, irregular shape, soft undermined edges, often multiple	Tender, regional, painful, erythematous, supperative nodes, usually unilateral	None
LGV	Small, painless vesicle/papule usually single, heals rapidly often not noticed	Painful, matted, firm, large nodes supperate with fistula tracts, usually unilateral	After genital lesions heal spread to regional lymph nodes
Donovanosis	Small, painless pustules, ulcers shallow, erythematous, sharply demarcated, may expand, deepen, become necrotic, can be dry or nodular	Inguinal adenopathy usually absent	Yes, but rarely Extragenital lesions via inoculation from genital sores may occur

Table 2. Characteristics of Genital Ulcers

3.3 Inguinal bubo

Inguinal buboes are frequently associated with LGV and chancroid. If genital ulcers accompany the buboes, patients should be managed using the genital ulcer syndromic management approach. Inguinal buboes not accompanied by genital ulcer presentation should be treated with a regimen effective against LGV and chancroid. The recommended syndromic treatment is ciprofloxacin, 500 mg orally twice daily for 3 days plus doxycycline, 100 mg orally twice daily for 14 days, or erythromycin, 500 mg orally four times daily for 14 days. Some cases may require longer treatment than 14 days if the buboes are not resolved. Fluctuant lymph nodes can be aspirated through healthy skin. Incision and drainage or excision of nodes may delay healing.

3.4 Scrotal swelling

There are multiple infectious causes for epididymitis as well as non-infectious causes such as trauma, testicular torsion, and tumor. Patients with testis that are rotated or elevated or with a history of trauma should be referred for surgical option. An STI is more likely the cause for men under 35 years of age than for older men. An epididymitis which is accompanied by urethral discharge should be treated with drugs for both gonococcal and chlamydial infection.

3.5 Vaginal discharge

An abnormal vaginal discharge in terms of quantity, color, or odor most commonly results from vaginal infection. *Trichomonas vaginalis* is the most common STI cause of vaginal infection, though bacterial vaginosis (BV) and yeast infections also produce vaginal discharge. All women presenting with vaginal discharge should be treated for trichomoniasis and BV, in the absence of specific diagnosis, with metronidazole, 400-500 mg orally twice daily for 7 days. Metronidazole is not recommended in the first trimester of pregnancy. Pregnant women should be treated with metronidazole, 200-250 mg orally 3 times daily for 7 days. In rare cases, vaginal discharge may result from a mucopurulent cervicitis due to infection with *N. gonorrhoeae* or *C. trachomatis*. Treatment for cervical infection in women presenting with vaginal discharge is dependent on the local prevalence of these STIs. Women in high risk areas for *N. gonorrhoeae* or *C. trachomatis* with vaginal discharge and evidence of cervicitis should be offered treatment for these STIs in addition to treatment for BV and trichomoniasis.

3.6 Lower abdominal pain

There are multiple causes of lower abdominal pain in sexually active women in addition to pelvic inflammatory disease (PID) caused by STIs. Women presenting with lower abdominal pain and a missed or overdue period, pregnant, recent delivery, abortion, or miscarriage, abdominal guarding and/or tenderness, abnormal vaginal bleeding, or abdominal mass, should be referred for surgical or gynecological assessment. In the absence of these signs women with lower abdominal pain accompanied by cervical excitation tenderness or lower abdominal tenderness and vaginal discharge should be managed for PID. The etiologic agents for PID include *N. gonorrhoeae*, *C. trachomatis*, *T. vaginalis*, anaerobic and facultative bacteria, and perhaps *Mycoplasma*. When diagnostic capacity to distinguish these agents is absent the treatment regimen must be effective against all these pathogens. The recommended syndromic treatment is a single dose therapy for gonorrhea, plus doxycyline, 100 mg orally twice daily, or tetracycline, 500 mg orally 4 times daily for 14 days, plus metronidazole, 400-500 mg orally twice daily for 14 days. Patients who do not respond to therapy within three days should be referred for a more complete diagnostic evaluation.

3.7 Neonatal conjunctivitis

Infants with neonatal conjunctivitis (ophthalmia neonatorum) present with eyes that are red, swollen and accompanied by discharge ("sticky eyes"). *Chlamydia trachomatis* and *N. gonorrhoeae* are the most significant pathogens which cause ophthalmia neonatorum in developing countries although infections from *Staphylococcus aureus*, *Streptococcus pneumoniae*, *Haemophilus* spp., and *Pseudomonas* spp. occur. The oropharynx, urogenital tract, and rectum of neonates may also be affected in *Chlamydia trachomatis* or *N. gonorrhoeae* infection. *Neisseria* conjunctivitis develops within a few days of birth whereas *C. trachomatis* conjunctivitis develops slower, 5-14 days after birth. Neonatal conjunctivitis caused by *N. gonorrhoeae* can lead to blindness when untreated. Coverage should be provided for both of these STIs in settings where definitive diagnosis is not possible, especially where there is evidence of a maternal STI. Treatment should include a single dose therapy for gonorrhea and multiple dose therapy for chlamydia. For gonorrhea a single intramuscular injection of ceftriaxone, 50 mg/kg to a maximum of 125 mg total, should be administered. If ceftriaxone is unavailable, single injections of kanamycin or spectinomycin at 25 mg/kg to a maximum dose of 75 mg total may be used. For chlamydia treatment, erythromycin syrup, 50 mg/kg per day orally, in 4 divided doses for 14 days or trimethoprim, 40 mg with sulfamethoxazole, 200 mg orally twice daily for 14 days are recommended. Gonococcal ophthalmia neonatorum is preventable if a 1% silver nitrate solution or 1% tetracycline ointment is applied at birth as a prophylactic measure.

4. Trichomoniasis

Trichomonas vaginalis infects the urogenital tract of men and women, causing trichomoniasis. *Trichomonas vaginalis* is a member of the Phylum Zoomastigina, Class Parabasalia, Order Trichomonadida, and Family Trichomonadidae. *Trichomonas vaginalis* has only one life stage, trophozoites, which display various shapes including pyriform, ameboid, ellipsoidal, ovoidal, and spherical. The organisms measure between 10 – 30 microns. The organism possesses four anterior flagella and a fifth flagellum located posteriorly along the undulating membrane. These flagella of the organism yield the characteristic quivering motion of *T. vaginalis*.

4.1 Epidemiology

Trichomoniasis is the most common, curable, non-viral sexually transmitted infection worldwide. An estimated 174 million new cases of trichomoniasis occur worldwide each year. The incidence of *Trichomonas vaginalis* infection varies in different countries throughout the world. Incidence in Asian countries varies from 0.7% in rural China to 15.1% in sex workers in Indonesia. In South America, studies report incidence ranging from 4-9%. In Brazil prevalence is thought to have a range of 20 up to 40%. Incidence in African countries ranges from 2-20%. The incidence of trichomoniasis is higher in sexually active women over 25 years of age than in younger women.

4.2 Clinical manifestations
The actual number of new or existing cases of trichomoniasis is not known with complete surety because trichomoniasis is not a reportable disease and because of the significant number of asymptomatic cases. Trichomoniasis is usually asymptomatic in men, although sometimes it can cause non-gonococcal, non-chlamydial urethritis, epididymitis, and prostatitis. Clinical trichomoniasis in women ranges from asymptomatic carriers to flagrant vaginitis. Women have symptomatic disease more often than men. One third of asymptomatic woman will become symptomatic within 6 months of the onset of infection. Symptoms can include a vaginal discharge, vulvovaginal irritation and itching, painful urination or intercourse, foul odor, and lower abdominal pain. The presence or absence and severity of these symptoms determine whether the infection is classified as acute, chronic, or asymptomatic.

4.3 Health sequelae
Trichomoniasis is associated with a higher risk for other infectious diseases and adverse pregnancy outcomes such as preterm birth, premature rupture of placental membranes, and low birth weight infants. One study has also found an association between T. vaginalis infection in pregnancy and mental retardation in children. Trichomonas vaginalis infection is associated with pelvic inflammatory disease, especially PID leading to sterility. Trichomoniasis is significantly associated with HSV infection. Trichomonas vaginalis infection also increases the risk of human immunodeficiency virus (HIV) acquisition and the Centers for Disease Control and Prevention (CDC) estimates that as much as 20% of HIV transmission in the African American population in the United States may be attributable to T. vaginalis infection. Trichomonas vaginalis infection also increases the risk of cervical neoplasia and prostate cancer. Exposure to T. vaginalis results in a 2-fold increase in the risk of diagnosis of extraprostatic prostate cancer and a 3-fold increase in the risk of cancer that led to cancer-specific death. Thus, although trichomoniasis itself is a curable disease, T. vaginalis infection may indirectly be a life threatening disease.

4.4 Diagnosis
Because of the high prevalence of trichomoniasis, any woman seeking medical care for vaginal discharge should be tested for T. vaginalis infection. Trichomoniasis is traditionally diagnosed microscopically (wet mount) by observing mobile protozoa in vaginal secretions, cervical samples, or from urethral or prostatic swabs. However, this method has a relatively low sensitivity and requires immediate evaluation of a wet preparation slide for optimal results. The low sensitivity of this diagnostic method leads to under-diagnosis. The current gold standard for diagnosis of trichomoniasis is culture in Diamonds media and is widely used. Rapid antigen based point-of-care tests and nucleic acid based diagnostic tools are also available. Both of these techniques have high sensitivity and specificity. Papanicolaou (Pap) smear allows for direct visualization in saline prep and can be performed within 10-20 minutes of sample collection but is not widely used. The Whiff test can be performed by mixing vaginal secretions with 10% potassium hydroxide (KOH) to yield a strong fishy odor. This test has a poor specificity due to the fact that bacterial vaginosis can yield a similar result. All of the above mentioned diagnostic methods are applicable for diagnosis in women. In men, culture testing of urethral swabs, urine, or semen and the nucleic acid amplification tests are more sensitive diagnostic tools.

4.5 Treatment

Metronidazole, 2 g orally in a single dose or 500 mg orally twice a day for 7 days, is the treatment of choice for trichomoniasis. An estimated 2.5-10% of *T. vaginalis* infections show some degree of resistance to treatment; a resistance rate of 17.4% has been reported in Papua New Guinea. Treatment failures are higher in HIV-positive individuals. Recalcitrant cases may be treated with tinidazole at 2 g orally in a single dose. Consumption of alcohol should be avoided during treatment and for 24 hrs after completion of metronidazole therapy or 72 hours after completion of tinidazole therapy.

5. Chlamydia

Chlamydia trachomatis is a small, obligate intracellular bacterium that typically infects non-ciliated epithelial cells of mucous membranes; urethral epithelial cells in males and columnar epithelial cells of the endocervix in women. However in the lymphogranuloma venereum serovars, macrophages appear to be the principal host cell. *Chlamydia* is organized into multiple serovars that cause a diverse variety of human disease. Serotypes A, B, Ba, and C are the agents of classic blinding trachoma. Serotypes D thru K can cause adult inclusion and neonatal conjunctivitis, pneumonia, urogenital infections and Reiter's syndrome. Serotypes L1, L2, and L3 infect tissues deeper to the epithelium and cause lymphogranuloma venereum (LGV).

5.1 Epidemiology

Chlamydia infection is the most common bacterial STI in the world and among STIs, only the prevalences of herpes and trichomoniasis are higher. *Chlamydia* infection is highest in sexually active young adults under 25 years of age. *Chlamydia trachomatis* causes 30-50% of nongonoccal urethritis in men and mucopurulent cervicitis in women. In men less than 35 years of age *Chlamydia* is the principal cause of epididymitis. Although there is no lasting immunity and re-infection is common, women do clear the infection faster with increasing age. Lymphogranuloma venereum (LGV) is an uncommon disease and relatively rare in developed countries. The disease is most common in sub-Saharan Africa and is also reported in areas of the Caribbean, Central America, and Southeast Asia and sporadically in developed nations.

5.2 Clinical manifestations

Symptoms of chlamydial infection typically appear 1-3 weeks post exposure. Asymptomatic infection is common among both men, approximately ~50%, and women, approximately 70-80%. When it occurs, symptomatic infection clears spontaneously about 50% of the time. However, both untreated and asymptomatic infections can persist for years; as many as 10% remain infected after 3 years. Symptomatic men might have a urethral discharge and dysuria with burning and itching around the urethral opening. Epididymitis and prostatitis are sometimes present causing pain and swelling of the testes, fever, and rarely sterility. *Chlamydial* infection of the rectum can cause pruritis, rectal pain, discharge, or bleeding. Chlamydia infected women may experience cervicitis, vaginal discharge and dysuria. Infection and inflammation in the cervix may spread to the fallopian tubes and uterus, leading to pelvic inflammatory disease (PID). *Chlamydia* is among the most frequent pathogens associated with PID and up to 40% of women with untreated chlamydia develop PID. Some women with PID report lower abdominal pain, lower back pain, nausea, fever, abnormal bleeding, and dysparenia but many women show no signs of infection. Untreated PID can result in chronic pelvic pain, tubal infertility in 10-20% of women, and occasionally potentially fatal ectopic pregnancy. Repeated infections increase the risk of adverse sequelae in both men and women. In rare cases persons with genital chlamydial infection can develop Reiter's syndrome, a triad of reactive arthritis accompanied by conjunctivitis and urethritis. Chlamydial infection, even asymptomatic disease, increases the risk of adverse pregnancy outcomes: premature rupture of membranes, preterm delivery and low birth weight. *Chlamydia* can easily pass to neonates during childbirth causing neonatal conjunctivitis and afebrile pneumonia in approximately 60% of those with infected mothers. The high levels of *Chlamydia* infection worldwide mean that there is substantial neonatal morbidity from perinatally transmitted chlamydial infection.

The *Chlamydia* serotypes which cause LGV are more virulent and more invasive than other chlamydial serotypes. The initial stage is a painless genital papule which heals rapidly and may be unrecognized. The organism then disseminates to regional lymph nodes, usually the inguinal nodes, where they replicate within macrophages and elicit a systemic response. This produces a painful inguinal lymphadenopathy, usually unilateral, by 2-6 weeks after the primary lesion often accompanied by fever, headache, and arthralgias. Rectal infection with LGV is characterized by a severe febrile proctocolitis, mimicking inflammatory bowel disease, with painful defecation, tenesmus, and less commonly a bloody mucopurulent discharge. Untreated LGV results in chronic inflammation with late fibrotic complications such as fistulas of the penis, urethra, and rectum, strictures, and genital lymphoedema and elephantiasis.

5.3 Diagnosis

Empirical evidence of *Chlamydia* infection is based on clinical presentation. The presence of greater than 10 polymorphonuclear leukocytes (PMNs) per 1000X field in vaginal discharge or 5 PMNs/field in urethral discharge is indicative of the cervicitis or urethritis characteristic of *Chlamydia* infection. There are currently no widely available point-of-care tests for *Chlamydia* infections. Most *Chlamydia* infections are detected through screening programs based on nucleic acid amplification testing (NAAT), antigen detection by ELISA, and DNA hybridization. Screening is useful for identifying asymptomatic infected individuals and in confirming symptomatic infections, but the delay in obtaining results means that initial diagnosis will be primarily based on clinical presentation. Traditional diagnostic techniques used for bacterial infections, culture and Gram stain, are of limited value for chlamydial infections. *Chlamydia* is an intracellular pathogen that requires tissue culture to propagate and so this approach is infrequently used even in developed countries. The unique cell wall structure of Chlamydia makes it very difficult to stain, although it is considered Gram negative. Direct fluorescent antibody staining can identify *Chlamydia* in clinical specimens but is not widely available. Where testing is available, all sexually active young adults under 25 years should be screened for *Chlamydia*. All pregnant women should be screened for *Chlamydia* as well.

5.4 Treatment

The recommended regimen for treatment of *Chlamydia* infection is azithromycin, 1 g orally in a single dose, or doxycycline, 100 mg orally twice daily for 7 days. Alternative 7 day regimens are 500 mg erythromycin base orally four times a day, 500 mg levofloxacin orally once daily, or 300 mg ofloxacin orally twice daily. The frequency of *Chlamydia* and gonococcal co-infection is high in many locales and dual treatment should be considered. The recommended treatment for LGV is doxycycline 100 mg orally twice a day for 21 days or alternatively, erythromycin base, 500 mg orally four times a day for 21 days. Azithromycin, 1 g orally once weekly for 3 weeks, may also be effective but clinical data is lacking. LGV buboes may require aspiration.

6. Gonorrhea

Neisseria gonorrheoae is an intracellular Gram-negative aerobic diplococcus that is the causative agent of gonorrhea. The adjacent sides of the diplococci pairs are flattened giving a characteristic kidney bean shape. Gonococci initially penetrate mucosal columnar epithelial cells and pass thru to establish infection in the subepithelial space. Cell destruction mediated by gonococci and the host inflammatory response is responsible for the disease pathology. Gonococci frequently change their surface antigens and lasting immunity does not develop. Therefore, re-infection is common.

6.1 Epidemiology

Gonorrhea is the second most common bacterial STI in the world with 62 million cases annually and is most prevalent in south and Southeast Asia with 27 million cases annually, and sub-Saharan Africa with 17 million cases annually. Gonococcal infection is most common among young persons, particularly those 15-24 years old. Women have a 60-80% risk of acquiring gonorrhea from a single act of vaginal intercourse with an infected man; men have only a 20-50% chance of acquiring infection from intercourse with infected women. Transmission among men who have sex with men is more efficient than a man's risk during heterosexual sex and gonorrhea prevalence is several fold higher in this demographic group. Pharyngeal and rectal gonococcal infection is also especially prevalent in this group. Co-infection with *Chlamydia* is common, occurring in up to 50% of gonococcal infections in some countries.

6.2 Clinical manifestations

Symptoms of infection in men usually appear 2-5 days after exposure with a range of 1-30 days. Women are less likely to have symptomatic infection, up to 70% are subclinical, but those who develop symptoms do so within 10 days of infection. The majority of men with gonococcal infection develop urethritis with a white, yellow, or greenish urethral discharge, dysuria, and sometimes painful and swollen testes. Erythema of the meatus is sometimes observed. Non gonococcal urethritis is usually characterized by less purulent and less copious discharge with little erythema of the meatus. The endocervical canal is the primary site of infection in women. Females with endocervicitis and urethritis experience dysuria, a purulent vaginal discharge, pelvic pain, and pain and bleeding brought on by sexual intercourse. Symptoms of rectal infection include itching, mucopurulent discharge, bleeding, tenesmus, and painful bowel movements. Pharyngeal infection is characterized by exudative pharyngitis and cervical lymphadenopathy. Untreated gonorrhea can lead to severe complications in both men and women. Gonorrhea can spread from the cervix and vagina to the fallopian tubes and uterus leading to chronic salpingitis or pelvic inflammatory disease, ectopic pregnancy, and infertility from scaring of the fallopian tubes. Pregnant women may experience chorioamnionitis and septic abortion. In men epididymitis, usually accompanied by unilateral testicular pain and swelling with fever, is relatively rare but can cause sterility. However a more likely cause of epididymitis in sexually active young men is *C. trachomatis*. Posterior urethritis, urethral stricture and prostatitis in men and Bartholin gland abscesses in women are additional complications of genital infection. In approximately 1- 3% of infected adults, with a higher occurrence in women, gonococci disseminates via the bloodstream to produce characteristic papulopustular lesions, and to infect joints, typically in fingers, wrists, toes, and ankles, causing septic arthritis. These manifestations are accompanied by fever and can range from mild to severe. Other less common complications of disseminated infection include a purulent conjunctivitis from autoinoculation, fatal septic shock, meningitis, perihepatitis, osteomyelitis, rapidly progressing endocarditis, especially of the aortic valve, and adult respiratory distress syndrome. Neonatal gonococcal infections are now an infrequent occurrence in developed countries but remain a serious problem in developing countries. Newborns infected during birth can develop conjunctivitis, known as ophthalmia neonatorum, which may lead to blindness. Neonates can also acquire pharyngeal or rectal infection and, rarely, develop gonococcal sepsis or pneumonia.

6.3 Diagnosis

There are currently five available tests for detection of gonorrhea; Gram stain, culture, nucleic acid amplification tests (NAAT), gonorrhea antigen detection tests, and nucleic acid hybridization tests. Clinical signs and symptoms of cervicitis or urethritis and the presence of Gram-negative intracellular diplococci within polymorphonuclear neutrophils from urethral, or less commonly, cervical discharge, are diagnostic for gonorrhea. The sensitivity of gram stain is very high in symptomatic men with urethritis but less so in infected women and in rectal infection. Stained smears are not recommended for diagnosis of pharyngeal gonococcal infection. Culture on specialized media can be used for urethral, cervical, pharyngeal, and rectal infection. This is the only testing technique that permits determination of gonococcal antibiotic sensitivity. In resource rich countries, diagnosis using very sensitive NAAT, gonorrhea antigen detection tests via immunoassay, and nucleic acid hybridization tests has become widespread. This has permitted screening of at risk populations and self referred testing in developed countries. NAAT tests are the most sensitive, and can be used on urine samples as well, but require hours to days to yield results. Rapid, point-of-care gonorrhea antigen detection tests and nucleic acid hybridization tests are in use, but are relatively expensive for settings in developing countries. Both of these tests are less sensitive than NAAT and are primarily designed for testing with cervical and urethral material. Some available NAAT, gonorrhea antigen detection tests, and nucleic acid hybridization tests can detect both *N. gonorrhoeae* and *Chlamydia* in the same sample and the NAAT test can be combined with Pap smears.

6.4 Treatment

The recommended treatment for gonococcal infections is ceftriaxone in a single 250 mg dose administered intramuscularly (IM). If unavailable cefixime, 400 mg orally in a single dose, or a single dose injectible cephalosporin plus azithromycin, 1 g orally in a single dose, or doxycycline, 100 mg orally twice a day for 7 days, may be used. Resistance to oral third generation cephalosporins has emerged recently and has been reported throughout Asia and in Australia and some European countries. The recent emergence in Japan of a strain, H041, which is extremely resistant to all cephalosporin-class antibiotics will pose a considerable public health challenge as this strain spreads throughout Asia and beyond.

Therapeutic use of sulfonamides, penicillin, erythromycin, and fluoroquinolones has been largely discontinued due to the development of widespread resistance to these agents. Azithromycin, 2 g orally, is effective but concerns over the prior ease of development of macrolide resistance in *N. gonorrhoeae* should limit its use to special circumstances. Gonococcal infections of the pharynx are more difficult to eliminate and are treated with ceftriaxone, 250 mg IM in a single dose, plus azithromycin, 1 g orally in a single dose, or doxycycline, 100 mg orally twice a day. Neonates born to infected mothers are given erythromycin ointment to the eyes to prevent blindness. Patients infected with *N. gonorrhoeae* are frequently co-infected with *Chlamydia*, and additional treatment for this infection may be appropriate, dependent on local prevalence of these STIs.

7. Syphilis

Treponema pallidum, a thin (0.1-0.18 μm by 6-15 μm) flagellated spirochete, is the etiologic agent of syphilis. *Treponema* spirochetes invade mucous membranes or penetrate through breaks in the skin. Although syphilis is typically acquired via sexual contact the disease can also be transmitted transplacentally and by exposure to blood or lesion exudates from infected persons in the primary and secondary stages of disease.

7.1 Epidemiology
Prior to the antibiotic era, syphilis was a very prevalent disease, particularly in large urban areas. Since then, the incidence has been steadily declining but there are still 12 million new cases each year around the world. Unlike many other STIs, the incidence of syphilis is higher in older individuals and is highest in men aged 30-45. Globally, congenital syphilis is a significant problem and it is estimated that neonatal mortality from syphilis exceeds that of neonatal tetanus, neonatal HIV infection, and mortality from malaria in pregnancy. There is no lasting immunity to syphilis and patients can be re-infected.

7.2 Clinical manifestations
Syphilis presents a wide spectrum of clinical manifestations as it progresses through the different stages of the disease: primary, secondary, latency, and tertiary. Syphilis, particularly the secondary stage, mimics many other infections and has been given the moniker, the "great imitator". The primary stage of syphilis is usually characterized by the appearance of a single sore (chancre) at the site of syphilis entry, although multiple lesions can be present. The chancre appears 10-90 days after infection, approximately 2-3 weeks on average. The chancre is typically a firm, round, and painless ulcer, 1-2 cm in size, which is highly infectious and will spontaneously resolve in 1-6 weeks. Chancres can also be present at non-genital sites, the anus, mouth, or perineum. Regional lymphadenopathy that is rubbery, painless, and bilateral is usually present.

Without treatment the systemic skin rash and mucocutaneous lesions of secondary syphilis appear 4-6 weeks after the primary lesion in approximately 25% of patients following dissemination of the disease throughout the body. Occasionally the symptoms of secondary syphilis will occur prior to resolution of the initial chancre. The red macropapular rash is symmetrical, non-pruritic, and present throughout the body including the palms of hands and soles of feet and may lead to hair loss. White, patchy, raised lesions on mucocutaneous surfaces, known as condylomata latum may also be present. The rash and lesions are accompanied by fever, malaise, and generalized lymphadenopathy. Rare manifestations of secondary syphilis include hepatitis, glomerulonephritis, and keratitis. Neurosyphilis can occur at any stage of syphilis but is classically associated with tertiary syphilis. Clinical manifestations of early neurosyphilis include acute syphilitic meningitis that typically involves cranial nerves III, VI, VII and VIII; or meningovascular syphilis, a stroke-like syndrome with seizures. Secondary syphilis is usually the fist clinical presentation in persons practicing receptive vaginal or anal intercourse as the primary lesions are often not noticed.

Whereas some secondary syphilis can spontaneously resolve, if untreated, approximately two thirds of secondary syphilis cases enter into a prolonged period of latency where symptoms of infection are absent. Relapses of secondary symptoms may occur in up to 25% of untreated patients, usually within the first year of infection. The latent stage can last for up to 25-30 years but if untreated, about one third of latent infections will progress to tertiary syphilis. Tertiary syphilis is rare in developed countries due to early diagnosis and treatment of syphilis. Tertiary syphilis is characterized by destructive lesions known as gummas, neurologic involvement, and cardiovascular lesions. Gummas, are highly destructive granulomas, usually in the skin, bone and mucosal areas but are sometimes found in other tissues such as genitals, lung, stomach, liver, spleen, spinal cord, breast, brain, and heart. Onset is 10-15 years after infection. Cardiovascular syphilis generally appears about 20-30 years after infection when lesions in the cardiac vasculature produce ascending aortic aneurysm, aortic insufficiency, or coronary ostial stenosis. In tertiary neurosyphilis focal endoarteritis in the blood vessels of the brain and spinal cord provokes signs and symptoms, usually decades after infection, which may resemble other neurologic diseases. Clinical manifestations typically include general paresis and tabes dorsalis. The presence of oral syphilitic lesions is common, particularly in primary and secondary syphilis, and in regions with a high prevalence of syphilis other health care workers, such as dentists, need to be aware of this risk.

7.3 Congenital syphilis

Worldwide each year over 2 million pregnant women, 1.5% of all pregnancies, test positive for syphilis. *Treponema* spirochetes can cross the placenta to infect the fetus resulting in severe adverse pregnancy outcomes. Untreated maternal syphilis will result in stillbirth, premature birth, neonatal death, or congenital infection in up to 80% of pregnancies in developing countries. An estimated 25% of all stillbirths and 11% of neonatal deaths in developing countries are due to fetal syphilis exposure. Symptoms of early congenital syphilis in children less than 2 year old include cutaneous and mucocutaneous lesions, macropapular rash, hepatosplenomegaly, lymphadenopathy, bone alterations from osteitis and osteochondritis, meningitis, pneumonia, and testicular masses. Hematologic abnormalities such as thrombocytopenia and anemia may occur. Early congenital syphilis is more common than late congenital syphilis. Late congenital syphilis in children >2 year old is characterized by Hutchinson's triad, Saddle nose, and bone deformations such as Saber shins. Hutchinson's triad includes tooth deformations where the crown of the incisors is wider in the cervical portion than at the incisor edge and a crescent-shaped notch is present at the incisor edge, interstitial keratitis which can lead to blindness, and eighth nerve deafness. Saddle nose refers to collapse of the bridge and resulting dorsal depression due to erosion of septal support, giving a saddled appearance. Saber shin is a malformation of the tibia with sharp anterior bowing. Interstitial keratitis is the most common manifestation of late congenital syphilis. These adverse pregnancy outcomes can be prevented by syphilis screening to identify and treat maternal infections prior to 24 weeks gestation.

7.4 Diagnosis

Initial diagnosis of syphilis is typically based on clinical presentation. *Treponema* spirochetes are Gram negative but they cannot be visualized using conventional light microscopy. Darkfield microscopy and direct fluorescent antibody test of spirochetes from lesion exudates and tissue provide definitive diagnosis of early syphilis. These tests however are not utilized in most settings. Presumptive diagnosis of syphilis relies on two types of testing for antibody in blood serum or cerebrospinal fluid. The Venereal Disease Research Laboratory (VDRL) and Rapid Plasma Reagin (RPR), Toluidine Red Unheated Serum (TRUST), and Unheated Serum Reagin (USR) tests utilize a non-treponemal antigen. The VDRL and RPR tests are the most widely used of these. VDRL and PRP testing is most sensitive in the middle stages of the disease, early syphilis and late stage disease may be missed. Detectable antibody titers are not attained until 1-4 weeks after appearance of the chancre and titers often decline to undetectable levels in latency. Non-treponemal tests are nonspecific and can give false-positive results and occasionally false negative results under conditions of antibody excess which can occur during secondary syphilis. Positive results are confirmed with a test utilizing treponemal antigens, such as the fluorescent treponemal antibody absorbed (FTA-ABS) test, treponemal enzyme immunoassay (EIA), microhemagglutination assay for *T. pallidum* antibodies (TPHA), and direct fluorescent antibody-*T. pallidum* test (DFA-TP). These tests are more sensitive than non-treponemal tests in detecting primary and tertiary syphilis. Non-treponemal test antibody titers usually correlate with disease activity and become non-reactive with time after treatment. Treponemal test antibody titers do not correlate disease activity and most (75-85%) will remain reactive for the rest of their lives. Commercially available point-of care tests for syphilis have been introduced recently although these are too expensive for most situations in the developing world.

7.5 Treatment

Benzathine penicillin G, 2.4 million units by intramuscular injection (IM) in a single dose for adults or 50,000 units/kg IM for children, is the preferred treatment for primary, secondary, and early latent stage syphilis. Alternatively, procaine penicillin at 1.2 million units IM daily for 10 days is used. Penicillin allergic non-pregnant patients may be treated with doxycycline, 100 mg orally twice daily for 2 weeks or tetracycline, 500 mg orally four times daily for 2 weeks. Penicillin allergic pregnant patients may receive erythromycin, 500 mg orally, 4 times daily for 14 days. Late latent stage syphilis and tertiary syphilis is treated with three doses benzathine penicillin G at 1 week intervals, 2.4 million units IM each dose for adults and 50,000 units/kg for children. Alternatively, procaine penicillin at 1.2 million units IM daily for 20 days is used. Penicillin allergic non-pregnant patients with late latent stage or tertiary syphilis may be treated with doxycycline, 100 mg orally twice daily for 4 weeks or tetracycline, 500 mg orally four times daily for 4 weeks. Penicillin allergic pregnant patients may receive erythromycin, 500 mg orally 4 times daily for 4 weeks. Neurosyphilis is treated with intravenous aqueous crystalline penicillin G, 3-4 million units every 4 hours (18-24 million units per day) for 10-14 days, or with daily IM injections of procaine penicillin, plus 500 mg probenecid orally 4 times daily, both for 10-14 days. Penicillin allergic non-pregnant patients with neurosyphilis are treated with doxycycline, 200 mg orally twice daily for 4 weeks or tetracycline, 500 mg orally four times daily for 4 weeks. Non-penicillin allergic pregnant women diagnosed with syphilis are treated with penicillin according to the stage of infection. Early congenital syphilis should be treated with intravenous aqueous crystalline penicillin G at 50,000 units/kg/dose every 12 hours for the first 7 days and every 8 hours for the next 3 days. Alternatively early congenital syphilis is treated with IM injections of procaine penicillin at 50,000 units/kg daily for 10 days. Late congenital syphilis is treated with intravenous or intramuscular aqueous crystalline penicillin G at 50,000 units/kg/dose every 4-6 hours for 10-14 days. For penicillin allergic children, after the first month of life, administer erythromycin, 7.5-12.5 mg/kg orally, 4 times daily for 4 weeks.

8. Chancroid

Haemophilus ducreyi, a fastidious Gram-negative facultative anaerobic coccobacillus, is the causative agent of chancroid. Chancroid is transmitted by vaginal, anal, or oral sex with an infected individual. The organism enters thru breaks in the epithelium and resides primarily in the extracellular spaces. *Haemophilus ducreyi* can resist phagocytosis and untreated lesions may take months to heal.

8.1 Epidemiology
Globally, chancroid is the most common cause of genital ulcer disease in regions where the disease is endemic. WHO estimates the annual global incidence to be about 6 million cases. Chancroid occurs in parts of Africa, south-east Asia and the Caribbean where it accounts for 23-56% of genital ulcer disease. Chancroid is more common in men than women and more common in areas where HIV prevalence is high (>8%). The incidence of chancroid is much lower in developed countries and sporadic outbreaks there are associated with travel, prostitution, and drug use. Chancroid, as are all genital ulcer producing STIs, is a risk factor for HIV transmission.

8.2 Clinical manifestations
After an incubation period of several days to two weeks, a tender erythematous papule develops at the site of inoculation which progresses to a pustular stage. The pustle ruptures within 2-3 days to form a painful genital ulcer with soft edges. Chancroid ulcerative lesions vary from 3-50 mm across but are typically 10-20 mm. Chancroid ulcers can be irregular, round, or oval in shape, are sharply circumscribed with an undermined edge, and contain a grey or yellow purulent exudate. Lesions will have a surrounding cutaneous erythema. One half of men have only a single ulcer and lesions typically appear on the penis: penile shaft, coronal sulcus, prepuce, urethral meatus, and glans. In women infection is often subclinical. Women have multiple ulcers more frequently than men that may merge to form large ulcers. Ulcers in women occur on the fourchette, labia majora, labia minora, cervix, perianal region, and inner thighs. "Kissing ulcers" may develop on the skin surfaces apposing the initial ulcer. Women may also experience dysuria and dyspareunia. Rectal sores in men or women may bleed or cause pain during defecation. Buboes, swelling of the inguinal lymph nodes, occur in one third to one half of infected individuals 1-2 weeks after the ulcers form and these may rupture, producing draining abscesses. The development of buboes is a more

common occurrence in men than women. Buboes are painful, tender, and fluctuant with underlying erythema, and are typically unilateral. Supperative adenopathy is almost pathognomonic for chancroid. The skin over the bubo does not become thickened and edematous or show furrows as in the adenopathy of LGV. Chancroid can also spread via self inoculation to other anatomical sites. Chancroid in HIV-infected patients may produce a larger number of ulcers, atypical ulcers, extra-genital lesions, and longer lasting ulcers even with treatment.

8.3 Diagnosis

Definitive diagnosis of chancroid requires cultivation of *H. ducreyi* on special culture media, which is not routinely carried in most laboratories. Culture on two media is recommended as not all *H. ducreyi* strains can be cultured using one medium. Culture also requires a humid environment, 5% CO_2, and incubation at 33-35 °C. Swabs for culture are collected from the undermined edge of the ulcer and the fastidious nature of *H. ducreyi* necessitates use of transport media if the organisms are not cultured within a few hours. Presumptive diagnosis by microscopy is possible if the organism load in ulcers is high and Gram-negative coccobacillus arranged in chains, paired chains or aggregates ("school of fish" appearance) are visualized. However the value of microscopy for diagnosis is limited by low sensitivity and specificity of this technique. Aspirates from buboes are less likely to yield positive results on microscopy or culture. In many cases chancroid is diagnosed clinically and treated without a definitive diagnosis. The combination of painful genital ulcer and suppurative inguinal lymphadenopathy is also supportive of a diagnosis of chancroid. Nucleic acid amplification tests for diagnosis have been developed but are not widely available.

8.4 Treatment

Azithromycin (1 g orally) or ceftriaxone (250 mg IM) offer the advantage of single-dose therapy. Alternatively ciprofloxacin (500 mg orally twice daily for 3 days) or erythromycin base (500 mg orally three times a day for 7 days) may be used. For reasons of cost, erythromycin is usually used for treatment in developing countries. Isolates with intermediate resistance to ciprofloxacin or erythromycin have been reported but data are rather limited on the current status of *H. ducreyi* drug resistance. Ulcerative lesions should be kept clean to avoid the chance of secondary infections. Fluctuant lymph nodes can be aspirated through healthy skin. Incision and drainage or excision of nodes may delay healing. Uncircumcised men and HIV-positive patients may not respond as well to treatment. Large ulcers may require weeks to resolve after treatment and patients should be followed until there is clear evidence of improvement or cure.

9. Human papilloma virus

Human papillomavirus (HPV) is a member of the papillomavirus family of viruses that infect only humans. HPVs can be divided into two general groups based on their preferred infection site: cutaneous and mucosal. Genital HPV, a member of the mucosal HPVs, is transmitted through sexual contact and infects the anogenital regions. There are more than 40 types of HPV that infect the genital area. Non-oncogenic or low risk HPV types are the causative agents of genital warts and recurrent respiratory papillomatosis. Oncogenic or high risk HPV types are the cause of cervical cancers and are associated with other anogenital cancers in men and women.

9.1 Epidemiology
Genital human papillomavirus is considered to be one of the most prevalent STIs in the world. It is estimated that more than 50% of sexually active individuals become infected at least once in their life. WHO estimates that 14.3% of women in developing regions and 10.3% of women in developed regions with normal cervical cytology are infected with HPV. Incidence of HPV in women increases significantly with severity of abnormal cervical cytology. Prevalence of HPV reaches to greater than 70% in women with cervical cancer.

9.2 Clinical manifestations
Asymptomatic genital HPV infection is common and usually self-limited. Seventy percent of infections are gone in 1 year, and 90% in 2 years. The most common symptom of genital HPV infection is genital warts, also known as condylomata acuminata. Genital warts appear as a small white bump or groups of bumps in the genital area. Genital warts are usually flat, papular, or pedunculated growths. However, they can be small or large, raised or flat. Genital warts are usually themselves asymptomatic, but can sometimes be painful and pruritic, depending on the size and anatomic location. Growths commonly occur around the introitus in women, under the foreskin of the uncircumcised penis, and on the shaft of the circumcised penis. Genital warts can also be found in or on the cervix, vagina, urethra, perineum, perianal skin, and scrotum. Intra-anal warts are most often observed in individuals who have had receptive anal intercourse, but may be present in men or women with no history of anal sexual contact.

9.3 Health sequelae
The correlation between persistent HPV infection and cervical cancer has been well established. Cervical cancer is the 2nd most common cancer among women, worldwide. Eighty-six percent of these cases occur in developing countries, making up 13% of the world female population. There is now increasing evidence linking HPV to anogenital cancers other than cervical cancer. These include anal, vulvar, vaginal, penile, and head and neck cancers. Anal cancer occurs rarely with about 99,000 cases in 2002, sixty percent of cases occurring in women and 40% in men. This type of cancer is more prevalent in populations of men who have sex with men and HIV-positive populations. Vulvar cancers make up about 3% of the gynecological cancers, with 40% of them occurring in developing countries. The majority of these cases occurring in the developed world suggest that HPV screening may not be an effective preventative method. Vaginal cancers make up 2% of gynecological cancers, with a majority of vaginal cancers (68%) occurring in developing countries. Penile cancer represents 0.5% of cancers in men. In western countries, incidence if penile cancer in men is less than 1 per 100,000, however, this rate increases in Latin America, India, and Thailand. Two-thirds of oral cancers occur in developing countries and about 15-20% of oral cancers are associated with HPV infection. Growing evidence suggests that HPV-related oral pharyngeal cancers are associated with the practice of oral sex.

9.4 Diagnosis
The presence of genital warts is a straight forward method for diagnosis of HPV. However, in the case of asymptomatic infections, there is no general diagnostic test used to screen normal patients for HPV. The Papanicolaou test (Pap smear or Pap test) is a cytological examination of cervical tissue sample that is used to screen for cervical cancer or

precancerous lesions. The Pap smear is more commonly used in developed countries. Abnormal results for a Pap smear usually result in screening of the tissue sample for the presence of HPV DNA. HPV DNA testing has been shown to have a higher sensitivity than cytology and a high negative predictive value for detecting cervical precancerous lesions. Other diagnostic strategies include visual inspection with acetic acid (VIA), self-vaginal sampling, and liquid based cytology (LBC). VIA has shown sensitivity similar to that seen with cytology, but has a lower specificity, which could lead to over treatment. However, its use has shown a decrease in the incidence of and mortality from cervical cancer, and may therefore be a useful method in resource poor areas. Developing countries have attempted to implement HPV screening programs with variable success. Successful implementation of these programs in some countries such as Taiwan, Japan, Singapore, and developed African countries has caused a decline in incidence and mortality of cervical cancer. In the remainder of the developing world either no screening programs currently exist or screening has had little success due to poor infrastructure and competing health priorities in these countries.

9.5 Treatment

Treatment is not recommended for subclinical genital HPV because these infections typically clear spontaneously. However, there are treatments for the diseases that are caused by HPV infection. Genital warts can resolve themselves or be removed by patient-applied or provider-administered therapy. Patient-applied therapy recommended by the CDC consists of podofilox 0.5% solution or gel, imiquimod 5% cream, or sinecatechins 15% ointment. Provider-administered therapy is cryotherapy with liquid nitrogen or cryoprobe applications ever 1-2 weeks, 10-25% podophyllin resin in a compound tincture of benzoin, 80-90% trichloroacetic acid (TCA) or bichloroacetic acid (BCA), or surgical removal by tangential scissor excision, tangential shave excision curettage, or electrosurgery. No evidence suggests that one treatment regimen is better than the other. Treatment against cervical lesions includes removal of precancerous lesions using cryotherapy and continuous preventative screening of cervical tissue.

A preventive strategy based on the development of vaccines against HPV is now widely available across the globe. A quadrivalent vaccine, Gardasil (Merck Co.) protects against 2 types of HPV that cause 75% of cervical cancer (HPV 16 &18) and the 2 types of HPV that cause 90% of genital warts (HPV 6 & 11). Gardasil can be used for both males and females ages 9-26. This vaccine is given in a series of 3 0.5 mL intramuscular injections at 0, 2, and 6 months. A bivalent vaccine, Cervarix (GlaxoSmithKline), protects against HPV 16 & 18 and is only approved for women ages 10-25. This vaccine is given in a series of 3 intramuscular 0.5 mL doses at 0, 1, and 6 months. Many countries have developed their own individual vaccine schedules. Both vaccines have been shown to be highly immunogenic and effective in prevention of incidence and persistent HPV infections that could lead to the development of precancerous lesions. It is recommended that vaccination begin at ages at which individuals have not yet become sexually active.

10. Herpes

Genital herpes is caused by herpes simplex viruses type 1 (HSV-1) or type 2 (HSV-2) with HSV-2 the primary genital STI. HSV-1 is acquired orally, usually in childhood, and typically causes cold sores and sometimes keratitis. HSV-1 can also cause genital infection but recurrent episodes during infection with HSV-1 are much less frequent. HSV-1 and HSV-2 are typically transmitted during sexual contact by virus shed from herpes sores but virus can also be released intermittently between outbreaks from skin without apparent sores. Herpes virus enters through mucous membranes or breaks in the skin and replicates locally in mucosal epithelial cells. Between outbreaks the herpes virus ascends peripheral sensory neurons to the dorsal root ganglia and becomes latent.

10.1 Epidemiology

Herpes is the most common STI in the world and HSV-2 infection is the main cause of genital ulcers in developing countries. An estimated one sixth to one third of the world's population has genital herpes caused by HSV-2. HSV-2 prevalence is greater than 60% in sub-Saharan Africa and East Asia and between 25-40% in Latin America, Eastern Europe, South Asia, and South-east Asia. HSV-2 prevalence rates are less than 20% in North America and Western Europe and below 10% in North Africa, the Middle East, Japan, Australia and New Zealand. Most herpes infections are asymptomatic and herpes is usually spread by people who are unaware they have the disease. Symptomatic genital herpes infection is approximately twice as common in women as in men. Transmission from an infected male to a female partner is more likely than transmission from infected female to a male partner during vaginal intercourse. Rates of herpes infection are also higher in men who have sex with men and in HIV-positive individuals. Herpes seroprevalence rates are as high as 80% among HIV-positive populations in North America, Europe and Africa.

10.2 Clinical manifestations

Most individuals have no or only minimal symptoms from herpes infection and do not realize they are infected. Herpes appears 2-7 days after infection as small, pruritic and painful, usually multiple, grouped vesicles (blisters) with a red base on or around the genitals and rectum or on the buttocks or thighs. The vesicles will ulcerate to leave shallow lesions that heal in 2-4 weeks. During the initial episode additional groups of sores may appear. Fever, malaise, and bilateral inguinal lymphadenopathy that is firm and tender may also be present. Infection in women usually involves the vulva, vagina, and cervix. In men lesions usually appear on the glans penis, prepuce, or penile shaft. After resolution of the primary infection herpes enters a latent state. However, outbreaks will re-occur from weeks to months after the initial infection, particularly during periods of stress or illness, and typically 4 or 5 outbreaks occur within the first year. About one half of patients experience prodromal symptoms of tingling or pain at the eruption site 1-2 days prior to the appearance of lesions. Although herpes infection persists indefinitely outbreaks diminish in number and severity with time. The duration and intensity of outbreaks are usually more severe in persons with suppressed immune systems. Persons with immune deficiencies such as HIV-infected persons may have persistent, extensive, and severe mucocutaneous lesions involving large areas of perianal, scrotal, or penile skin. Complications of herpes infection include an aseptic meningitis in as many as 10% with primary infection, transverse myelitis, and perinatal transmission. Pregnant women experiencing primary genital herpes during birth can transmit a potentially fatal herpes infection to their infant and a caesarean delivery may be appropriate in these cases. The risk of transmission during birth is very low in women with recurrent disease. Infected neonates can experience disseminated disease with organ failure, severe neurologic damage, ocular involvement, cutaneous and mucocutaneous sores, and even death.

10.3 Diagnosis

There are four types of testing employed in herpes diagnosis, DNA testing, antibody testing, antigen testing, and herpes culture. Nucleic acid amplification tests are very sensitive and can detect herpes DNA in samples from herpetic sores even when virus is in low copy number, such as in older lesions or in cerebrospinal fluid samples. It is the method of choice to detect HSV meningitis, encephalitis, and keratitis. HSV antibody tests are available to measure both IgM antibody, which can detect primary herpes infection after first several days of infection, and IgG antibody, which indicates prior HSV infection. The presence of HSV-2 antibody indicates anogenital infection but the presence of HSV-1 antibody does not distinguish genital infection from oral infection. Rapid antibody tests are available that detect antibodies to HSV-2 in blood from a finger stick within 10-15 minutes. The relatively quick turnaround and ease of this antibody tests makes it ideal for herpes screening for persons with undiagnosed disease as well as disease diagnosis. Fluorescently labeled antibody is used in antigen tests to detect markers expressed on herpes infected cells. Herpes culture is very specific but prone to false negative results, especially for recurrent infection, and requires several days to a week for results. Material from the base of the ulcer in fresh primary lesions is best for any herpes diagnosis as viral shedding decreases as lesions age and heal and in subsequent outbreaks. However, the requirement for tissue culture of host cells to grow herpes limits the utilization of this technique. Herpes can also be diagnosed by visual examination for the characteristic vesicles and sores although signs and symptoms of herpes can vary, making diagnosis problematic in some patients.

10.4 Treatment

There is no effective treatment for genital herpes but antiviral medications can lessen the duration and severity of outbreaks. Antiviral prophylaxis also reduces the chances of transmission from infected individuals to uninfected partners. Clinical episodes can be treated by acyclovir in a 7 day regimen for the initial episode or a 5 day regimen for subsequent episodes at 200 mg orally 5 times daily or 400 mg orally 3 times daily. Ideally treatment should begin within one day of the appearance of the herpes vesicles. Suppressive therapy uses acyclovir, 400 mg orally twice daily, continuously. Alternatively the acyclovir analogues valaciclovir and famciclovir can be used for treatment and prophylaxis although the dosages and regimens may vary. The acyclic nucleoside drugs are effective and well tolerated in most patients. Immunosuppressed individuals such as HIV-positive patients may respond poorly to treatment and require larger doses and longer treatment schedules or even parenteral drug administration.

11. Granuloma inguinale (Donovanosis)

Calymmatobacterium granulomatis is an intracellular Gram-negative facultative aerobic coccobacillus that is the causative agent of granuloma inguinale. Other designations for this disease include granuloma venereum and donovanosis, named for the discoverer of the infectious agent. A close phylogenetic relationship with *Klebsiella* spp. has led some to call for a reclassification of *Calymmatobacterium* into the genus *Klebsiella*. Some *C. granulomatis* strains are capsulated. *Calymmatobacterium granulomatis* resides in the cytoplasm of mononuclear phagocytes or histiocytes in tissue.

11.1 Epidemiology
The incidence of granuloma inguinale has decreased in recent years but it still endemic in certain tropical and subtropical regions; south-east India, Indonesia, Papua New Guinea, South Africa, Guyana, Peru, Argentina, Brazil, and among aborigines of Central Australia. It is only occasionally reported in developed countries. Most infections occur in sexually active people 20-40 years of age and men are more than twice as likely to have disease. Granuloma inguinale is spread primarily thru vaginal or anal intercourse, infection via oral sex is rare. Non-sexual transmission via contact with infected material from lesions or by fecal contamination is possible.

11.2 Clinical manifestations
The infection begins approximately 10-50 days after exposure with the appearance of small, relatively painless, erythematous pustules or subcutaneous nodules. These will ulcerate to produce shallow and sharply demarcated lesions. Four types of lesions are described: ulcerogranulomatous ulcers, the most common, oozing lesions with a beefy red friable base that bleeds when touched, hypertropic ulcers with a raised irregular edge, sometimes completely dry, deep necrotic ulcers with an offensive smell from decaying tissue, and sclerotic ulcers with fibrous and scar tissue. In early stages the ulcers resemble chancroid, in later stages granuloma inguinale may resemble LGV. The lesions slowly expand destroying adjacent tissue. Anatomical areas most commonly infected in men include the sulcus, subprepucial region, and the anus. Women are most affected in the labia minor, fourchette, and occasionally in the cervix and upper genital tract. Extra-genital lesions occur in a minority of patients, these are secondary to the genital lesions. Oral lesions are the most frequent, loss of teeth indicates oral bone involvement, but lesions are possible on any surface. Very rarely disseminated donovanosis may occur, spreading to cause lesions in the liver, other organs, and bone, particularly tibia. Disseminated disease may be fatal as a diagnosis of donovanosis is rarely considered. Inguinal lymphadenopathy is generally absent. Untreated disease results in the destruction of genital tissue with scarring.

11.3 Diagnosis
Granuloma inguinale is diagnosed by clinical signs, particularly the presence of persistent spreading lesions, and the demonstration of intracellular Donovan bodies in the cytoplasm of mononuclear phagocytes or histiocytes present in scrapings or punch biopsies stained with Giemsa, silver, or Wright's stain. Specimens from just below the surface of the ulcer are most likely to yield positive results. Culture is difficult to perform as it requires growth of host cells and is not readily available.

11.4 Treatment
WHO guidelines recommend azithromycin, 1 g orally followed by 5500 mg daily or doxycycline, 100 mg orally twice daily but do not state the duration of therapy. Typically therapy is given for 3-6 weeks or until lesions are healed. Alternative regimens are erythromycin, 500 mg orally 4 times daily or tetracycline, 500 mg orally 4 times daily or trimethoprim 80 mg/sulfamethoxazole 400 mg, 2 tablets orally twice daily for a minimum

of 14 days. WHO recommends the addition of a parenteral aminoglycoside, such as gentamicin, for the therapy of HIV-positive patients. Treatment should be continued until complete healing is achieved. The intracellular residence of *C. granulomatis* makes it somewhat resistant to treatment.

12. STIs among travelers and immigrants from the tropics

Travel is known to be a major factor in the spread of STIs around the world, particularly in developing countries where STIs are endemic and very high rates are encountered in commercial sex workers. The rapid spread of antibiotic resistance around the world for a number of STIs and the spread of HIV infection are cases in point. It is difficult to assess the risk of acquiring STIs during travel in which sexual acts occur. Poverty and lack of legal enforcement certainly facilitate access to sexually compliant individuals in the developing world. In addition, risk-taking behavior increases when on vacation and often vacations involve higher risk activities than the traveler typically encounters at home. Studies have shown that engaging in sexual activity is the specific reason for travel, i.e. 'sex vacations', in some travelers. Reports of lower condom rate usage and higher rates of engagement in anonymous sex by travelers support a conclusion of increased risk. Travel clinics and physicians advising overseas travelers should counsel travelers about the risks and proper prophylactic regimens available. Travelers should also be strongly encouraged to be tested for STIs upon return if they have engaged in sexual activity. There are high rates of asymptomatic infection for many STIs and long incubation periods can also occur before there is an onset of symptoms. Immigrants and refugees pose a problem to the health care system in developed countries as well. STIs uncommon in the developed world such as chancroid, LGV, and donovanosis present a diagnostic challenge to the physician unfamiliar with these diseases. Incorrect diagnosis and subsequent incorrect treatment can delay resolution of the disease and increase the risk to the patient and sex partners, even permitting local mini-epidemics of new STIs. Health care providers should be aware of uncommon STIs present in their patient's country of origin when evaluating symptoms of genital infection in this population.

13. Prevention and control

Prompt diagnosis and treatment of infected individuals and public education of sexually active populations on proper prevention and prophylactic measures for STIs are the foundation of STI prevention and control. To be successful this approach should be supplemented with screening programs to identify individuals with subclinical infections as many, if not most, STIs are transmitted by individuals who do not know they are infected. However, the lack of adequate diagnostic capacity in most tropical settings severely compromises diagnosis and screening for STIs. This is the biggest barrier to addressing the STI epidemic in the developing world. Provision of a minimal diagnostic capacity, both equipment and trained individuals, at the initial point of contact with STI patients would yield enormous benefits. The development of affordable point-of care tests for STIs would also significantly advance efforts for controlling STIs in these countries. Public health education initiatives for STIs should encourage safe sex behavior and emphasize the advantages of prompt access to healthcare for suspected infections. Education is key to changing sexual behavior in high risk groups, especially adolescents and young adults who are disproportionately afflicted by STIs. Some health care advisors have advocated a policy of treating all sexually active adolescents and adults in a village or locale as a means to controlling STIs, an approach similar to mass treatment with anti-helminthics utilized to control the endemic of intestinal worm disease. This approach may be the single most cost effective mechanism for managing the STI epidemic in developing countries and should be given careful consideration. Although perhaps not applicable for all STIs, certainly for highly prevalent STIs with drugs that are inexpensive, safe, efficacious, and well tolerated, such as metronidazole for treating trichomoniasis, this approach has much merit.

On an individual basis the only truly reliable protection is abstinence from sexual activity. People in long term monogamous relationships also have greatly reduced risk of STIs and HIV. Vaccines are available for the prevention of HPV infection and potential HIV vaccines are in clinical trials. Protective measures for sexually active individuals include reducing the number of sexual partners and the use of latex condoms and other barriers during sexual activity. Consistent and proper use of condoms has been shown to reduce the transmission of STIs and HIV. Male circumcision has also been shown to be significantly protective against transmission of HIV and STIs. STI treatment should include sexual partners of the index case whenever possible to prevent re-infection and to reduce disease transmission. Due to compliance issues and difficulties in following patients in many locales, directly observed single dose therapies are preferred for the treatment of STIs.

14. The future: Vaccines for STIs

Vaccination offers the ultimate tool for control of STIs; prevention before exposure. Safe and efficacious vaccines could eliminate the vast majority of STI-associated morbidity and mortality. Unfortunately this goal has only been attained relative to HPV infection (section 9.5) and prospects for additional STI vaccines in the immediate future are remote. In part, this is because the precise correlates of protective immunity have not been well-defined for these STIs. However, some progress has been made in the development of vaccines for genital herpes and *Chlamydia* infection. Three types of herpes vaccines have shown efficacy in animal models: (i) HSV-2 subunit vaccines combined with adjuvant; (ii) gene delivery vehicles, such as vaccinia virus, *Listeria* or *Salmonella typhimurium*, expressing HSV-2 proteins; and (iii) attenuated (replication-defective) HSV-2 viruses. Subunit vaccines based on herpes glycoproteins gD and gB have failed in two human clinical trials. Live attenuated viruses have not been tested in humans to date although they have shown the most promise in animal models. Recent progress in identification of T-cell epitopes mediating asymptomatic versus symptomatic disease manifestation should enhance future development of a herpes vaccine. *Chlamydia* candidate vaccines containing *Chlamydia* major outer membrane protein (MOMP) with HPV major capsid membrane protein L1, recombinant MOMP with cholera toxin, co-expressed *Chlamydia* Porin B and polymorphic membrane protein-D proteins in a *Vibrio cholerae* ghost delivery system, MOMP-based DNA vaccines, and live attenuated *Chlamydia* organisms have each shown efficacy in animal models but none have advanced to human trials.

Although the lack of progression to disease in some individuals infected with gonorrhea, syphilis, chancroid, and granuloma inguinale and the ability of immune responses to contain and clear infections in others in the absence of treatment indicates the theoretical feasibility of vaccination, progress on the development of a vaccine for these STIs has lagged. The syphilis spirochete, *Treponema pallidum*, has a unique molecular architecture and the cell envelope consists of a dual membrane structure. The outer membrane is poorly immunogenic, lacking lipopolysaccharide and possessing few integral membrane proteins that could serve as surface antigenic targets for the host immune system. The strong antibody response observed in syphilis is principally generated by lipopolysaccharide and protein immunogens located in the inner membrane where they are inaccessible to this antibody response. To date, research on a syphilis vaccine has not progressed past the identification of these rare outer membrane proteins as candidate vaccine antigens. Development of a gonococcal vaccine has been hampered by the ability of *N. gonorrhoeae* to change surface antigens, especially Type IV pili, deficiencies in current animal models, and the lack of target capsular polysaccharides such as are present in *N. meningitidis*. Two candidate gonorrhea vaccines, utilizing killed whole gonococcal cells or pilus and pilus-associated proteins, have been tested in human clinical trials but neither produced protection. Recent work on gonococcal vaccines has been focused on the identification of potential B- and T-cell epitopes for candidate antigens. The relatively low incidence of chancroid and donovanosis in most developed countries is mirrored by limited research interest towards development of vaccines for *Haemophilus ducreyi* and *Calymmatobacterium granulomatis* infections and there is little in the way of published work or progress on vaccines for these organisms.

15. References

Barh, D., Misra, A. N., Kumar, A. & Azevedo V. (2010). A novel strategy of epitope design in *Neisseria gonorrhoeae*. *Bioinformation*, 5, 77-82, ISSN 0973-2063

Barry, P. M. & Klausner, J. D. (2009). The use of cephalosporins for gonorrhea: the impending problem of resistance. *Expert Opin. Pharmacother.*, 10, 555-577, ISSN 1465-6566

Bharadwaj, M., S. Hussain, V. Nasare, V. & Das, B. C. (2009). HPV & HPV vaccination: issues in developing countries. *Indian J. Med. Res.*, 130, 327-333, ISSN 0019-5359

Celum, C. (2010). Sexually transmitted Infections and HIV: epidemiology and interventions. *Top. HIV Med.*, 18, 138-142, ISSN 1542-8826

Centers for Disease Control and Prevention. (2010). Sexually transmitted diseases treatment guidelines, 2010. *Morb. Mort. Wkly. Rep.*, 59(RR-12), 1-110, ISSN 1057-5987

Corey, L. (2002). Challenges in genital herpes simplex virus management. *J. Infect. Dis.*, 186 (Suppl 1), S29-S33, ISSN 0022-1899

Cox, D. L., Luthra, A., Dunham-Ems, S., Desrosiers, D. C., Salazar, J. C., Caimano, M. J. &Radolf, J. D. (2010). Surface immunolabeling and consensus computational framework to identify candidate rare outer membrane proteins of *Treponema pallidum*. *Infect. Immun.*, 78, 5178-5194, ISSN 0019-9567

Cunningham, K. A. & Beagley, K. W. (2008). Male genital tract chlamydial infection: implications for pathology and infertility. *Biol. Reprod.*, 79, 180-189, ISSN 0006-3363

Da Ras, C. T. & da Silva Schmitt, C. (2008). Global epidemiology of sexually transmitted diseases. *Asian J. Androl.*, 10, 110-114, ISSN 1008-682X

Dasgupta, G., Chentoufi, A. A., Nesburn, A. B., Wechsler, S. L. & BenMohamed, L. (2009). New concepts in herpes simplex virus vaccine development: notes from the battlefield. *Expert Rev. Vaccines*, 8, 1023-1035, ISSN 1476-0584

Domantay-Apostol, G. P.; Handog, E. B. & Gabriel, M. T. G. (2008). Syphilis: the international challenge of the great imitator. *Dermatol. Clin.*, 26; 191-202, ISSN 0733-8635

Eduardo, P.; Velho, N. F.; de Souza, E. M. & Belda, Jr., W. (2008). Donovanosis. *Brazil J. Infect. Dis.*, 12, 521-525, ISSN 1413-8670

Edwards, J. L. & Butler, E. K. (2011). The pathobiology of *Neisseria gonorrhoeae* lower female genital tract infection. *Front. Microbiol.*, 2, 102, ISSN 1664-302X

Grm, H. S., Bergant, M. & Banks L. (2009). Human papillomavirus infection, cancer and therapy. *Indian J. Med. Res.*, 130, 277-285, ISSN 0019-5359

Haggerty, C. L.; Gottlieb, S. M.; Taylor, B. D.; Low, N.; Xu, F. & Ness, R. B. (2010). Risk of sequelae after *Chlamydia trachomatis* genital infection in women. *J. Infect. Dis.*, 201(S2), S134-S155, ISSN 0022-1899

Halford, W. P., Püschel, R., Gershberg, E., Wilber, A., Gershberg, S. & Rakowski B. (2011). A live-attenuated HSV-2 ICPO⁻ virus elicits 10 to 100 times greater protection against genital herpes than a glycoprotein D subunit vaccine. *PLOS One*, 6, e17748, ISSN 1932-6203

Hilber, A. M., Francis, S. C., Chersich, M., Scott, P., Redmond, S., Bender, N., Miotti, P., Temmerman, M. & Low, N. (2010). Intravaginal practices, vaginal infections and HIV acquisition: systemic review and meta-analysis. *PLOS One*, 5, e9119, ISSN 1932-6203

Johnston, V. J. & Mabey, D. C. (2008). Global epidemiology and control of *Trichomonas vaginalis*. *Curr. Opin. Infect. Dis.*, 21, 56-64, ISSN 0951-7375

Joint United Nations Programme on HIV/AIDS (UNAIDS). (2010). UNAIDS report on the global AIDS epidemic 2010. UNAIDS, ISBN 9789291738717, Geneva

Kamb, M. L.; Newman, L. M.; Riley, P. L.; Mark, J.; Hawkes, S. J.; Malik, T. & Broutet, N. (2010). A road map for the global elimination of congenital syphilis. *Obstet. Gynecol. Int.*, 2010: 312798, 1-6, e-ISSN 1687-9597

Lewis, D. A. (2003). Chancroid: clinical manifestations, diagnosis, and management. *Sex. Transm. Infect.*, 79, 68-71, ISSN 1472-3263

Looker K. J., Garnett, G. P. & Schmid, G. P. (2008). An estimate of the global prevalence and incidence of herpes simplex virus type 2 infection. *Bull. World Health Org.*, 86, 805-812, ISSN 0042-9686

Low. N.; Broutet ,N.; Adu-Sarkodie, Y.; Barton, P.; Hossain, M. & Hawkes, S. (2006). Global control of sexually transmitted infections. *Lancet*, 368, 2001-2016, ISSN 0140-6736

McClelland, R. S., Sangare, L., Hassan, W. M. Lavreys, L., Mandaliya, K., Kiarie, J., Ndinya-Achola, J., Jaoko, W. & Baeten, J. M. (2007). Infection with *Trichomonas vaginalis* increases the risk of HIV-1 acquisition. *J. Infect. Dis.*, 195, 698-702 ISSN 0022-1899

McGill, M. A., Edmondson, D. G., Carroll. J. A., Cook, R. G., Orkiszewski, R. S. & Norris, S. J. (2010). Characterization and serologic analysis of the *Treponema pallidum* proteome. *Infect. Immun.*, 78, 2631-2643, ISSN 0019-9567

Memish, Z. A. & Osoba, A. O. (2006). International travel and sexually transmitted diseases. *Trav. Med. Infect. Dis.*, 4, 86-93, ISSN 1477-8939

Mohammed, T. T. & Olumide, Y. M. (2008). Chancroid and human immunodeficiency virus infection – a review. *Int. J. Dermatol.*, 47, 1-8, ISSN 0011-9059

Newman, L. M.; Moran, J. S. & Workowski, K. A. (2007). Update on the management of gonorrhea in adults in the United States. *Clin. Infect. Dis.*, 44, S84-S101, ISSN 1058-4838

Nikolic, D. S. &Piguet V. (2010). Vaccines and microbicides preventing HIV-1, HSV-2, and HPV mucosal transmission. *J. Invest. Dermatol.*, 130, 352-361, ISSN 0022-202X

Nusbaum, M. R., Wallace, R. R., Slatt, L. M. & Kondrad E. C. (2004). Sexually transmitted infections and increased risk of co-infection with human immunodeficiency virus. *J Am. Osteopath. Assoc.* 104, 527-35, ISSN 0098-6151

O'Farrell, N. (2002). Donovanosis. *Sex. Transm. Infect.*, 78, 452-457, ISSN 1472-3263

Palefsky, J. M. (2010) Human papillomavirus-related disease in men: not just a women's issue. *J. Adolescent Health*, 46, S12-S19, ISSN 1054-139X

Schautteet, K., De Clercq, E. & Vanrompay, D. (2011). *Chlamydia trachomatis* vaccine research through the years. *Infect. Dis. Obstet. Gynecol.* 2011, 963513, ISSN 1098-0997

Ward, H. & Rönn, M. (2011). The contribution of STIs to the sexual transmission of HIV. *Curr. Opin. HIV AIDS*, 5, 305-310, ISSN 1746-630X

World Health Organization. (2001). *Global prevalence and incidence of selected curable sexually transmitted infections: Overview and estimates*, WHO Press, Geneva

World Health Organization. (2003). *Guidelines for the management of sexually transmitted infections*, WHO Press, ISBN 9241546263, Geneva,

World Health Organization. (2005). *Sexually transmitted and other reproductive tract infections*, WHO Press, ISBN 9241592656, Geneva,

World Health Organization. (2007a). *Global Strategy for the prevention and control of sexually transmitted infections: 2006-2015*, WHO Press, ISBN 9789241563475, Geneva

World Health Organization. (2007b). *Training modules for the syndromic management of sexually transmitted infections, 2nd edition*, WHO Press, ISBN 9241593407, Geneva

World Health Organization. (2011). *Global health sector strategy on HIV/AIDS 2011-2015*, WHO Press, ISBN 9789241501651, Geneva

Zhu, W., Chen, C.-J., Thomas, T. E., Anderson, J. E., Jerse, A. E. & Sparling P. F. (2011). Vaccines for gonorrhea: can we rise to the challenge. *Front. Microbiol.*, 2, 124, ISSN 1664-302X

13

Re-Emergence of Malaria and Dengue in Europe

Rubén Bueno Marí and Ricardo Jiménez Peydró

Laboratorio de Entomología y Control de Plagas, Inst. Cavanilles de Biodiversidad y Biología Evolutiva, Universitat de València

Spain

1. Introduction

Currently, the emergence/reemergence of several vector-borne diseases in Europe is one of the most important threats for Public Health. In recent years, it is well known that global change have led to drastic modifications in the eco-epidemiology of various tropical and subtropical diseases. Global change can be defined as the impact of human activity on the fundamental mechanisms of biosphere functioning. Therefore, global change includes not only climate change, but also habitats transformation, water cycle modification, biodiversity loss, synanthropic incursion of alien species into new territories or introduction of new chemicals in nature. Consequently a holistic approach is a key factor to assessing the likelihood of vector-borne diseases transmission in Europe. Among these vectors, culicid mosquitoes are probably the most important because of its large vectorial capacity and its high degree of opportunism (Table 1).

Vector species	Distribution	Indigenous/exotic	Vectorial capacity
Ae. aegypti	Madeira (Portugal), The Netherlands	Exotic (recently imported)	Dengue (DEN), Yellow Fever (YF), Chikungunya (CHIK), West Nile (WN), Japanese encephalitis (JE), Saint-Louis encephalitis (SLE), La Crosse encephalitis (LACE), Murray valley encephalitis (MVE), Western equine encephalitis (WEE), Eastern equine encephalitis (EEE), Venezuelan equine encephalitis (VEE), Myxomatosis (MYX), Avian Malaria (AMAL), Dirofilariasis (DF)
Ae. albopictus	Mediterranean area, Central Europe	Exotic (first reported in Albania in 1979)	DEN, YF, CHIK, WN, JE, SLE, LACE, WEE, EEE, VEE, Jamestown Canyon (JC), Sindbis (SIN), Tahyna (TAH), DF

Vector species	Distribution	Indigenous/exotic	Vectorial capacity
Ae. vexans	All over Europe	Indigenous	WN, TAH, Tularaemia (TU), DF
Ae. vittatus	Spain, Portugal, France, Italy	Indigenous	DEN, YF, CHIK, AMAL
An. algeriensis	Mediterranean area, Eastern Europe, Central Europe, United Kingdom	Indigenous	Malaria (MAL)
An. claviger s.l.	All over Europe	Indigenous	MAL, WN, Batai (BAT), TAH, MYX, Anaplasmosis (ANA), Borreliosis (BO), TU, DF
An. maculipennis s.l.	All over Europe	Indigenous	MAL, WN, BAT, TAH, MYX, TU, DF
An. plumbeus	All over Europe	Indigenous	MAL, WN, DF
An. sergentii	Sicily (Italy)	Indigenous	MAL
An. superpictus	Southeastern Europe	Indigenous	MAL, DF
Cx. pipiens s.l.	All over Europe	Indigenous	WN, SIN, Usutu (USU), TAH, AMAL, DF
Oc. atropalpus	Italy, France, The Netherlands.	Exotic (first reported in Italy in 1996)	WN, JE, SLE, LACE, MVE, WEE, EEE
Oc. caspius	All over Europe	Indigenous	WN, TAH, MYX, TU, DF
Oc. japonicus	France, Belgium, Switzerland, Germany	Exotic (recently imported)	WN, JEV, SLE, LACE, EEE
Oc. triseriatus	Intercepted in a batch of used tyres imported from Louisiana (USA) to France in 2004	Exotic (not yet known as established)	DEN, YF, WN, SLE, LACE, WEE, EEE, VEE, JC

Table 1. Mosquito vectors in Europe with indication of distribution, indigenous or exotic status and vectorial capacity in each case.

2. Malaria

Malaria was a widespread disease in the whole of Europe until the second half of 20th century. The anthroponosis, often called "marsh fever" in the past, was particularly devastating between XVI and XIX centuries in Southern Europe due to the boom of irrigation techniques based on long flooding periods (e.g. rice fields). Several environmental modifications (mainly the drainage of swamps, moats, ditches and other stagnant waters), but particularly the availability of efficient synthetic antimalarial drugs and improved mosquito control activities including DDT spraying after World War II, have led to the disappearance of malaria from Europe (Bruce-Chwatt & de Zulueta, 1980). However, although *Anopheles* populations were significantly reduced by different control methods, in most cases, the vectors were not eradicated.

Today malaria annually affects 500 million people and threatens directly or indirectly 40% of world population (World Health Organization [WHO], 2007). However it is well known that these morbidity and mortality data show an asymmetric distribution, mainly depending on the economical, social and sanitary level of each country or region. The disease is endemic in much of Africa and several countries of Asia, Central America and South America. In Europe, the cycles of malaria transmission are relatively common in Georgia, Azerbaijan, Kyrgyzstan, Tajikistan, Uzbekistan and Turkey (WHO, 2010). This mosquito-borne parasitaemic disease is caused by protozoa of the genus *Plasmodium*. Although the simian parasite *Plasmodium knowlesi* (Knowles and Das. Gupta 1932) has been found recently as a cause of human malaria in Southeastern Asia (Luchavez et al., 2008), other four plasmodia species are the most recognized to infect humans in nature conditions: *Plasmodium falciparum* (Welch, 1897), *Plasmodium vivax* (Grassi & Feletti, 1890), *Plasmodium malariae* (Feletti & Grassi, 1889) and *Plasmodium ovale* (Stephens, 1922). About 90% of malaria mortality is caused by tropical strains of *P. falciparum* (most pathogenic species), which is also the species of *Plasmodium* most frequently imported to Europe (European Network on Imported Infectious Disease Surveillance [TropNetEurop], 2010). Furthermore, *P. vivax* shows the largest distribution range because it may also develop in temperate climates, being consequently the only species currently present in the cycles of transmission in Europe. Finally, *P. malariae* and *P. ovale* are characterized by its narrow distribution range and low parasitemia. Regarding to malaria vectors, there are about 40 *Anopheles* species with an important role in disease transmission (Kiszewski, 2004).

2.1 Malariogenic potential of Europe

The increasing of imported malaria cases in last decades, together with the high presence of anophelines in many Southern Europe regions (Romi et al., 1997; Ponçon et al., 2007; Bueno Marí & Jiménez Peydró, 2010a), has enabled the appearance of several autochthonous malaria cases, as recently has occurred in countries like Italy (Baldari et al., 1998), Greece (Kampen et al., 2002), France (Doudier et al., 2007) or Spain (Santa-Olalla Peralta et al., 2010). This situation forces us to investigate the possible reemergence of malaria in the current context of global change. One of the best methods to deep into the knowledge of possible malaria reemergence is the study of the malariogenic potential, which can be analyzed from the study of the receptivity, infectivity and vulnerability parameters (Romi et al., 2001; Bueno Marí & Jiménez Peydró, 2008).

2.1.1 Receptivity

Receptivity could be analyzed by the presence, density, and biological characteristics of vectors. At respect, the estimation of the Vectorial Capacity (VC) is postulated as a very useful tool to assess the receptivity of a determined territory in a concrete moment (Carnevale & Robert, 2009). The VC could be estimated by the MacDonald formula (MacDonald, 1957) according to the modifications proposed by Garrett-Jones (1964):

$$VC = ma2\, p^n \, / \, -\ln p$$

Where, m represents the relative vector density (number of vectors per man), a refers to human-biting frequency (number of human blood meals per vector and per day), p is the daily survival rate (life expectancy of the female mosquito) and n alludes to duration of the sporogonic cycle (length in days of the latent period of the parasite in the mosquito, i.e. extrinsic incubation cycle). It is important to note that ma is usually measured by collecting mosquitoes during an entire night using human bait. Consequently VC could be defined as the future daily sporozoite inoculation rate arising from a currently infective human case, on the assumption that all female mosquitoes biting that person become infected (Githeko, 2006). Of course VC changes from site to site, from vector to vector, and within and between transmission seasons.

2.1.1.1 Malaria receptivity in Southern Europe

Because of climatic conditions, the Southern Europe represents the territory of the Old Continent where disease cycles can be completed more likely. In terms of receptivity, of twenty species of *Anopheles* described in Europe twelve are confined in its distribution to Southern areas (Table 2). In the Iberian Peninsula rice cultivation was clearly associated with malaria endemicity until the beginning of the 20th century (Cambournac & Hill, 1938; Cambournac, 1939, Blázquez, 1974; Bueno Marí & Jiménez Peydró, 2010b). In these larval biotopes the species *Anopheles atroparvus* and, to a much lesser extent and only in the more arid areas, *Anopheles labranchiae* were supposed to be the major malaria vectors (Bruce-Chwatt & de Zulueta, 1977), although some other species, such as *Anopheles maculipennis* or *Anopheles claviger* may locally also have contributed to disease transmission (Bueno Marí, 2010). Currently *An. atroparvus* remains widespread in rice fields and other potential *Anopheles* breeding sites of Portugal and Spain (Capinha et al. 2009; Sainz-Elipe et al. 2010), since the most important western Mediterranean malaria vector *An. labranchiae* is considered dissapeared. *An. labranchiae* was found to be abundant in a restricted area of the contiguous Alicante and Murcia Provinces (South-eastern Spain) in 1946 (Clavero & Romeo Viamonte, 1948), but had disappeared by 1973 (Blázquez & de Zulueta, 1980) probably due to abandonment of rice cultivation in this area (Eritja et al., 2000). Recent surveys carried out in this area have revealed again the absence of *An. labranchiae* as well as high populations of the secondary vector *Anopheles algeriensis* also characterized by high domiciliation degrees (Bueno Marí, 2011). This was the only area where *An. labranchiae* has been able to establish itself in the Iberian Peninsula (Blázquez & de Zulueta, 1980). Though abundant along the African coastline between Ceuta and Tangiers, *An. labrachiae* has been unable to obtain a toe-hold in 15 km distant coastal plains of southern Spain, where rice fields support large populations of *An. atroparvus* (Ramsdale & Snow, 2000). It is important to note that the most important vector of the Iberian Peninsula *An. atroparvus* is suspected of being the vector of an autochthonous case of *Plamodium vivax* which recently occurred in Northeastern Spain (Santa-Olalla Peralta et al., 2010) and even also in other case of *Plamodium ovale* which happened in Central Spain, although airport malaria cannot be discarded in this last case due to the proximity of the patient's residence to two international airports (Cuadros et al., 2002).

Anopheles Species	European distribution	Malaria outbreaks
An. algeriensis	Brit, Ire, Fra, Cors, Spain, Bala, Port, Ger, Aust, Ital, Sard, Sic, Croa, Alb, Gree, Turk, Hung, Bulg, Moldv, Ukr, EurRus, Est	Argelia (non demonstrated vector in Europe)
An. atroparvus	Brit, Ire*, Swe, Den, Fra, Spain, Port, Belg, Neth, Ger, Aust, Czech, Slovk, Pol, Switz[a], Ital, Ser-Mon, Croa, Bosn, Slovn, Mace, Hung, Rom, Bulg, Moldv, Ukr, Bela, EurRus, Lith, Latv	Northern Europe, Central Europe, Eastern Europe, Mediterranean Europe
An. beklemishevi	Swe, Fin, EurRus	-
An. cinereus	Spain, Port	-
An. claviger	Brit, Ire, Nor, Swe, Den, Fra, Cors, Spain, Port, Belg, Neth, Lux, Ger, Aust, Czech, Slovk, Pol, Switz, Ital, Sic, Ser-Mon, Croa, Bosn, Slovn, Mace, Alb, Gree, Turk, Cypr, Hung, Rom, Bulg, Moldv, Ukr, Bela, EurRus, Lith, Latv, Est	Eastern Mediterranean countries, Central Asia
An. daciae [b]	Brit, Rom	-
An. hyrcanus	Fra, Cors, Spain, Ital, Sard, Sic, Ser-Mon, Croa, Mace, Alb, Gree, Turk, Hung, Rom, Bulg, Moldv, Ukr, EurRus	Asia (as An. hyrcanus s.l.)
An. labranchiae	Cors, Ital, Sard, Sic, Croa	France (Corsica), Italy (Peninsular Italy, Sardinia and Sicily), Southeastern Spain (disappeared since 1973)
An. maculipennis	Nor, Swe, Den, Fra, Cors, Spain, Port, Belg, Neth, Lux*, Ger, Aust, Czech, Slovk, Pol, Switz[a], Ital, Sic, Ser-Mon, Croa, Bosn, Slovn, Mace, Alb, Gree, Turk, Hung, Rom, Bulg, Moldv, Ukr, Bela, EurRus, Lith, Latv, Est	Coastal areas in the Balkans, Asia Minor, Northern Iran
An. marteri	Cors, Spain, Port, Ital, Sard, Sic, Alb, Gree, Turk, Bulg	-
An. melanoon [c]	Fra, Cors, Spain, Ital, Rom, EurRus	-
An. messeae	Brit, Ire[a], Nor, Swe, Den, Fra, Cors, Belg, Neth, Ger, Aust, Czech, Slovk, Pol, Switz[a], Ital, Ser-Mon, Croa, Bosn, Slovn, Mace, Alb, Gree, Hung, Rom, Bulg, Moldv, Ukr, Bela, EurRus, Lith, Latv, Est	Eastern Europe

An. multicolor	Spain	-
An. petragnani	Fra, Cors, Spain, Port, Ital, Sard, Sic	-
An. plumbeus	Brit, Ire, Swe, Den, Fra, Cors, Spain, Port, Belg, Neth, Lux, Ger, Aust, Czech, Slovk, Pol, Switz, Ital, Sic, Ser-Mon, Croa, Bosn, Slovn, Mace, Alb, Gree, Turk, Hung, Rom, Bulg, Ukr, Bela, EurRus, Lith, Est	England, Germany, Caucasus
An. pulcherrimus [d]	Turk	Middle East
An. sacharovi	Cors, Ser-Mon, Croa, Mace, Alb, Gree, Turk, Bulg, EurRus	Near East
An. subalpinus [c]	Fra, Cors, Port, Ser-Mon, Croa, Mace, Alb, Gree, Turk, Bulg, EurRus	Albania, Greece
An. sergentii	Sic	Mediterranean Africa
An. superpictus	Cors, Ital, Sic, Ser-Mon, Croa, Mace, Alb, Gree, Turk, Bulg, EurRus	Middle East

Note 1: Countries with anophelines records considered as doubtful or sporadic were not included. If it is thought that the species has been eradicated, the country is also not listed. Note 2: Brit (Britain), Ire (Ireland), Nor (Norway), Swe (Sweden), Den (Denmark), Fra (France), Cors (Corsica), Spain, Bala (Balearic Islands), Port (Portugal), Belg (Belgium), Neth (Netherlands), Lux (Luxemburg), Ger (Germany), Aust (Austria), Czech (Czech Republic), Slovk (Slovakia), Pol (Poland), Switz (Switzerland), Ital (Italy), Sard (Sardinia), Sic (Sicily), Malt (Malta), Ser-Mon (Serbia-Montenegro), Croa (Croatia), Bosn (Bosnia), Slovn (Slovenia), Mace (Macedonia), Alb (Albania), Gree (Greece), Turk (Turkey), Cypr (Cyprus), Hung (Hungary), Rom (Romania), Bulg (Bulgaria), Moldv (Moldavia), Ukr (Ukraine), Bela (Belarus), EurRus (Eropean Russia), Lith (Lithuania), Latv (Latvia), Est (Estonia).
[a] Records referred to Anopheles maculipennis s.l.
[b] Species recently described by molecular and morphological techniques.
[c] There is confusion with these two species.
[d] Present in Asiatic Turkey.

Table 2. Anopheles species with endemic presence in Europe and indication of historical data about its vectorial role (Ramsdale & Snow, 2000; Schaffner et al., 2001; Beck et al., 2003; Nicolescu et al., 2004; Linton et al., 2005; Becker et al., 2010; European Mosquito Taxonomists [MOTAX], 2010).

In France, the same two species mentioned above for the Iberian Peninsula, are also considered to be primary malaria vectors because of their abundance and their potential anthropophily: An. atroparvus in continental France and An. labranchiae in Corsica. In a former malaria-endemic area of Southern France, intensive samplings conducted recently in rice fields showed that Anopheles hyrcanus seems to be the only potential vector likely to play a role in malaria transmission in view of its abundance and anthropophily (Ponçon et al., 2007). Since 1994 several cases of vivax and falciparum malaria with no history of international travels, blood transfusion or injection drug use have been reported in Southern France (Delmont et al., 1994; Baixench et al., 1998; Doudier et al., 2007). In Corsica, where An. labranchiae still present in high densities in different regions (Toty et al., 2010), autochthonous P. vivax malaria transmission has been diagnosed, probably via the bite of a local Anopheles mosquito infected with P. vivax from a patient who had acquired infection in Madagascar (Armengaud et al., 2006). The second most important malaria vector of Corsica, Anopheles sacharovi, has not been detected in the island since 2002 (Toty et al., 2010).

Until the beginning of dichlorodiphenyltrichloroethane (DDT) application, the main malaria vectors in Italy were *An. superpictus* as well as two species of the *Anopheles maculipennis* complex: *An. labranchiae* and *An. sacharovi* (Hackett & Missiroli 1935). Despite *An. labranchiae* used to breed in various types of waters, such as marshes, streams, small pools or irrigation channels, the rice fields established in the 1970s currently represent its most important larval habitats in Central Italy (Bettini et al., 1978; Romi et al., 1992). Even in Western province of Grosseto *An. labranchiae* has replaced *Anopheles melanoon*, species that in 1970 represented for 100% of the anophelines fauna (Majori et al., 1970). Precisely in Grosseto region occurred the last autochthonous malaria case in Italy in August 1997 (Baldari et al., 1998). Nowadays of the anopheline species that have been vectors of malaria in Italy, only *An. labranchiae* and *An. superpictus* are still present in epidemiologically relevant densities (Romi et al., 1997). Moreover *An. atroparvus* is also present in Italy at low densities and *An. sacharovi* is currently considered disappeared, since last specimens of the vector were found 50 years ago (Sepulcri, 1963).

In Balkan countries (Bulgaria, Romania, Croatia, Serbia, Bosnia-Herzegovina, Montenegro and Albania, among others) the species *An. sacharovi* used to be the main malaria vector in coastal areas while *An. superpictus* and *An. maculipennis* were the primary vectors in inland areas due to the specific adaptations of their preimaginal stages (Hackett, 1937; Hadjinicolaou & Betzios, 1973; Bruce-Chwatt & de Zulueta, 1980). Larvae of *An. sacharovi* are tolerant against brackish water but not against salt water. On the other hand *An. superpictus* breeds in slowly flowing waters in hilly areas while *An. maculipennis* breeds in stagnant inland waters (Jetten & Takken, 1994). However, when sporadically *An. maculipennis* has colonized coastal areas of Balkans, Asia Minor and Northern Iran, it has also showed an important role in malaria transmission (Postiglione et al., 1973; Zaim, 1987; Manouchehri et al., 1992; Schaffner et al., 2001). Of the three most important vectors of Balkans, *An. superpictus* was never collected in Romania. Therefore in this country in addition to *An. sacharovi* and *An. maculipennis*, also *Anopheles messeae* and *An. atroparvus* have contributed to the endemism of malaria. Generally *An. messeae* has played a prominent role as a malaria vector in the Danube Valley and Delta, while *An. maculipennis* was mainly responsible for malaria transmission in the Romanian plains and *An. sacharovi* and *An. atroparvus* have been primary vectors at the Black Sea coast (Zotta, 1938; Zotta et al., 1940; Ciuca, 1966). All these issues represent the concept of "malaria stratification", which indicates a good relation between the distribution of the different anophelines species and the great "malaria geographic lines" (Nicolescu, 1996). Moreover a new species of the *An. maculipennis* complex, named *Anopheles daciae*, was recently first described in Romania (Nicolescu et al., 2004). It seems likely that *An. daciae* could be widespread in Eastern Europe and the Balkan States, and also could be responsible for malaria transmission in these regions that is currently attributed to *An. messeae*.

In order of relevance, *An. sacharovi*, *An. superpictus* and *An. maculipennis* were considered the main malaria vectors in Greece (Belios, 1955, 1978). During the recent years several autochthonous cases of *P. falciparum*, *P. malariae* and *P. vivax* have been diagnosed in Northern Greece (Kampen et al., 2002). At respect, it is important to note the proximity of this region to an unstable malaria country as Turkey. In Turkey malaria is still one of the most important vector-borne diseases in Turkey (Kasap et al., 2000; Alten et al., 2003), even remaining some endemic areas with hundreds of vivax cases yearly. The most important vectors in Turkey are *An. sacharovi* and *An. superpictus* (Kuhn et al., 2002), taking *An. maculipennis*, *An. claviger* and *Anopheles hyrcanus* a secondary role in malaria transmission.

If we analyze the VC of European anophelines we can extract several conclusions. In Spain the populations of *An. atroparvus* were deeply studied by several authors basically during the endemic period (Buen de, 1931, 1932; Buen de & Buen de, 1930, 1933; Torres Cañamares, 1934; Olavarria & Hill, 1935; Lozano Morales, 1946; Zulueta de, 1973; Blázquez, 1974). The estimation of VC shows that *An. atroparvus* was an important malaria vector in different wetlands of Spain mainly during summer months. The VC was especially high for *P. vivax* (in August VC=0.7–21.2) which has a shorter sporogonic cycle than *P. falciparum* (in August VC=0.2-5.3). In September VC values were lower for both *P. vivax* (VC=0.2–9.2) and *P. falciparum* (VC=0.04-2.3) and in October VC values were drastically reduced, but still relevant in the case of *P. vivax* (VC *P. vivax*=0.01-2.1 / VC *P. falciparum*=0.00007-0.02) (Bueno Marí & Jiménez Peydró, 2012). These results are similar to others derivates from different entomological researches carried out in Italy more recently. During August 1994 in Tuscany (Grosseto Province) were reported for *An. labranchiae* VC values ranging from 8.3-32.5 for *P. vivax* and 7.3-26 for *P. falciparum* (Romi et al., 1997). However VC was very low in early July, constituting no real risk for malaria transmission (<0.01 for both *P. vivax* and *P. falciparum*). Subsequently during 1998 in the same province but in areas where only natural anopheline breeding sites were reported, the VC of *An. labranchiae* from mid-July through the end of August ranged from 0.96-3.3 for *P. vivax* and 0.8-2.9 for *P. falciparum* (Romi, 1999). In other Mediterranean areas (North of Morocco), VC of *An. labranchiae* for *P. vivax* also showed high values during summer months (in July VC=17.2; in August=34; in September=18.3), while values from April to June were lower ranging from 0.5-3.7 (Faraj et al., 2008). On the other hand the average VC of *An. sacharovi* was found to be 0.22 (VC ranging from 0.63-0.014) in an endemic area of Southeastern Turkey (Tavşanoğlu & Çağlar, 2008). These last low VC values were probably related with very low percentages of human blood meals by anophelines.

Accordingly, although of course all these values of VC are purely theoretical, it is important to note that can be numerically shown that summer (from July to September, but especially in August) is an excellent season for malaria transmission, at least at receptivity level, in Southern Europe.

2.1.1.2 Malaria receptivity in Northern Europe

Endemic northern malaria reached to 68°N latitude in Europe during the 19th century, where the summer mean temperature only irregularly exceeded 16°C. It is important to note that precisely 16°C is considered the lower limit needed for sporogony of *P. vivax* (Garnham, 1988). In Finland *Anopheles beklemishevi* has a northern distribution, while the other common species, *An. messeae*, is dominant in the southern part of the country (Gutsevich et al., 1974; Lokki et al., 1979; Kettle, 1995). Both species are known as an important malaria vectors (White, 1978). Despite other potential vectors, such as *An. claviger* and *An. maculipennis* have been observed (Utrio, 1979; Dahl, 1997), it is not possible to define certainly which mosquito species was most important for the malaria transmission in Finland. This is because temperature conditions of Finland, as well as in other northern countries, should have caused that malaria transmission have mainly occurred in indoor conditions due to transmission of sporozoites throughout the winter by semiactive hibernating mosquitoes (Huldén et al., 2005), since it is well known that in warm conditions the overwintering females of *Anopheles* can take several blood meals (Ekblom & Ströman, 1932; Encinas Grandes, 1982). Therefore, the best malaria vectors in Northern Europe will be those anthropophilic and endophagic anophelines which present hibernating females with semiactive winter habits but not a complete diapause. In conclusion, northern malaria existed in a cold climate by means of summer dormancy of *P. vivax* hypnozoites in addition to the indoor feeding activity of overwintering *Anopheles* females previously mentioned.

In other Scandinavian countries such as Sweden or Denmark, besides the anophelines which has been mentioned above, there have been described other potential malaria vectors: *An. atroparvus* and *Anopheles plumbeus* (Ramsdale & Snow, 2000). Although *An. messeae* was probably the main vector during the malaria epidemics in Sweden, some authors proposed that *An. atroparvus* may have maintained malaria endemicity in certain coastal localities in the south of the country (Jaenson et al., 1986). Regarding to *An. plumbeus* there are several aspects that should be pointed to understand the increasing epidemiological importance of the species in Central Europe. *An. plumbeus* is the only hole breeding species of the genus *Anopheles* in Europe. Although it is a strictly dendrolimnic species, during dry periods females can also lay the eggs in small domestic and peridomestic containers, as well as other artificial breeding sites below the ground such as catch basins and septic tanks with water contaminated with organic waste (Bueno Marí & Jiménez Peydró, 2011). There are several reports in Europe about the presence of larvae in a biotope different from the tree cavity (Aitken, 1954; Senevet et al., 1955; Rioux, 1958; Tovornik, 1978; Bueno Marí & Jiménez Peydró, 2010a). Moreover, remarkable populations can also be found in urban situations, where the larvae develop in tree holes in gardens and parks, especially in Central Europe where *An. plumbeus* has increased in numbers during the last decades and can be a major nuisance species (Becker et al., 2010). This is a very important issue, because the continuous development of this species in urban environments could increase considerably the possibilities of interaction between malaria vectors and humans. In fact, *An. plumbeus* has been suspected to be responsible for two recorded cases of locally transmitted malaria in London, United Kingdom (Blacklock, 1921; Shute, 1954) and other two cases recently reported in Duisburg, Germany (Krüger et al., 2001). Of the five *Anopheles* species present in Britain only two, *An. atroparvus* and *An. plumbeus*, have been confirmed as malaria vectors in United Kingdom (James, 1917; Shute, 1954), while *An. messae* and *An. atroparvus* were the vectors involved in vivax epidemics occurred in Germany during the 20th Century (Kirchberg & Mamlok, 1946).

Therefore, it exists in Europe a latitudinal gradient in relation to the distribution of the species of the *An. maculipennis* complex. Without ignoring the possible participation of several species in malaria transmission cycles, the fact is that in Northern Europe (including European Russia) at 68°N *An. beklemishevi* prevails as vector, being this species replaced by *An. messae* partially at 63°N and fully about 59°N. Around 56°N *An. atroparvus* begins to acquire an important role in disease transmission and already in Mediterranean countries the situation of malaria receptivity is basically governed by *An. atroparvus*, *An. labranchiae* and *An. sacharovi* in Eastern, Central and Western Mediterranean respectively. As was previously pointed, this situation can be locally modified by the presence of other potential vectors widely distributed in Europe such as *An. claviger*, *An. hyrcanus*, *An. maculipennis* or *An. plumbeus*. Of course climate change could drastically modify not only the distribution of European anophelines, but also their phenology and overwintering patterns. However the changes in agricultural practices have a greater effect on the risk of malaria than an elevation in temperature of approximately 2°C (Becker, 2008), which is considered the average increasing temperature in Europe in next 50 years. Hence habitat modification is probably the factor with more influence in possible changes in malaria receptivity all over Europe.

2.1.2 Infectivity

Infectivity is defined as the degree of susceptibility of *Anopheles* mosquitoes to different *Plasmodium* species, i.e. refers to the possibilities that the sporogonic cycle of parasite could be completed within a concrete vector species. It is well known that mosquito populations of the same species but different geographic areas can differ drastically at infectivity level due to genetic reasons (Frizzi et al., 1975).

Infectivity tests carried out on European populations of species of the *An. maculipennis* complex showed that *An. atroparvus* can transmit Asian strains of *P. vivax* and African strains of *P. ovale* but is refractory to African strains of *P. falciparum* (James et al., 1932; Garnham et al., 1954; Ramsdale & Coluzzi, 1975; Teodorescu, 1983; Ribeiro et al., 1989). However, more recent studies have shown the ability of *An. atroparvus* to generate oocysts of *P. falciparum* (Marchant et al., 1998), but not to complete sporogony. Information about *An. labranchiae* is quite confusing due to the scanty and old infectivity tests conducted. Moreover laboratory studies have revealed that *An. labranchiae* can transmit *P. ovale* (Constantinescu & Negulici, 1967) but populations of the vector collected in Italy were refractory to African strains of *P. falciparum* (Ramsdale & Coluzzi, 1975; Zulueta de et al., 1975). Nevertheless recent researches with populations from Corsica have indicated that *P. falciparum* cycle can be successfully completed in *An. labranchiae* (Toty et al., 2010). Furthermore *An. labranchiae* has been involved in transmission of autochthonous vivax malaria cases and in Corsica (France), Greece and Italy (Sautet & Quilici, 1971; Zahar, 1987; Baldari et al., 1998) and even several outbreaks of *P. falciparum*, *P. malariae* and *P. vivax* in Morocco (Houel & Donadille, 1953). Under laboratory conditions, *An. sacharovi* has been demonstrated as an excellent vector of *P. vivax* (Kasap, 1990) and *An. messeae* was reported, not only as being the main vector of malaria over a large part of European Russia several decades ago (Detinova, 1953), but also the responsible of disease resurgence in Russia and Ukraine more recently (Nikolaeva, 1996). With regard to *An. maculipennis* it is known that in certain coastal areas in the Balkans, Asia Minor and Northern Iran (Postiglione et al., 1973; Zaim, 1987; Manouchehri et al., 1992), the species has participated actively in malaria transmission cycles. Due to its recent description, *An. daciae* yet must be tested on its susceptibility to *Plasmodium* species

Outside the species of the *An. maculipennis* complex is remarkable that European populations of *An. plumbeus* can produce sporozoites of tropical strains of *P. falciparum* (Marchant et al., 1998; Eling et al., 2003), as well as also Eurasiatic strains of *P. vivax* (Shute & Maryon, 1974). Even some authors suggest that *An. plumbeus* is capable of transmitting the four Plasmodium species (Shute & Maryon, 1969). However this hypothesis should be confirmed with modern molecular techniques. Respect to *An. algeriensis* and *An. claviger*, it is important to note that in natural populations it has been shown the presence of oocysts of *P. vivax* at intestinal level (Blacklock & Carter, 1920; Horsfall, 1972). In the case of *An. algeriensis*, even has been successfully tested the transmission of *P. falciparum* in laboratory conditions (Becker et al., 2010). *An. superpictus* can transmit *P. vivax* (Kasap, 1990) but its susceptibility to *P. falciparum* has not been tested, although this anopheline is probably sensitive, as it belongs to the subgenus *Cellia*, to which the principal African malaria vectors also belong. Another species of the subgenus *Cellia* poorly represented in Europe, such as *Anopheles multicolor* and *Anopheles sergentii*, have been also found parasitized by *P. vivax* and *P. falciparum* in natural conditions (Kenawy et al., 1990). Finally, there is no infectivity information about *An. marteri*, *An. cinereus* and *An. petragnani*. Anyway the epidemiological role of these species it seems secondary due to their zoophylic behaviour and rural distribution.

2.1.3 Vulnerability

Vulnerability is determined by the number of gametocyte carriers (malaria patients) during the suitable period for malaria transmission. If we analyze the data about imported malaria in Europe in recent years we can extract several conclusions. Malaria represents about 77% of tropical diseases imported in Europe (TropNetEurop, 2010). A total of 65.596 cases were reported in Europe between 2000 and 2009 (Table 3). However this number is clearly underestimated, since in last years the number of malaria reporting sites in Europe has increased significantly. Most of these cases are referred to immigrants (48.5%), and *P. falciparum* (81%) was the dominant species in analytic results. A high percentage of malaria cases in immigrants correspond to Visiting Friends and Relatives (VFR). This group of special epidemiological significance refers to those people who, once are established in their host countries, often travel to their origin countries to visit family or friends. Travels that these people can do to their origin countries exponentially increase the chances of disease contracting, since usually these areas are endemic regions and the stay within resident population and their customs is often long and intense (Gascón, 2006). Therefore this is an important collective to promote the need to take appropriate prophylactic measures during travels to endemic areas. Several studies have revealed that only 16% of VFR search for medical advice pre-travel, being malaria prophylaxis practically nonexistent in this collective (Leder et al., 2006). The European countries with higher number of imported malaria cases reported yearly are France and Germany, usually followed by other like Spain, Italy or Belgium. As it was shown before, malaria receptivity is remarkable in concrete regions of these countries.

	2000	2001	2002	2003	2004	2005	2006	2007	2008	2009	Total
Cases (sites reporting)	1120 (32)	3313 (38)	4555 (47)	5561 (44)	6536 (47)	7411 (50)	8544 (50)	8904 (52)	9509 (57)	10.143 (59)	65.596
P. falciparum	78.4%	70.0%	77.6%	82.4%	81.2%	81.6%	87.8%	82.8%	83.9%	84.0%	81%
P. vivax	11.5%	13.9%	11.7%	10.4%	11.2%	10.2%	7.5%	8.3%	8.2%	8.6%	10.1%
P. ovale	5.2%	5.3%	3.4%	3.1%	3.5%	4.4%	2.8%	4.3%	3.9%	3.1%	3.9%
P. malariae	2%	5.9%	4.3%	1.5%	1.5%	1.7%	1%	1.2%	1.5%	2.3%	2.3%
Unkn./Coinf.	2.9%	4.9%	3.1%	2.7%	2.4%	2.2%	0.9%	3.4%	2.7%	4.4%	2.7%
Imm./Refu.	30.5%	35.4%	44.8%	50.2%	54%	54.6%	52.8%	50.8%	55.2%	56.7%	48.5%
For. Vis.	11.8%	14.6%	7.5%	9.1%	7%	9.2%	10.3%	3.3%	5.1%	9.2%	8.7%
Eur. E.C.	53.8%	44.4%	38.9%	30.6%	30%	26.1%	26.2%	35.2%	34%	26.4%	34.5%
Eur. Exp.	3.9%	5.6%	8.8%	11.1%	9%	10.1%	10.7%	10.7%	5.7%	7.7%	8.3%

Note 1: Unkn./Coinf. (Plasmodium species unknown or coinfection of various species), Imm./Refu. (Immigrants/Refugees), For. Vis. (Foreign Visitors), Eur. E.C. (Europeans living in EC), Eur. Exp. (European Expatriates).

Table 3. Imported malaria in Europe between 2000-2009 (TropNetEurop, 2010).

The temporal distribution analysis of imported malaria cases indicates that high-risk months for disease transmission (between July and September) also coincides with the period of the most cases reported in Europe. Therefore most of cases occur during the epoch theoretically favorable for malaria transmission. In regard to the diagnostic delay, i.e. the average time between appearance of symptoms and malaria diagnosis (when therapy began), it shows disparate values according to each country. For example, in Eastern Spain the diagnostic delay of imported malaria was estimated in 13.7 days (Bueno Marí & Jiménez Peydró, 2012), while in other European countries like Sweden, France or Italy values are clearly lower, ranging from 3 to 8.2 days (Romi et al., 2001; Askling et al., 2005; Chalumeau et al., 2006). From an epidemiological point of view it is very important to reduce the diagnostic delay, because this is the period when malaria patients could be a source of infection for *Anopheles* females. Additionally, from an exclusively clinical perspective, delay to diagnosis leads of course to high parasitemia, which itself leads to severe forms of malaria.

3. Dengue fever and yellow fever

There are many similarities between dengue fever and yellow fever:
- Both are viruses of the genus Flavivirus (family Flaviviridae) and are strictly primatophilic, infecting only primates, including man.
- In their original habitat, both are zoonotic infections transmitted by forest mosquitoes.
- Their importance as human pathogens can be related with two forest mosquitoes characterized by high ecological plasticity that have become closely associated with the peridomestic environment.
- Both diseases have a history of transmission in temperate regions, including Europe, and share essentially the same selvatic and urban vectors.
- Transovarian transmission in female mosquitoes has been demonstrated for both viruses.
- The viruses and their urban vectors have a worldwide distribution due to transportation of goods and people.
- Both arboviruses are characterized by short incubation period and can provoke similar clinical symptoms, including hemorrhagic illness in humans, often with fatal consequences. However mortality rate is higher in yellow fever (20%) than in dengue (5%).

In the case of dengue fever its annual incidence has increased dramatically around the world in recent decades. It is estimated that over 2500 millions people who live in over 100 tropical and non-tropical countries, are currently at risk from dengue viruses globally. The rise in dengue incidence has been marked by geographic expansion of the virus and the vectors due to globalization, habitat modifications, lack of effective mosquito control programs and climate change. Although the major disease burden occurs in South East Asia, the Americas and the western Pacific, dengue was also a common disease in Europe in the past centuries. Large epidemics of dengue and yellow fever occurred in European ports of Spain, Portugal, France, Italy and even Wales and Ireland as the more northern countries of the continent (Eager, 1902; Monath, 2006). Last dengue epidemic in Europe, estimated at one million cases, occurred in Greece in 1927-28 (Papaevangelou & Halstead, 1977; Rosen, 1986).

Dengue is the most frequent tropical arboviruses imported in Europe and together with schistosomiasis both are considered, after malaria, the most important tropical diseases in quantitative terms in Old continent. Of the hundreds of dengue imported cases reported yearly en Europe (Table 4), the vast majority are represented by tourists (about 84%). A difference to what happens with malaria, immigration (9%) seems to have comparatively little influence on dengue importation. This could be explained, of course by distinct perspectives and approaches of European tourists (e.g. travels to urbanized areas) and immigrants who come to Europe (e.g. Africa, where malaria is much prevalent than dengue, is the main origin from immigrants who arrive to Europe), but also by differences between incubation periods and existing prophylactic measures in both diseases. All dengue cases reported have shown the typical symptomatology of disease, including febrile symptoms in more than 90% of cases (TropNetEurop, 2010). However, it is important to note that the majority of imported dengue infections remain undiagnosed, with a ratio between symptomatic and asymptomatic travelers estimated in 1/3.3 (Cobelens et al., 2002). In general terms, it is estimated that about 80% of all dengue infections are asymptomatic (Farrar, 2008). This high asymptomatic, added to the fact that dengue is not a notifiable disease in much of European countries (Bueno Marí & Jiménez Peydró, 2010c; 2010d), allow us to consider that the knowledge of dengue virus circulation is very limited.

	2001	2002	2003	2004	2005	2006	2007	2008	2009	Total
Cases (sites reporting)	477 (37)	664 (47)	742 (46)	852 (48)	1023 (51)	1167 (50)	1273 (53)	1419 (57)	1553 (61)	9170
Imm./Refu.	10%	5.5%	8.2%	12.9%	6.8%	10.5%	9%	6.8%	11.3%	9%
For. Vis.	0.8%	0.5%	1%	0%	1.2%	4.8%	2.2%	0.8%	2.4%	1.5%
Eur. E.C.	86.7%	91.3%	79.6%	81.9%	87.7%	77.1%	81.3%	87.3%	83.9%	84.1%
Eur. Exp.	2.5%	2.7%	11.2%	5.2%	4.3%	7.6%	7.5%	5.1%	2.4%	5.4%

Note 1: Imm./Refu. (Immigrants/Refugees), For. Vis . (Foreign Visitors), Eur. E.C. (Europeans living in EC), Eur. Exp. (European Expatriates).

Table 4. Imported dengue in Europe between 2001-2009 (TropNetEurop, 2010).

Aedes aegypti is the primary urban vector of dengue and yellow fever basically because it exist a 'domesticated' form of the species that is rarely found more than 100 m from human habitation and feeds almost exclusively on human blood (Reiter, 2010). Both factors allow that *Ae. aegypti* will be considered as an excellent urban vector of viruses. Its distribution was traditionally limited by latitude between 45° N and 35° S according to the existence of January and July 10° C isotherms. Although records out of this latitude range are very rarely, it must be pointed that European northernmost collection of the species occurred in Brest (France) at 48° N (Christopher, 1960). Moreover recent studies have demonstrated that *Ae. aegypti* larvae can withstand temperatures of 2.5° C (Chang et al., 2007). In Eastern Europe it was also seen at its temperature limit at Odessa (Ukraina) at 46° N. (Korovitzkyi and Artemenko, 1933). Despite the species was relatively common in Mediterranean countries, it disappeared from the entire region in the mid-20th century, for reasons that currently are not clear but probably related with thermic tolerance and intensive mosquito control campaigns with the employment of DDT. *Ae. aegypti* was common in the Iberian Peninsula mainly introduced from North Africa and was present in this Southern European region up to 1956 (Ribeiro & Ramos, 1999). Since the eradication of the species in Europe, its sporadic presence has been recognized in several countries, namely Britain, France, Italy, Malta, Croatia, Ukraine, Russia and Turkey (Snow & Ramsdale, 1999). However it must be pointed that the species has been reported in Madeira (Portugal) in 2005 (Margarita et al., 2006) and it seems that *Ae. aegypti* is now deeply established in this region because of continuous collections in later years (Almeida et al., 2007). This is the first report of the establishment of the species in Europe since mid-20th century. More recently *Ae. aegypti* has been also captured in The Netherlands (Scholte et al., 2010). In summary, we must pay some attention to surveillance and behavior of *Ae. aegypti* because globalization is provoking the arrival of the species to Europe and global warming could allow the definitive establishment of the species again in Southern areas.

On the other hand the situation is clearly divergent in regard to the secondary vector of dengue and yellow fever, *Aedes albopictus*, usually known as Asian tiger mosquito, due to its quick expansion in Europe in last years. There are several ecological factors that can help us to understand the different importance of *Ae. aegypti* and *Ae. albopictus* as primary and secondary vectors of human viruses respectively. Unlike patterns of oviposition and feeding exhibited by *Ae. aegypti*, Asian tiger mosquito is often abundant in the peridomestic environment, particularly in areas with plentiful vegetation, and feeds freely on humans and other animals. Consequently *Ae. albopictus* can also exist far from human habitation. Additionally *Ae. aegypti* has been globally dispersed from Africa by humans activities since several centuries ago while *Ae. albopictus* was firstly report out of its original Asiatic distribution range in 1979 in Albania (Adhami & Reiter, 1998). Current data indicate that *Ae. albopictus* has been detected much farer north than *Ae. aegypti* and one major difference between both species is that Asian tiger mosquito has the ability to adapt to cold temperatures by becoming dormant during the winter of temperate regions. The ability of *Ae. albopictus* to resist cold temperatures is partially related with its ability to synthesize a high amount of lipids, especially to produce larger amounts of yolk lipid in cold temperatures. At respect, it was demonstrated that larval lipogenesis of *Ae. albopictus* is much more efficient than that of *Ae. aegypti* (Briegel & Timmermann, 2001). Although *Ae. albopictus* occurs in both temperate and tropical areas, only temperate population, but not tropical ones, show a photoperiodic diapauses (Hawley, 1988). During the shortening daylight hours in late summer/early autumn, the reduced photoperiod stimulates the females of *Ae. albopictus* to produce eggs that enter facultative diapause (Estrada-Franco & Craig 1995). These eggs can resist hatching stimuli until the following spring and remain in a state of reduced morphogenesis as fully formed first instar larvae, exhibiting increased resistance to environmental extremes. Although the diapause occurs in the egg stage, only adults and pupae are known to be photoperiodically sensitive stages (Wang, 1966; Imai & Maeda, 1976; Mori et al, 1981).

Ae. albopictus has been found to be capable to transmit 26 viruses (Moore & Mitchell, 1997; Gratz, 2004; Paupy et al., 2009) and to be experimentally susceptible to several filariasis of veterinary interest (Cancrini et al., 1995; Nayar & Knight, 1999). Globalization has allowed the arrival of this species to Europe, mainly through the transport of eggs and larvae in used tires and gardening products (Reiter & Sprenger, 1987; Madon et al., 2002). The presence of Asian tiger mosquito has been confirmed in 16 European countries, but only in Southern ones the species is deeply established. Particularly interesting is the situation of Italy, where the species was firstly detected in 1990 (Sabatini et al., 1990) and nowadays has colonized more than 2/3 parts of the territory, even having different areas of the country with mosquitoes densities in considerable epidemiological levels. Precisely these locally high densities have allowed the appearance of first cases of human viruses in Europe transmitted by *Ae. albopictus*. Specifically, in the province of Ravenna (Northeastern Italy) occurred an outbreak of Chikungunya virus in 2007. This virus is very similar to dengue and yellow fever (same vectors, bioecology and symptomatology), but much less pathogenic. Just in two and a half months, a total of 205 cases of Chikungunya were reported in two small towns of Ravenna where the infection of *Ae. albopictus* was also confirmed (Rezza et al., 2007). This outbreak of Chikungunya infection, outside a tropical country, was probably begun by a man from India, country that previous year had suffered an epidemic with more than 1 million cases (Ravi, 2006). The Indian man developed a febrile syndrome two days after his arrival in Italy and also had high titres of antibodies against Chikungunya. The phylogenetic analysis showed that the strain that caused Italian outbreak was similar to the strains detected on the Indian subcontinent (Yergolkar et al., 2006), showing in all cases a better adaption to *Ae. albopictus* than other variants. However most worrying scenario took place in 2010 with the re-appearance of first autochthonous cases of dengue in Europe transmitted by *Ae. albopictus*. In this year, two cases of autochthonous dengue fever were diagnosed in Nice (Southeast France) (La Ruche et al., 2010), region where *Ae. albopictus* is established at least since 2004 (Delaunay et al., 2007). Just days after two indigenous cases of Chikungunya in the districts of Alpes-Maritime and Var (also in Southeastern France) were detected through a routinely surveillance of dengue and Chikungunya (ECDC, 2010), which is yearly conducted since 2006 due to the establishment of *Ae. albopictus* in this region. In Greece, other Mediterranean country where *Ae. albopictus* is established at least since 2004 (Klobucar et al., 2006), two cases of indigenous dengue were diagnosed also in 2010 (Schmidt-Chanasit et al., 2010; Gjenero-Margan et al., 2011). The identification of these cases of dengue fever and Chikungunya occurred in 2010, which were in all cases well clustered in space and time, is strongly suggestive that autochthonous transmission of tropical viruses in Europe is ongoing.

According to these epidemiological perspectives it seems evident that there is a need to be able to predict the potential distribution and activity of *Ae. albopictus* in Europe to asses about possible re-emergence of dengue and other tropical arboviruses. At respect several Geographic Information Systems (GIS) have been developed in order to predict the number of weeks of activity of *Aedes albopictus* (ECDC, 2009). These GIS models have revealed that throughout much of Europe, more than 23 weeks are predicted to elapse between egg hatching in spring (in response to at least 11.25 hours of daylight and 10.5° C of mean temperature) and adult die-off in autumn (below critical temperature threshold of 9.5° C). Assuming that immature development takes about 2–4 weeks, this constitutes more than 20 weeks of adult activity in Central Europe and Southern United Kingdom, even increasing this activity to more than 40 weeks in southern areas (mainly Greece, Turkey and south of Iberian and Italic Peninsula), depending on availability of surface water for breeding. If these predictions would be fulfilled in Southern Europe, consequently could increase the speed of spread of the species, could also extend the episodes of medical and social alerts derivates from its feeding behavior in urban areas, and even could change the eco-epidemiology of viruses that *Ae. albopictus* can transmit.

It must be pointed that *Ae. albopictus* and *Ae. aegypti* are not the only aedine vectors with invasive behavior in Europe. Other exotic mosquitoes, such as *Ochlerotatus japonicus* and

Ochlerotatus atropalpus, have been also reported. *Oc. japonicus* is an Asian species and a competent vector of several arboviruses, including West Nile virus and Japanese encephalitis virus and is considered a significant public health risk (Sardelis & Turell, 2001; Sardelis et al., 2002a; 2002b; 2003). *Oc. japonicus* has been collected only in France, Belgium, Switzerland and Germany (Schafther et al., 2003; 2009; Becker et al., 2011). On the other hand *Oc. atropalpus* is endemic to North America and has been observed in Italy, France and Netherlands (Romi et al., 1997; Adege-EID Méditerranée, 2006; Scholte et al., 2009). Although in the field, *Oc. atropalpus* has not been evidenced as an important vector of infectious diseases, under laboratory conditions, the species has been proven as a competent vector for West Nile virus, Japanese encephalitis virus, Saint-Louis encephalitis virus La Crosse encephalitis virus, among other arboviruses (King, 1960; Turell et al., 2001). Globalization, especially traffic of used tires, has led the arrival of *Oc. japonicus* and *Oc. atropalpus* to Europe. Out of these exotic vectors, we can not forget or ignore the presence of potential indigenous vectors of dengue and yellow fever in Europe. For example, *Aedes vittatus* is an important vector of yellow fever in different parts of Africa (Lewis, 1943; Satti & Haseeb, 1966) and also a potential vector of Chikungunya and four dengue serotypes (Mourya & Banerjee, 1987; Mavale et al., 1992). Although the species is deeply distributed in Mediterranean region (Spain, Portugal, France and Italy), the studies about its biology and phenology have been scanty in Europe. Anyway it seems unlikely that *Ae. vittatus* could start a cycle of virus transmission to humans because of its high degree of ruralism. Moreover *Ochlerotatus geniculatus* is a dendrolimnic species endemic to Europe that can efficiently transmit yellow fever, but this possibility has been evidenced only in laboratory conditions (Roubaud et al., 1937).

3.1 New challenges: The development of dengue vaccines

Although a vaccine based on live attenuated virus of the strain 17D is available for yelow fever since years, currently we haven´t any vaccine to be used with full warranty against dengue. However, the need for a dengue vaccine is clear. The most effective measures of an integrated mosquito control program (including changes in human habitation and behavior, the use of insecticides, and long-lasting modification of natural and man-made mosquito habitats) are difficult to implement and largely unsuccessful in most poverty-stricken settings, and consequently have not been carried out comprehensively enough to limit dengue's spread. While vector control is an integral part of any dengue prevention strategy, it is not enough on its own.

In recent years it has been obtained a better understanding of the disease and its etiopatogenicity, as well as of the necessary aspects to develop a vaccine that provides an effective and lasting protection against the virus. Dengue vaccine development is a very difficult task due to the possible participation of four related serotypes, since immunity to one serotype does not confer immunity to the remaining three. Complicating the scenario further is immune enhancement, which can result in severe dengue hemorrhagic fever or dengue shock syndrome in anyone who has been infected with one of the serotypes and subsequently becomes infected with another. Most of researchers agree that only effective solution is a tetravalent vaccine that simultaneously protects against all four serotypes. Regarding to this, it must be noted that tetravalent vaccines against dengue are currently in last phases of trials and is expected to be available for human population in the next following years.

4. Conclusions

Although malaria's receptivity is still high in different parts of Europe, we may conclude that the malariogenic potential of the Old Continent is low. Fortunately socio-economic and sanitary conditions of most European countries also support this assertion. While it is true that infectivity studies should be further promoted, percentages of imported malaria cases remain very low. However we must pay some attention to the increasing trend of malaria importation in last years, as well as also awareness among tourists and VFR's for to take corresponding prophylactic measures during their travels to endemic areas. Anyway, sporadic and local cases of autochthonous transmission mainly transmitted by *An. atroparvus, An. labranchiae, An. sacharovi* and/or *An. plumbeus*, can not been discarded in next years.

On the other hand, the answer to the question about if should be expected the re-emergence of dengue and other mosquito-borne tropical viruses in Europe in next years is indubitable: definitively yes. The arrival, establishment and expansion of dengue urbanite vectors due to global changes such as globalization, climate change and the lack of effective mosquito control programs, together with the increasing of imported cases in humans provokes that local and intense transmission of dengue could be a reality in next years in Southern Europe. To cope this possibility is necessary to enhance the entomological surveillance in potential areas of mosquitoes importation, such as airports or seaports, strength the monitoring of tropical viruses imported and awareness among citizens about their role in mosquito control and best prophylactic measures to take during the travels to tropical regions.

5. Acknowledgments

We wish to acknowledge that current work was partially funded by the Research Project CGL 2009-11364 (BOS), supported by the Ministry of Science and Innovation of Spain (Ministerio de Ciencia e Innovación del Gobierno de España).

6. References

Adege-EID Méditerranée. (2006). *Éléments entomologiques relatifs au risque d'apparition du virus Chikungunya en métropole* . Entente interdépartementale pour la démoustication du littoral (EID) Méditerranée, Montpellier, France.

Adhami, J.R. & Reiter, P. (1998). Introduction and establishment of *Aedes (Stegomyia) albopictus* Skuse (Diptera: Culicidae) in Albania. *Journal of American Mosquito Control Association*, Vol.14, No.3, (September 1998), pp. 340-343, ISSN 1046-3607.

Aitken, T.G.H. (1954). The Culicidae of Sardinia and Corsica (Diptera). *Bulletin of Entomological Research*, Vol.45, No.3, (September 1954), pp. 437-494, ISSN 0007-4853.

Almeida, A.P.; Gonçalves, Y.M.; Novo, M.T.; Sousa, C.A.; Melim, M. & Gracio AJ. (2007). Vector monitoring of *Aedes aegypti* in the Autonomous Region of Madeira, Portugal. *Euro Surveillance*, Vol.12, No.46, (November 2007), ISSN 1560-7917, Available online in: http://www.eurosurveillance.org/ViewArticle.aspx?ArticleId=3311

Alten, B.; Çağlar, S.S.; Şimşek, F.M. & Kaynas, S. (2003). Effect of insecticide-treated bednets for malaria control in Southeast Anatolia - Turkey. *Journal of Vector Ecology*, No.28, Vol.1, (June 2003), pp. 97-107, ISSN 1081-1710. Date of submission:

Armengaud, A.; Legros, F.; Quatresous, I.; Barre, H.; Valayer, P.; Fanton, Y.; D' Ortenzio, E. & Schaffner, F. (2006). A case of autochthonous *Plasmodium vivax* malaria, Corsica, August 2006. *Euro Surveillance*, Vol.11, No.46, (November 2006), ISSN 1560-7917, Available online in: http://www.eurosurveillance.org/ViewArticle.aspx?ArticleId=3081

Askling, H.H.; Ekdahl, K.; Janzon, R.; Henric Braconier, J.; Bronner, U.; Hellgren, U.; Rombo, L. & Tegnell, A. (2005). Travellers returning to Sweden with falciparum malaria: pre-travel advice, behaviour, chemoprophylaxis and diagnostic delay. *Scandinavian Journal of Infectious Diseases*, Vol.37, No.10, (October 2005), pp. 760-765, ISSN 0036-5548.

Baixench, M.T.; Suzzoni-Blatger, J.; Magnaval, J.F.; Lareng, M.B. & Larrouy, G. (1998). Two cases of inexplicable autochthonous malaria in Toulouse, France. *Medecine tropicale : revue du Corps de sante colonial*, Vol.58, No.1, (January 1998), pp. 62–64, ISSN 0025-682X.

Baldari, M.; Tamburro, A.; Sabatinelli, G.; Romi, R.; Severini, C., Cuccagna, P.; Fiorilli, G.; Allegri, M.P.; Buriani, C. & Toti, M. (1998). Introduced malaria in Maremma, Italy, decades after eradication. *The Lancet*, Vol.351, No.9111, (April 1998), pp. 1246-1248, ISSN 0140-6736.

Beck, M.; Galm, M.; Weitzel, T.; Fohlmeister, V.; Kaiser, A.; Arnold, A. & Becker, N. (2003). Preliminary studies on the mosquito fauna of Luxembourg. *European Mosquito Bulletin*, Vol.14, (January 2003), pp. 21-24. ISSN 1460-6127.

Becker, N. (2008). Influence of climate change on mosquito development and mosquito-borne diseases in Europe. Parasitology Research, Vol.103, No.1, (January 2008), 103:19–28, ISSN 0932-0113.

Becker, N.; Petric, D.; Zgomba, M.; Boase, C.; Madon, M.; Dahl, C. & Kaiser, A. (2010). *Mosquitoes and Their Control*. 2 nd ed. Springer, ISBN 978-3-540-92873-7, Berlin, Deutschland.

Becker, N.; Huber, K.; Pluskota, B. & Kaiser, A. (2011). Ochlerotatus japonicus japonicus – a newly established neozoan in Germany and a revised list of the German mosquito fauna. *European Mosquito Bulletin*, Vol.29 (April 2011), pp. 88-102, ISSN 1460-6127.

Belios, G.D. (1955). Recent course and current pattern of malaria in relation to its control in Greece. *Rivista di Malariologia*, Vol.34, pp. 1-24, ISSN 0370-565X.

Belios, G.D. (1978). From malaria control to eradication: problems and solutions. *Archeion Hygiene Athens*, Vol.27, pp. 54-59.

Bettini, S.; Gradoni, L.; Cocchi, M. & Tamburro, A. (1978). Rice culture and *Anopheles labranchiae* in Central Italy. WHO unpublished document, WHO/MAL 78.897, WHO/VBC series 78.686, Geneva, Switzerland.

Blacklock, B. (1921). Notes on a case of indigenous infection with *P. falciparum*. *Annals of Tropical Medicine and Parasitology*, Vol.15, pp. 59-72, ISSN 0003-4983.

Blacklock, B. & Carter, H.F. (1920). The experimental infection in England of *Anopheles plumbeus*, Stephens, and *Anopheles bifurcatus*, L., with *Plasmodium vivax*. *Annals of Tropical Medicine and Parasitology*, Vol.13, No.4, (March 1920), pp. 413-420, ISSN 0003-4983.

Blázquez, J. (1974). Investigación entomológica sobre anofelismo en el delta del Ebro. *Revista de Sanidad e Higiene Pública*, Vol.48, No.4 (April 1974), pp. 363-377, ISSN 0034-8899.

Blázquez, J. & Zulueta de, J. (1980). The disappearance of *Anopheles labranchiae* from Spain. *Parassitologia*, Vol.22, No.1-2, (January 1980), pp. 161-163, ISSN 0048-2951.

Briegel, H. & Timmermann, S.E. (2001). *Aedes albopictus* (Diptera: Culicidae): physiological aspects of development and reproduction, *Journal of Medical Entomology*, vol.38, No.4, (July 2001), pp. 566–571, ISSN 0022-2585.

Bruce-Chwatt, L.J. & Zulueta de, J. (1977). Malaria eradication in Portugal. *Transactions of the Royal Society of Tropical Medicine and Hygiene*, Vol. 71, No.3, (March 1977), pp. 232-240, ISSN 0035-9203.

Bruce-Chwatt, L.J. & Zulueta de, J. (1980). *The Rise and Fall of Malaria in Europe*. Oxford University Press, ISBN 978-0198581680, New York, USA.

Buen de, E. (1931). Algunos estudios sobre biología del *Anopheles maculipennis* en lo que se refiere a la casa habitada por el hombre o animales. *Medicina de los Países Cálidos*, Vol.4, (September 1931), pp. 400-414.

Buen de, E. (1932). Algunos datos sobre la biología del *A. maculipennis* (*claviger*) en su fase de adulto. *Medicina de los Países Cálidos*, Vol.5, (November 1932), pp. 449-485.

Buen de, S. & De Buen, E. (1930). Notas sobre la biología del *A. maculipennis*. *Medicina de los Países Cálidos*, Vol.3, (September 1930), pp. 1-17.

Buen de, S. & Buen de, E. (1933). El *Anopheles maculipennis* y la casa; sus relaciones con la epidemiologia del paludismo en España. *Medicina de los Países Cálidos*, Vol.6, (July 1933), pp. 270-299.

Bueno Marí, R. (2011). El anofelismo en la Comunidad Valenciana: un ejemplo de estudio del potencial malariogénico de España. *Boletín de la Asociación española de Entomología*, Vol.35, No.1-2 (June 2011), pp. 47-83, ISSN 0210-8984.

Bueno Marí, R. (2010). *Bioecología, diversidad e interés epidemiológico de los culícidos mediterráneos (Diptera, Culicidae)*. Servei de Publicacions de la Universitat de València, ISBN 978-84-370-7987-5, Valencia, Spain.

Bueno Marí, R. & Jiménez Peydró, R. (2008). Malaria en España: aspectos entomológicos y perspectivas de futuro. *Revista Española de Salud Pública*, Vol.82, No.5, (September 2008), pp. 467-489, ISSN 1135-5727.

Bueno Marí, R & Jiménez Peydró, R. (2010a). New anopheline records from the Valencian Autonomous Region of Eastern Spain (Diptera: Culicidae: Anophelinae). *European Mosquito Bulletin*, Vol.28, (September 2010), pp. 148-156, ISSN 1460-6127.

Bueno Marí, R. & Jiménez Peydró, R. (2010b). Crónicas de arroz, mosquitos y paludismo en España: el caso de la provincia de Valencia (s. XVIII-XX). *Hispania* Vol.70, No.236, (September 2010), pp. 687-708, ISSN 0018-2141.

Bueno Marí, R. & Jiménez Peydró, R. (2010c). Situación actual en España y eco-epidemiología de las arbovirosis transmitidas por mosquitos culícidos (Diptera: Culicidae), Vol.84, No.3, (May 2010), pp. 255-269, ISSN 1135-5727.

Bueno Marí, R. & Jiménez Peydró, R. (2010d). ¿Pueden la malaria y el dengue reaparecer en España?, Vol.24, No.4, (July 2010), pp. 347-353, ISSN 0213-9111.

Bueno Marí, R & Jiménez Peydró, R. (2012). Study of the Malariogenic Potential of Eastern Spain. *Tropical Biomedicine*, in press.

Bueno Marí, R & Jiménez Peydró, R. (2011). *Anopheles plumbeus* Stephens, 1828: a neglected malaria vector in Europe. *Malaria Reports*, Available online in: http://www.pagepressjournals.org/index.php/malaria/article/view/malaria.2011.e2. ISSN 2039-4381.

Cambournac, F.J.C. (1939). A method for determining the larval *Anopheles* population and its distribution in rice fields. *Rivista di Malariologia* Vol.18, pp. 17-22, ISSN 0370-565X.

Cambournac, F.J.C. & Hill, R.B. (1938). The Biology of *Anopheles maculipennis* var. *atroparvus* in Portugal. *Transactions of 3rd International Congress of Tropical Medicine & Malaria.* Vol.2, pp. 178-184.

Cancrini, G.; Pietrobelli, M.; Frangipane di Regalbono, A.F.; Tampieri, M.P. & della Torre, A. (1995). Development of *Dirofilaria* and *Setaria* nematodes in *Aedes albopictus*. *Parassitologia,* Vol. 37, No.2-3, (December 1995), pp. 141–145, ISSN: 0048-2951.

Capinha, C.; Gomes, E.; Reis, E.; Rocha, J.; Sousa, C.A.; Rosário, V.E..; Almeida, A.P. (2009). Present habitat suitability for *Anopheles atroparvus* (Diptera, Culicidae) and its coincidence with former malaria areas in mainland Portugal. *Geospatial Health* Vol.3, No.2, (May 2009), pp. 177-187, ISSN 1827-1987.

Carnevale, P. & Robert, V. (2009). *Les anophèles: Biologie, transmission du Plasmodium et lutte antivectorielle*, Bondy, IRD, ISBN 978-2-7099-1662-2, Montpellier, France.

Chalumeau, M.; Holvoet, L.; Chéron, G.; Minodier, P.; Foix-L'Hélias, L.; Ovetchkine, P.; Moulin, F.; Nouyrigat, V.; Bréart, G. & Gendrel, D. (2006). Delay in diagnosis of imported *Plasmodium falciparum* malaria in children. *European Journal of Clinical Microbiology & Infectious Diseases*, Vol.25, No.3, (March 2006), pp. 186-189, ISSN 0934-9723.

Chang, L.H.; Hsu, E.L.; Teng, H.J. & Ho C.M. (2007). Differential survival of *Aedes aegypti* and *Aedes albopictus* (Diptera: Culicidae) larvae exposed to low temperatures in Taiwan. *Journal of Medical Entomology*, vol.44, No.2, (March 2007), pp. 205-210, ISSN 0022-2585.

Christopher, S.R. (1960). *Aëdes aegypti (L.) the yellow fever mosquito, its life history, bionomics and structure*, Cambridge University Press, New York, United States of America..

Ciuca, M. (1966). *L'eradication de Paludisme en Roumanie.* Editions Medicales, Bucarest, Romania.

Clavero, G. & Romeo Viamonte, J.M. (1948). El paludismo en las huertas de Murcia y Orihuela. Ensayos de aplicación de los insecticidas modernos, D.D.T. y 666, en la lucha antipalúdica. *Revista de Sanidad e Higiene Pública* Vol. 22, pp. 199-228, ISSN 0034-8899.

Cobelens, F.G.; Groen, J.; Osterhaus, A.D.; Leentvaar-Kuipers, A.; Wertheim-Van Dillen, P.M. & Kager, P.A. (2002). Incidence and risk factors of probable dengue virus infection among Dutch travellers to Asia. *Tropical Medicine and International Health*, Vol.7, No.4, (April 2002), pp. 331-338, ISSN 1360-2276.

Constantinescu, P. & Negulici, E. (1967). The experimental transmission of *Plasmodium malariae* to *Anopheles labranchiae atroparvus. Transactions of the Royal Society of Tropical Medicine and Hygiene*, Vol.61, No.2, pp. 182-188, ISSN 0035-9203.

Cuadros, J.; Calvente, M.J.; Benito, A.; Arévalo, J.; Calero, M.A.; Segura J. & Rubio, J.M. (2002). *Plasmodium ovale* Malaria acquired in Central Spain. *Emerging Infectious Diseases*, Vol.8, No.12, (December 2002), pp. 1506-1508, ISSN 1080-6040.

Dahl, C. (1997). *Diptera Culicidae, Mosquitoes.* In: *Aquatic Insects of northern Europe-A Taxonomic Handbook.* Vol.II, Nilsson, A.N. (Eds.), 163-186, Apollo Books, ISBN 8788757552, Stenstrup, Denmark.

Delaunay, P.; Mathieu, B.; Marty, P.; Fauran, P. & Schaffner, F. (2007). Historique de l' installation d'*Aedes albopictus* dans les Alpes-Maritimes (France) de 2002 à 2005. *Medecine tropicale*, Vol.67, No.3, (June 2007), pp. 310-311. ISSN 0025-682X.

Delmont, J.; Brouqui, P.; Poullin, P. & Bourgeade, A. (1994). Harbour-acquired *Plasmodium falciparum* malaria. *The Lancet*, Vol.344, No. 8918, (July 1994), pp. 330–331, ISSN 0140-6736.

Detinova, T.S. (1953). Age composition and epidemiological importance of the population of Anopheles maculipennis in the Province of Moscow. *Meditsinskaya Parazitologiya i Parazitarnie Bolezni*, Vol.22, pp. 486-495.

Doudier, B.; Bogreau, H.; De Vries, A.; Ponçon, N.; Stauffer, W.M. & Fontenille, D. (2007). Possible autochthonous malaria from Marseille to Minneapolis. *Emerging Infectious Diseases*, Vol.13, No.8, (August 2007), pp. 1236-1238, ISSN 1080-6059.

Eager JM. (1902). Yellow fever in France, Italy, Great Britain and Austria and bibliography of yellow fever in Europe. *Yellow Fever Institute Bulletin*, Vol.8, pp. 25-35.

European Center of Disease Control (ECDC). *EWRS Message: ID: 20100924FR0001*. 2010, Accessed 14th March 2011 Available online in: https://ewrs.ecdc.europa.eu/Pages/Secure/Messages/ViewMessage.aspx?id=201 00924FR0001

European Center of Disease Control (ECDC). *Development of Aedes albopictus risk maps*. 2009, Accessed 14th March 2011 Available online in: http://ecdc.europa.eu/en/publications/Publications/0905_TER_Development_of _Aedes_Albopictus_Risk_Maps.pdf

Ekblom, T. & Ströman, R. (1932). Geographical and biological studies of *Anopheles maculipennis* in Sweden from an epidemiological point of view. *Kungliga Svenska Vetenskapsakademiens handling*, Vol.11, No.1, pp. 1-113.

Eling, W.; Van Gemert, G.J.; Akinpelu, O.; Curtis, J. & Curtis, C.F. (2003). Production of *Plasmodium falciparum* sporozoites by *Anopheles plumbeus*. *European Mosquito Bulletin*, Vol.15, (June 2003), pp. 12-13, ISSN 1460-6127.

Encinas Grandes, A. (1982). *Taxonomía y biología de los mosquitos del área salmantina (Diptera, Culicidae)*, Universidad de Salamanca, ISBN 8400050673, Salamanca, Spain.

Eritja, R.; Aranda, C.; Padrós, J.; Goula, M.; Lucientes, J.; Escosa, R.; Marquès, E. & Cáceres, F. (2000). An annotated checklist and bibliography of the mosquitoes of Spain (Diptera: Culicidae). *European Mosquito Bulletin*, Vol.8, (November 2008), pp. 10-18, ISSN 1460-6127.

Estrada-Franco, J.G. and Craig, G.B. (1995). *Biology, disease relationships, and control of Aedes albopictus*, Pan American Health Organization, ISBN 9275130426, Washington, United States of America.

European Mosquito Taxonomists (MOTAX). *Chart of European Mosquitoes*. 2010, Accessed 14th March 2011 Available online in: http://www.sove.org/motax/chart.htm

European Network on Imported Infectious Disease Surveillance (TropNetEurop). *Friend and observers Sentinel Surveillance Report*. 2010, Accessed 14th March 2011 Available online in: http://www.tropnet.net/reports_friends/reports_friends_index.html

Faraj, C.; Ouahabi, S.; Adlaoui, E.; Boccolini, D.; Romi, R. & El Aouad, R. (2008). Risque de réémergence du paludisme au Maroc étude de la capacité vectorielle d'*Anopheles labranchiae* dans une zone rizicole au nord du pays. *Parasite,* Vol.15, No.4, (December 2008), pp. 605–610, ISSN 1252-607X.

Farrar, J. (2008). *Clinical features of dengue.* In: *Dengue,* Halstead, S.B. (Ed.), 171-191, Imperial College Press, ISBN: 978-1-84816-228-0, London, United Kingdom.

Frizzi, G.; Rinaldi, A. & Bianchi, L. (1975). Genetic studies on mechanisms influencing the susceptibility of Anopheline mosquitoes to plasmodial infections. *Mosquito News,* Vol.35, No.4, (December 1975), pp. 505-508, ISSN 0027-142X.

Garnham, P.C.C.; Bray, R.S.; Cooper, W.; Lainson, R.; Awad, F.I. & Williamson, J. (1954). Pre-erythrocytic stages of human malaria: *Plasmodium ovale. Transactions of the Royal Society of Tropical Medicine and Hygiene,* Vol.49, No.1, (January 1954), pp. 158-167, ISSN 0035-9203.

Garnham, P.C.C. (1988). *Malaria parasites of man: life-cycles and morphology (excluding ultrastructure).* In *Malaria: principles and practice of malariology,* Wernsdorfer W.H. & McGregor, I. (Ed), Vol. I, 61-96, Churchill Livingstone, ISBN 0443024170, Edinburgh, United Kingdom.

Garrett-Jones, C. (1964). Prognosis for Interruption of Malaria Transmission Through Assessment of the Mosquito's Vectorial Capacity. *Nature* Vol.204, (December 1964), pp. 1173-1175, ISSN 0028-0836.

Gascón, J. (2006). Paludismo importado por inmigrantes. *Anales del Sistema Sanitario de Navarra,* Vol.29, No.1, (January 2006), pp. 121-125, ISSN 1137-6627.

Githeko, A.K. (2006). *Entomological correlates of epidemiological impacts: how do we know it is working?* In: *Bridging Laboratory and Field Research for Genetic Control of Disease Vectors,* Knols, B.G.J., Louis, C. & Bogers, R.J. (Eds.), 215-219, Springer, ISBN 1-4020-3799-6, Dordrecht, Netherlands.

Gjenero-Margan, I.; Aleraj, B.; Krajcar, D.; Lesnikar, V.; Klobučar, A.; Pem-Novosel, I.; Kurečić-Filipović, S.; Komparak, S.; Martić, R.; Đuričić, S.; Betica-Radić, L.; Okmadžić, J.; Vilibić-Čavlek, T.; Babić-Erceg, A.; Turković, B.; Avšić-Županc, T.; Radić, I.; Ljubić, M.; Šarac, K.; Benić, N. & Mlinarić-Galinović, G. (2011). Autochthonous dengue fever in Croatia, August–September 2010. *Euro Surveillance,* Vol.16, No.9, (March 2011), ISSN 1560-7917, Accessed 14th March 2011, Available online in:
http://www.eurosurveillance.org/ViewArticle.aspx?ArticleId=19805

Gratz, N.G. (2004). Critical review of the vector status of *Aedes albopictus. Medical and Veterinary Entomology,* Vol.18, No.3, (September 2004), pp. 215–227, ISSN 0269-283X.

Gutsevich, A.V.; Monchadskii, A.S. & Shtakelberg, A.A. (1974). *Fauna of the USSR. Diptera. Mosquitoes. Family Culicidae.* Vol.3, No.4., Keter Publishing House Jerusalem Ltd, ISBN 7065 1475, Jerusalem, Israel.

Hackett, L.W. (1937). *Malaria in Europe: An Ecological Study.* Oxford University Press, London, United Kingdom.

Hackett, L.W. & Missiroli, A. (1935). The varieties of *Anopheles maculipennis* and their relation to the distribution of malaria in Europe. *Rivista di Malariologia,* Vol.14, pp. 45-109, ISSN 0370-565X.

Hadjinicolaou, J. & Betzios, B. (1973). Resurgence of *Anopheles sacharovi* following malaria eradication. *Bulletin of the World Health Organization,* Vol.48, No.6, pp. 699-703, ISSN 0042-9686.

Hawley, W.A. (1988). The biology of Aedes albopictus. Journal of the American Mosquito Control Association, Vol.4, No.1, (March 1988), pp. 1–39, ISSN 1046-3607.

Horsfall, W.R. (1972). Mosquitoes: their bionomics and relation to disease. Hafner, New York, United States of America.

Huldén, L.; Huldén, L. & Heliövaara, K. (2005). Endemic malaria: an 'indoor' disease in northern Europe. Historical data analysed. Malaria Journal, Vol.4, No.4, (April 2005), ISSN 1475-2875, Accessed 14th March 2011 Available online in: http://www.malariajournal.com/content/4/1/19

Imai, C. & Maeda, O. (1976). Several factors effecting on hatching on Aedes albopictus eggs. Japanese Journal of Sanitary Zoology, Vol.27, pp. 363-372, ISSN 0424-7086.

Jaenson, T.G.T.; Lokki, J.; Saura, A. (1986). Anopheles (Diptera: Culicidae) and malaria in Northern Europe, with special reference to Sweden. Journal of Medical Entomology, Vol.23, No.1, (January 1986), pp. 68-75, ISSN 0022-2585.

James, S.P. (1917). Note recording the proof that Anopheles maculipennis is an efficient host of the benign tertian malaria parasite in England. Journal of the Royal Army Medical Corps, Vol.29, pp. 615, ISSN 0035-8665.

James, S.P.; Nicol, W.D. & Shute, P.G. (1932). P. ovale passage through mosquitoes and successful transmission by their bites. Annals of Tropical Medicine and Parasitology, Vol.26, pp. 139-145, ISSN 0003-4983.

Jetten, T.H. & Takken, W. (1994). Anophelism Without Malaria in Europe: A review of the ecology and distribution of the genus Anopheles in Europe. Wageningen Agricultural University Papers, Wageningen, The Netherlands, ISBN 906754373X.

Kampen, H.; Maltezos, E.; Pagonaki, M.; Hunfeld, K.P.; Maier W.A. & Seitz, H.M. (2002). Individual cases of autochthonous malaria in Evros Province, northern Greece: serological aspects. Parasitology Research, Vol.88, No.3, (March 2002), pp. 261-266, ISSN 0932-0113.

Kasap, H. (1990). Comparison of experimental infectivity and development of Plasmodium vivax in Anopheles sacharovi and An. superpictus in Turkey. American Journal of Tropical Medicine and Hygiene, Vol.42, No.2, (February 1990), pp. 111-117, ISSN 0002-9637.

Kasap, H.; Kasap, M.; Alptekin, D.; Lüleyap, U. & Herath, P.R.J. (2000). Insecticide resistance in Anopheles sacharovi Favre in southern Turkey. Bulletin of the World Health Organization, Vol.78, No.5, pp. 686-692, ISSN 0042-9686.

Kenawy, M.A.; Beier, J.C.; Asiago, C.M.: Said el S.E. & Roberts C.R. (1990). Interpretation of low-level Plasmodium infection rates determined by ELISA for anophelines (Diptera: Culicidae) from Egyptian oases. Journal of Medical Entomology, Vol.27, No.4, (July 1990), pp. 681-685, ISSN 0022-2585.

Kettle, D.S. (1995). Medical and veterinary entomology. 2nd edition. CAB International, ISBN: 0-851-98968-3, Cambridge, United Kingdom.

King, W.L.; Bradley, G.H.; Smith, C.N. & McDuffie, W.C. (1960). A handbook of the mosquitoes of the southeastern United States. Handbook 173. US Department of Agriculture, Washington, United States of America.

Kirchberg, E. & Mamlok, E. (1946). Malariabekämpfung in Berlin im Jahre 1946. Ärztl Wochenschr, Vol.1, pp. 119–122, ISSN 0365-6403.

Kiszewski, A.; Mellinger, A.; Spielman, A.; Malaney, P.; Sachs, S.E. & Sachs, J. (2004). Global Index. Representing the Stability of Malaria Transmission. American Journal of

Tropical Medicine and Hygiene, Vol.70, No.5, (May 2004), pp. 486-498, ISSN 0002-9637.

Klobucar, A.; Merdic, E.; Benic, N.; Baklaic, Z. & Krcmar, S. (2006). First record of *Aedes albopictus* in Croatia. *Journal of the American Mosquito Control Association*, Vol.22, No.1, (March 2006), pp. 147-148, ISSN 1046-3607.

Korovitzkyi, L.K. & Artemenko, V.D. (1933). Zur Biologie des *Aedes aegypti*. *Magasin de parasitologie de l'Institut zoologique de l'Acad'emie des Sciences de l'URSS*, Vol.2, pp. 400-406.

Krüger, A.; Rech, A.; Su, X.Z. & Tannich, E. (2001). Two cases of autochthonous *Plasmodium falciparum* malaria in Germany with evidence for local transmission by indigenous *Anopheles plumbeus*. *Tropical Medicine & International Health*, Vol.6, No.12, (December 2001), pp. 983-985, ISSN 1360-2276.

Kuhn, K.G.; Campbell-Lendrum, D.H. & Davies, C.R. (2002). A continental risk map for malaria mosquito (Diptera: Culicidae) vectors in Europe. *Journal of Medical Entomology*, Vol.39, No.4, (June 2002), pp. 621-630, ISSN 0022-2585.

Houel, G. & Donadille, F. (1953). Vingt ans de lutte antipaludique au Maroc. *Bulletin de l'Institut d'Hygiène du Maroc*, Vol.13, pp. 3–51.

La Ruche, G.; Souarès, Y.; Armengaud, A.; Peloux-Petiot, F.; Delaunay, P.; Desprès, P.; Lenglet, A.; Jourdain, F.; Leparc-Goffart, I.; Charlet, F.; Ollier, L.; Mantey, K.; Mollet, T.; Fournier, J.P.; Torrents, R.; Leitmeyer, K.; Hilairet, P.; Zeller, H.; Van Bortel, W.; Dejour-Salamanca, D.; Grandadam, M. & Gastellu-Etchegorry, M. (2010). First two autochthonous dengue virus infections in metropolitan France, September 2010. *Euro Surveillance*, Vol.15, No.39, (September 2010), ISSN 1560-7917, Accessed 14th March 2011, Available online in:
http://www.eurosurveillance.org/ViewArticle.aspx?ArticleId=19676

Leder, K.; Tong, S.; Weld, L.; Kain, K.C.; Wilder-Smith, A.; von Sonnenburg, F.; Black, J.; Grown, G.V. & Torresi, J. (2006). Ilness in travelers visiting friends and relatives: a review of the GeoSentinel Surveillance Network. *Clinical Infectious Diseases*, Vol.43, No.9, (November 2006), pp. 1185-1193, ISSN 1058-4838.

Lewis, D.J. (1943). Mosquitoes in relation to yellow fever in the Nuba Mountains Anglo-Egyptian Sudan. *Annals of Tropical Medicine and Parasitology*, Vol37, No.1, pp. 65-76, ISSN 0003-4983.

Linton, Y.M.; Lee, A.S. & Curtis, C. (2005). Discovery of a third member of the Maculipennis Group in SW England. *European Mosquito Bulletin*, Vol.19, (April 2005), pp. 5-9, ISSN 1460-6127.

Lokki, J.; Saura, A.; Korvenkontio, P. & Ulmanen, I. (1979). Diagnosing adult *Anopheles* mosquitoes. *Aquilo Seriologica Zoologica*, Vol.20, pp. 5-12.

Lozano Morales, A. (1946). Contribución al estudio de la biología del *A. maculipennis var. atroparvus* en función del ambiente. *Revista de Sanidad e Higiene Pública*, Vol.20, pp. 239-250, ISSN 0034-8899.

Luchavez, J.; Espino, F.; Curameng, P.; Espina, R.; Bell, D.; Chiodini, P.; Nolder, D.; Sutherland, C.; Lee, K.S. & Singh, B. (2008). Human Infections with *Plasmodium knowlesi*, the Philippines. *Emerging Infectious Diseases* Vol.14, No.5, (May 2008), pp. 811-813, ISSN 1080-6040.

MacDonald, G. (1957). *The epidemiology and control of malaria*. Oxford University Press, London, United Kingdom.

Madon, M.B.; Mulla, M.S.; Shaw, M.W.; Kluh, S. & Hazelrigg, J.E. (2002). Introduction of *Aedes albopictus* (Skuse) in southern California and potential for its establishment. *Journal of Vector Ecology*, Vol.27, No.1, (June 2002), pp. 149-154, ISSN 1081-1710.

Majori, G.; Maroli, M.; Bettini, S. & Pierdominici, G. (1970). Osservazioni sull'anofelismo residuo nel Grossetano. *Rivista di Parassitologia*, Vol.31, No.2, pp. 147-154, ISSN 0035-6387.

Manouchehri, A.V.; Zaim, M. & Emadi, A.M. (1992). A review of malaria in Iran, 1975–90. *Journal of the American Mosquito Control Association*, Vol.8, No.4, (December 1992), pp. 381-385, ISSN 1046-3607.

Marchant, P.; Rling, W.; Van Gemert, G.J.; Leake, C.J. & Curtis, C.F. (1998). Could British mosquitoes transmit falciparum malaria? *Parasitology Today*, Vol.14, No.9, (September 1998), pp. 344-345, ISSN 0169-4758.

Margarita, Y., Santos Grácio, A.J.; Lencastre, I.; Silva, A.C.; Novo, T.; Sousa, C.; Almeida, A.P.G. & Biscoito, M.J. (2006). Mosquitos de Portugal: primeiro registo de *Aedes (Stegomia) aegypti* Linnaeus, 1762 (Diptera, Culicidae) na Ilha da Madeira. *Acta Parasitológica Portuguesa*, Vol. 13, No.1, pp. 59-61, ISSN 0872-5292.

Mavale, M.S.; Ilkal, M.A. & Dhanda, V. (1992). Experimental studies on the susceptibility of *Aedes vittatus* to dengue viruses. *Acta Virologica*, Vol.36, No.3, (August 1992), pp. 412–416, ISSN 0001-723X.

Monath, T.P. (2006). Yellow fever as an endemic/epidemic disease and priorities for vaccination. *Bulletin de la Societe de Pathologie Exotique*, Vol.99, No.5, (December 2006), pp. 341-347, ISSN 0037-9085.

Moore, C.G. & Mitchell, C.J. (1997). *Aedes albopictus* in the United States: ten-years presence and public health implications. *Emerging Infectious Diseases*, Vol.3,No.3, (July 1997), pp. 329–334, ISSN 1080-6059.

Mori, A.; Oda, T. & Wada, Y. (1981). Studies on the egg diapause and overwintering of *Aedes albopictus* in Nagasaki. *Tropical Medicine*, Vol.23, No.2, (June 1981), pp. 79-90, ISSN 0385-5643.

Mourya, D.T. & Banerjee, K. (1987). Experimental transmission of chikungunya virus by *Aedes vittatus* mosquitoes. *Indian Journal of Medical Research*, Vol.86, (August 1987), pp. 269–271, ISSN 0971-5916.

Nayar, J.K. & Knight, J.W. (1999). *Aedes albopictus* (Diptera: Culicidae): an experimental and natural host of *Dirofilaria immitis* (Filarioidea: Onchocercidae) in Florida, U.S.A. *Journal OF Medical Entomology*, Vol.36, No.4, (July 1999), pp. 441–448, ISSN 0022-2585.

Nikolaeva, N. (1996). Resurgence of malaria in the former Soviet Union (FSU). Society of Vector Ecology News, Vol.27, pp. 10–11.

Nicolescu, G. (1996). George Zotta (1886-1942). An early concept of malaria stratification. *Romanian Archives of Microbiology and Immunology*, Vol.55, No.2, (April 1996), pp. 173-79, ISSN 1222-3891.

Nicolescu, G.; Linton, Y.M.; Vladimirescu, A.; Howard, T.M. & Harbach, R.E. (2004). Mosquitoes of the *An. maculipennis* group (Diptera; Culicidae) in Romania, with the discovery and formal recognition of a new species based on molecular and morphological evidence. *Bulletin of Entomological Research*, Vol.94, No.6, (December 2004), pp. 525-535, ISSN 0007-4853.

Olavarria, J. & Hill, R.B. (1935). Algunos datos sobre las preferencias hemáticas de las *A. maculipennis*. *Medicina de los Países Cálidos*, Vol.8, pp. 169–173.

Papaevangelou, G. & Halstead, S.B. (1977). Infections with two dengue viruses in Greece in the 20th century. Did dengue hemorrhagic fever occur in the 1928 epidemic? *Journal of Tropical Medicine & Hygiene*, Vol.80, No.3, (March 1977), pp. 46-51, ISSN 0022-5304.

Paupy, C.; Delatte, H.; Bagny, L.; Corbel, V. & Fontenille, D. (2009). *Aedes albopictus*, an arbovirus vector: From the darkness to the light. *Microbes and Infection*, Vol.11, No.14-15, (December 2009), pp. 1177-1185, ISSN 1286-4579.

Ponçon, N.; Toty, C.; L'Ambert, G.; Le Goff, G.; Brengues, C.; Schaffner, F. & Fontenille, D. (2007). Biology and dynamics of potential malaria vectors in Southern France. *Malaria Journal*, Vol.6, No.18 (February 2007), ISSN 1475-2875, Accessed 14th March 2011, Available online in: http://www.malariajournal.com/content/6/1/18

Postiglione, M., Tabanli, B. & Ramsdale, C.D. (1973). The Anopheles of Turkey. *Rivista di Parassitologia*, Vol.34, No.2, pp. 127-159. ISSN 0035-6387.

Ramsdale, C.D. & Coluzzi, M. (1975). Studies on the infectivity of tropical African strains of *Plasmodium falciparum* to some southern European vectors of malaria. *Parassitologia*, Vol.17, No.1-3, (January-December 1975), pp. 39-48, ISSN 0048-2951.

Ramsdale, C. & Snow, K. (2000). Distribution of the genus Anopheles in Europe. *European Mosquito Bulletin*, Vol.7, (July 2000), pp. 1-26, ISSN 1460-6127.

Ravi, V. (2006). Re-emergence of Chikungunya virus in India. *Indian journal of medical microbiology*, Vol.24, No.2, (April 2006), pp. 83-84, ISSN 0255-0857.

Reiter, P. & Sprenger, D. (1987). The used tire trade: a mechanism for the worldwide dispersal of container breeding mosquitoes. *Journal of the American Mosquito Control Association*, Vol.3, No.3, (September 1987), pp. 494-501, ISSN 1046-3607.

Reiter. P. (2010). Yellow fever and dengue: a threat to Europe? *Euro Surveillance*, Vol.15, No.10, (March 2010), ISSN 1560-7917, Accessed 14th March 2011, Available online in: http://www.eurosurveillance.org/ViewArticle.aspx?ArticleId=19509

Rezza, G.; Nicoletti, L.; Angelini, Romi, R.; Finarelli A.C.; Panning, M.; Cordioli, P.; Fortuna, C.; Boros, S.; Magurano, F.; Silvi, G.; Angelini, P.; Dottori, M.; Ciufolini, M.G.; Majori, G.C. & Cassone, A.. (2007). Infection with chikungunya virus in Italy: an outbreak in a temperate region. *The Lancet*, Vol.370, No.9602, (December 2007), pp. 1840-1846, ISSN 0140-6736.

Ribeiro, H.; Batista, J.L.; Ramos, H.C.; Pires, C.A.; Champalimaud, J.L.; Costa, J.M.; Araújo, C.; Mansinho, K. & Pina, M.C. (1989). An attempt to infect *Anopheles atroparvus* from Portugal with African *Plasmodium falciparum*. *Revista Portuguesa de Doenças Infecciosas*, Vol.12, pp. 81-82, ISSN 1646-3633.

Ribeiro, H. & Ramos, H.C. (1999). Identification keys of the mosquitoes of Continental Portugal, Açores and Madeira. *European Mosquito Bulletin*, Vol.3, (January 1999), pp. 1-11, ISSN 1460-6127.

Rioux, J.A. (1958). *Les Culicidés du Midi méditerranéen. Encyclopédie Entomologique XXXV*. Paul Lechevalier, Paris, France.

Romi, R. (1999). *Anopheles labranchiae*, an important malaria vector in Italy, and other potential malaria vectors in Southern Europe. *European Mosquito Bulletin*, Vol.4, (June), pp. 8-10, ISSN 1460-6127.

Romi, R.; Severini, C.; Cocchi, M.; Tamburro, A.; Menichetti, D.; Pierdominici, G. & Majori, G. (1992). Anofelismo residuo in Italia: distribuzione nelle aree risicole delle provincie di Grosseto e Siena. *Annali Dell Istituto Superiore Sanita*, Vol.28, No.4, (December 1992), pp. 527-531, ISSN 0021-2571.

Romi, R.; Pierdominici, G.; Severini, C.; Tamburro, A.; Cocchi, M.; Menichetti, D.; Pili, E. & Marchi, A. (1997). Status of malaria vectors in Italy. *Journal of Medical Entomology*, Vol.34, No.3, (May 1997), pp. 263-271, ISSN 0022-2585.

Romi, R.; Sabatinelli, G.; Giannuzzi Savelli, L.; Raris, M.; Zago, M. & Malatesta, R. (1997). Identification of a North American mosquito species, *Aedes atropalpus* (Diptera: Culicidae), in Italy. *Journal of the American Mosquito Control Association*, Vol.13, No.3, (September 1997), pp. 245-246, ISSN 1046-3607.

Romi, R.; Sabatinelli, G. & Majori, G. (2001). Could malaria reappear in Italy? *Emerging Infectious Diseases*, Vol.7, No.6, (June 2001), pp. 915-919, ISSN 1080-6059.

Rosen, L. (1986). Dengue in Greece in 1927 and 1928 and the pathogenesis of dengue hemorrhagic fever: new data and a different conclusion. *American Journal of Tropical Medicine and Hygiene*, Vol.35, No.3, (May 1986), pp. 642-653, ISSN 0002-9637.

Roubaud, E.; Colas-Belcour, J. & Stefanopoulo, G. (1937). Transmission de fièvre jaune rar un moustique paléarctique répandu dans la region parisiennes, l'*Aedes geniculatus* Olivier. *Compte Rendus Hebdomadaires des Seances de l'Academie des Sciences*, Vol.202, pp. 182-183, ISSN 0567-655X.

Sabatini, A.; Raineri, V.; Trovato, G. & Coluzzi, M. (1990). Aedes albopictus in Italia e possible diffusione del la especie nell' area mediterranea. *Parassitologiu*, Vol.32, No.3, (December 1990), pp. 301-304, ISSN 0048-2951.

Sainz-Elipe, S.; Latorre, J.M.; Escosa, R.; Masià, M.; Fuentes, M.V.; Mas-Coma, S.; Bargues, M.T. (2010). Malaria resurgence risk in southern Europe: climate assessment in an historically endemic area of rice fields at the Mediterranean shore of Spain. *Malaria Journal*, Vol.9, No.7, (July 2010), ISSN 1475-2875, Accessed 14th March 2011. Available online in: http://www.malariajournal.com/content/9/1/221

Santa-Olalla Peralta, P.; Vazquez-Torres, M.C.; Latorre-Fandós, E.; Mairal-Claver, P.; Cortina-Solano, P.; Puy-Azón, A.; Adiego Sancho, B.; Leitmeyer, K.; Lucientes-Curdi, J. & Sierra-Moros, M.J. (2010). First autochthonous malaria case due to *Plasmodium vivax* since eradication, Spain, October 2010. *Euro Surveillance*, Vol.15, No.41, (October 2010), ISSN 1560-7917, Accessed 14th March 2011. Available online in: http://www.eurosurveillance.org/ViewArticle.aspx?ArticleId=19684

Sardelis, M.R. & Turell, M.J. (2001). *Ochlerotatus j. japonicus* in Frederick County, Maryland: discovery, distribution, and vector competence for West Nile virus. *Journal of the American Mosquito Control Association*, Vol.17, No.2, (June 2011), pp. 137-141, ISSN 1046-3607.

Sardelis, M.R.; Dohm, D.J.; Pagac, B.; Andre, R.G. & Turell, M.J. (2002a). Experimental transmission of eastern equine encephalitis virus by *Ochlerotatus j. japonicus* (Diptera: Culicidae). *Journal of Medical Entomology*, Vol.39, No.3, (May 2002), pp. 480-484, ISSN 0022-2585.

Sardelis, M.R.; Turell, M.J. & Andre, R.G. (2002b). Laboratory transmission of La Crosse virus by *Ochlerotatus j. japonicus* (Diptera: Culicidae). *Journal of Medical Entomology*, Vol.39, No.4, (July 2002), pp. 635-639, ISSN 0022-2585.

Sardelis, M.R., Turell, MJ. & Andre, R.G. (2003). Experimental transmission of St. Louis encephalitis virus by *Ochlerotatus j. japonicus*. *Journal of the American Mosquito Control Association*, Vol.19, No.2, (June 2003), pp. 159–162, ISSN 1046-3607.

Satti, M.H. & Haseeb, M.A. (1966). An outbreak of yellow fever in the Southern Fung and Upper Nile province, Republic of the Sudan. *Journal of Tropical Medicine and Hygiene*, Vol.69, No.1, pp. 36-44, ISSN 0022-5304.

Sautet, J. & Quilici, R. (1971). A propos de quelques cas de paludisme autochtone contractés en France pendant l'été. *Presse Médicale*, Vol.79, pp. 524, ISSN 0755-4982.

Schaffner, F.; Angel, G.; Geoffroy, B.; Hervy, J.O. & Rhaeim, A. (2001). The mosquitoes of Europe / Les moustiques d' Europe [CD-ROM]. IRD Éditions and EID Méditerranée, Montpellier, France.

Schafther, F.; Chouin, S. & Guilloteau, J. (2003). First record of *Ochlerotatus (Finlaya) japonicus japonicas* (Theobald, 1901) in metropolitan France. *Journal of the American Mosquito Control Association*, Vol.19, No.1, (March 2003), pp. 1-5, ISSN 1046-3607.

Schaffner, F., Kaufmann, C. &Mathis, A. (2009). The invasive mosquito *Aedes japonicus* in Central Europe. *Medical and Veterinary Entomology*, Vol.23, No.4, (December 2009), pp. 448-451, ISSN 0269-283X.

Schmidt-Chanasit, J.; Haditsch, M.; Schöneberg, I.; Günther, S.; Stark, K. & Frank, C. (2010). Dengue virus infection in a traveller returning from Croatia to Germany. *Euro Surveillance*, Vol.15, No.40, (October 2010), ISSN 1560-7917, Accessed 14th March 2011. Available online in:
http://www.eurosurveillance.org/ViewArticle.aspx?ArticleId=19677

Scholte, E.J.; Den Hartog, W.; Braks, M.; Reusken, C.; Dik, M. & Hessels, A. (2009). First report of a North American invasive mosquito species *Ochlerotatus atropalpus* (Coquillett) in the Netherlands, 2009. Euro Surveillance, Vol.14, No.45, (November 2009), ISSN 1560-7917, Accessed 14th March 2011. Available online in:
http://www.eurosurveillance.org/ViewArticle.aspx?ArticleId=19400

Scholte, E.J.; Den Hartog, W.; Dik, M.; Schoelitsz, B.; Brooks, M.; Schaffner, F.; Foussadier, R.; Braks, M. & Beeuwkes, J. (2010). Introduction and control of three invasive mosquito species in the Netherlands, July-October 2010. *Euro Surveillance*, Vol.15, No.45, (November 2010) ISSN 1560-7917, Accessed 14th March 2011. Available online in:
http://www.eurosurveillance.org/ViewArticle.aspx?ArticleId=19710

Senevet, G.; Andarelli, L. & Adda, R. (1955). Presence of *Anopheles plumbeus* St. in Algerian shores. *Archives de l'Institut Pasteur d'Algérie*, Vol.33, No.2, (June 1955), pp. 138-139, ISSN 0020-2460.

Sepulcri, P. *La malaria nel Veneto.* (1963). Istituto Interprovinciale per la Lotta Antimalarica nelle Venezie, Venice, Italy

Shute, P.G. (1954). Indigenous *P. vivax* malaria in London believed to have been transmitted by *An. plumbeus. Monthly Bulletin of the Ministry of Health and the Public Health Laboratory Service*, Vol.13, pp. 48-51, ISSN: 0368- 881X.

Shute, P. & Maryon, M. (1969). Imported Malaria in the United Kingdom. *British Medical Journal*, Vol.28, (June 1969), pp. 781–785, ISSN 0959-8138.

Shute, P. & Maryon, M. (1974). Malaria in England past, present and future. *Journal of the Royal Society of Health*, Vol.94, (February 1974), No.1, pp. 23-29, ISSN 1466-4240.

Snow, K. & Ramsdale, C. (1999). Distribution chart for European mosquitoes. *European Mosquito Bulletin*, Vol.3, (January 1999), pp. 14-31, ISSN 1460-6127.

Tavşanoğlu, N. & Çağlar, S.S. (2008). The vectorial capacity of *Anopheles sacharovi* in the malaria endemic area of Şanlıurfa, Turkey. *European Mosquito Bulletin*, Vol. 26, (December 2008), pp. 18-23, ISSN 1460-6127.

Teodorescu C. (1983). Experimental infection of an indigenous strain of *Anopheles atroparvus* with imported species of *Plasmodium*. *Archives roumaines de pathologie experimentale et de microbiologie*, Vol.42, No.4, (October 1983), pp. 365-370, ISSN 0004-0037.

Torres Cañamares, F. (1934). Observaciones sobre los *A. maculipennis* y sus razas en Camporredondo (Jaén). *Medicina de los Países Cálidos*, Vol.7, (February 1934), pp. 53-72.

Toty, C.; Barré, H.; Le Goff, G.; Larget-Thiéry, I.; Rahola, N.; Couret, D. & Fontenille, D. (2010). Malaria risk in Corsica, former hot spot of malaria in France. *Malaria Journal*, Vol.9, No.8, (August 2010), ISSN: 1475-2875, Accessed 14th March 2011 Available online in: http://www.malariajournal.com/content/9/1/231

Tovornik, D. (1978). An atypical breeding place of the *Anopheles plumbeus* Stephens, 1828, in an unfinished house. *Biološki vestnik*, Vol.26, pp. 41-46, ISSN 0502-1969

Turell, M.J.; O'Guinn, M.L.; Dohm, D.J. & Jones, J.W. (2001). Vector competence of North American mosquitoes (Diptera: Culicidae) for West Nile virus. *Journal of Medical Entomology*, vol.38, No.2, (March 2001), pp. 130-134, ISSN 0022-2585.

Utrio, P. (1979). Geographic distribution of mosquitoes (Diptera, Culicidae) in eastern Fennoscandia. *Notulae Entomologicae*, Vol.59, pp. 105-123, ISSN 0029-4594.

Wang, K.C. (1966). Observations on the influence of photoperiod on egg diapause in *Aedes albopictus*. Acta Entomologica Sinica, Vol.15, pp. 75-77 ISSN 0970-3721

White, G.B. (1978). Systematic reappraisal of the *Anopheles maculipennis complex*. *Mosquito Systematics*, Vol.7, No.1, (January 1978), pp. 303-344, ISSN 0091-3669.

World Health Organization (WHO). *Malaria*. Fact sheet N° 94, May 2007, Accessed 14th March 2011 Available online in:
http://www.who.int/mediacentre/factsheets/fs094/en/print.html/

World Health Organization (WHO), Regional Office for Europe. (n.d.). *Centralized information system for infectious diseases (CISID) database. Malaria.*, Accessed 14th February 2011, Available online in: http://data.euro.who.int/cisid/

Yergolkar, P.N; Tandale, B.V.; Arankalle, V.A.; Sathe, P.S.; Sudeep, A.B.; Gandhe, S.S.; Gokhle, M.D.; Jacob, G.P.; Hundekar, S.L. & Mishra, A.C. (2006). Chikungunya outbreaks caused by African genotype, India, *Emerging Infectious Diseases*, Vol.12, No.10, (October 2006), pp. 1580–1583, ISSN 1080-6040.

Zahar, A.R. (1987). *Vector bionomics in the epidemiology and control of malaria. Part II: The WHO European Region and the WHO Eastern Mediterranean Region*. VBC/88.5. World Health Organization, Geneva, Switzerland. Accessed 14th March 2011 Available online in: http://whqlibdoc.who.int/hq/1990/VBC_90.1_eng.pdf

Zaim, M. (1987). Malaria control in Iran: present and future. *Journal of the American Mosquito Control Association*, Vol.3, No.3, (September 1987), pp. 392-396, ISSN 1046-3607.

Zotta, G. (1938). Contribution à l'etude de la distribution des races d'*A. maculipennis* en Roumanie. *Archives Roumaines de Pathologie Experimentale et de Microbiologie*, Vol.11, pp. 209-246. ISSN 0004-0037.

Zotta, G.; Georgesco, M.; Ionesco, V.; Lupasco, G.; Mardare, I. & Teodoresco, A.M. (1940). Nouvelle carte de la distribution des races d'*Anopheles maculipennis* en Roumanie. *Bulletin de la Section Scientifique de l'Académie Roumaine*, Vol.23, pp. 73-87.

Zulueta de, J.; Blazquez, J. & Maruto, J.F. (1973). Aspectos entomológicos sobre la receptividad del paludismo en la zona de Navalmoral de la Mata. *Revista de Sanidad e Higiene Pública*, Vol.47, No.10, (October 1973), pp. 853-870, ISSN 0034-8899.

Zulueta de J.; Ramsdale, C.D. & Coluzzi M. (1975). Receptivity to malaria in Europe. *Bulletin of the World Health Organization*, Vol. 52, No.1, pp. 109-11, ISSN 0042-9686.

14

Associations Between Nutritional Indicators Using Geoadditive Latent Variable Models with Application to Child Malnutrition in Nigeria

Khaled Khatab

Institute of Occupational and Social Medicine, Medical School, RWTH Aachen University
Germany

1. Introduction

Childhood undernutrition is amongst the most serious health issues facing developing countries. It is an intrinsic indicator of well-being, but it is also associated with morbidity, mortality, impaired childhood development, and reduced labor productivity (Svedberg 1996; UNICEF 1998; Sen 1999)

To assess nutritional status, the 2003 DHS obtained measurements of height and weight for all children below five years of age.(Survey 2003) Researchers distinguish between three types of malnutrition: wasting or insufficient weight for height indicating acute malnutrition; stunting or insufficient height for age indicating chronic malnutrition; and underweight or insufficient weight for age which could be a result of both stunting and wasting.

These three anthropometric variables are measured through z-scores for wasting, stunting and underweight, defined by

$$Z_i = \frac{AI_i - MAI}{\sigma},\tag{1}$$

where AI refers to the individual anthropometric indicator (e.g. height at a certain age), MAI refers to the median of a reference population, and σ refers to the standard deviation of the reference population. Each of the indicators measures somewhat different aspects of nutritional status. Note that higher values of a z-score indicate better nutrition and vice versa. Therefore, a decrease of z-scores indicates an increase in malnutrition. This has to be taken into account when interpreting the results. The reference standard typically used for the calculation is the NCHS-CDC Growth Standard that has been recommended for international use by WHO. (WHO 1999) The reference population are children from the USA. More precisely, the children, up to the age of 24 months are from white parents with a high socio-economic status, while children older than 24 months are from a representative sample of all US children. The selection of the reference populations can affect the results, for example a higher z-score can be caused by the change of the reference population.

Latent variable model: Previous analyses are often based on Demographic and Health Surveys (DHS) as a well-established data sources with reliable information on childhood undernutrition, and they rely on statistical inference with various forms of regression models. Because of methodological restraints, it is difficult to detect nonlinear covariate effects adequately, for example, age, and it is impossible to recover small-scale, district-specific spatial effects with common linear regression or correlation analysis. Recent research has therefore applied geoadditive regression models (Fahrmeir L 2001; Fahrmeir 2004) .They have been used in regression studies of risk factors for acute or chronic undernutrition (e.g., Kandala et al., 2001; Adebayo 2003; Khatab, 2007) and   for morbidity.(Kandala 2001; Adebayo 2003; Kandala, Magadi et al. 2006; Kandala, et al. 2007; Khatab 2007) These models can account for nonlinear covariate effects and geographical variation while simultaneously controlling for other important risk factors.

However, in all these studies regression analyses are carried out separately for certain types of undernutrition such as stunting, wasting or underweight, neglecting possible association among these response variables and without aiming at the detection of common latent risk factors. Because of common and overlapping risk factors, separate analyses may fail to give a comprehensive picture of the epidemiology for the malnutrition and the joint effects of childhood malnutrition at population level.

To asses the association between the the nutritional indicators, we applied the recently developed latent variable model. This model gives us the opportunity to study the association or interrelationship between the three types of malnutrition as indicators for nutritional status. The factor loadings describe the association between these indicators and their impact on the nutritional status of a child. Latent variable model permits modeling of covariate effects on the latent variables through a flexible geoadditive predictor

The objective of this study is to determine the associations between nutritional indicators among Nigerian children under 5 and also to examine the impact of socioeconomic and public health factors on the nutritional status.

Nutritional status is known to have various risk factors including geographical locations as a proxy of socioeconomic and environmental factors that affect the disease prevalence and incidence.

Spatial heterogeneity in these factors influences the nutritional status pattern. Consequently, efforts to reduce the burden of childhood undernutrition should include investigations into the influence of the associations between the different measurements of the malnutrition status of children and their distribution among the locations on child health.

Two approaches of latent variable models (joint model) analysis of malnutrition have emerged: the measurement model which accommodates and describes the effect of the latent variables and a set of observed covariates (e.g. child's sex, mother's educational attainment, working status, etc) on the nutritional indicators such as stunting, wasting and underweight.

The structural model is linking a set of observed covariates which have indirect effects (such as child and mother's age, etc), with the latent variables.

In the latent variables overall specific risks are estimated having adjusted for covariates, and in addition, the correlation of risk between measurements of the malnutrition can be quantified.

In this study, we considered the latent variable model to jointly analyse childhood stunting, wasting and underweight, with the objective of highlighting spatial patterns of these indicators.

To build a regression model for undernutrition, we first have to define a distribution for the response variable. In this application, it is reasonable to assume that z-score is Gaussian distributed; thus in principle, could be applied.

The analysis started by employing a separate geoadditive Gaussian model to continuous response variables for wasting, stunting and underweight. The author then applied geoadditive latent variable models, based on these separate analyses results, which were reported in Khatab, 2007, where the three undernutrition variables were taken as indicators for the nutritional status of a child.

All computations have been carried out with R Programs using the MCMC package; see(Raach 2005; Khatab 2007)

2. Data & methods

DHS collects information on household living conditions such as housing characteristics, on childhood morbidity, malnutrition and child health from mothers in reproductive ages (15-49). There were 6029 children's records in the 2003 survey of Nigeria. Each record consists of information on childhood malnutrition and diseases and the list of covariates that could affect the health and nutritional status of children. In the following, we provide some more information about the nutritional indicators, which were used as response variables and information about the covariates considered in this study.

Stunting. Stunting is an indicator of linear growth retardation relatively uncommon in the first few months of life. However it becomes more common as children get older. Children with *height-for-age* z-scores below minus two standard deviations from the median of the reference population are considered short for their age or stunted.

Wasting. Wasting indicates body mass in relation to body length. Children whose *weight-for-height*'s z-scores are below minus two standard deviations (z-scores $< -2SD$) from the median of the reference population are considered wasted (i.e. too thin for their height) which implies that they are acutely undernourished otherwise they are not wasted.

Underweight. Underweight is a composite index of stunting and wasting. This means children may be underweight if they are either stunted or wasted, or both. In a similar manner to the two previous anthropometric incidences, children may be underweight when their z-score is below minus two standard deviations and they are severely or moderately so if their z-score is lower than two standard deviations. The included variables in Table 1 were considered in the analysis to study child nutritional status.

3. Statistical analysis

In the following, we focus on geoadditive Gaussian models for continuous response variables to analyze the effects of metrical, categorical, and spatial covariates on stunting, wasting and underweight response variables in latent variable analyses. Furthermore, we use "nutritional status" as the indicator in the analysis of the latent variable models as mentioned.

3.1 Geoadditive gaussian model
In this analysis, we apply a noval approach by exploring regional patterns of childhood malnutrition and possible nonlinear effects of the factor within latent model framework using geoadditive Bayesian gaussian model for continuous response variable.The model

Factor	N(%)	Coding effect
Place of residence		
Urban	2237(33.58%)	1
Rural	4424(66.42%)	-1.ref
Child's sex		
Male	3487(52.35%)	1
Female	3174(47.65%)	-1.ref
Working		
Yes	1209(18.15%)	1
No	5452(81.85%)	-1.ref
Mother's Education		
No,		
Incomp.prim,		
Comp.prim,		
Incomp.sec	4194(62.97%)	1
Compl.sec,		
Higher	2467(37.04%)	-1.ref
Pregnancy's treatment		
Yes	697(10.46%)	1
No	5964(89.54%)	-1.ref
Drinking water		
Controlled	5374(80.68%)	1
Not controlled	1287(19.32%)	-1.ref
Missing	1%	
Had radio		
Yes	5374(80.68%)	1
No	1559(19.32%)	-1.ref
Has electricity		
Yes	6203(93.12%)	1
No	458(6.88%)	-1.ref
Toilet facility		
Own flush toile facility	1768(28%)	1
Other and no toilet facility	4511(71.8%)	-1.ref
Missing	1%	
Antenatal visit		
Yes	4181(63%)	1
No	2342(35%)	-1.ref
Missing	2%	

Table 1. Factors analyzed in malnutrition study

used for this investigation has been described else where.(Raach 2005; Khatab 2007) .
Basicaly in the early stage of this study we used the geoadditive Bayesian gaussian model
for the separate analysis. In this model we replace the strictly linear predictor

$$\eta_{ij}^{lin} = x_{ij}'\beta_j + w_{ij}'\gamma_j \quad j = 1,..,3, \tag{2}$$

With geoadditive predicator, to have geoadditive model

$$\eta_{ij}^{geo} = \beta_{0j} + f_1(Chage_i) + f_2(BMI_i) + f_3(Mageb_i) + f_{spat_i}(s) + w_{ij}'\gamma_j \tag{3}$$

where w includes the categorical covariates in effect coding. The function f_1, f_2 and f_3
are non-linear smooth effects of the metrical covariates (body mass index, child, and
mother's age) which are modelled by Bayesian P-splines, and f_{spat} is the effect of the spatial
covariate $s_i \in 1;...;S$ labeling the districts in Nigeria. Regression models with predictors are
referred to as geoadditive models. However, in this work we have used **geoadditive latent
variable models** to overcome the drawbacks of separate analysis.

3.2 A bayesian geoadditive LVM (latent varaible models)
A latent variable model with covariates consists of two main approaches: the measurment
model for continuous response with covaraites influencing the indicators directly (direct
effects); and the structural model explaining the modificatio of the latent variables by
covariates (indirect effects) (Fharmeir and Raach, 2007; Khatab, 2007)

3.2.1 Mesurment model

$$y_{ij} = \lambda_0 + a_j'w_i + \lambda_j\upsilon_i + \varepsilon_{ij}, i = 1,..,n, j = 1,...,p, \tag{4}$$

Where υ_i represents the nutritional status with independent and identically distributed
Gaussian errors $\varepsilon_{ij}\sim N(0,\sigma^2)$. In this model, υ_i is the unobservable value of υ for
individual i, λ_j is the "factor loading", and $\lambda_j\upsilon_i$ is the effect of υ_i. In addition, w_i are the
direct effects which affect the observed variables directly and a_j is the vector of regression
coefficients. The restriction to $\sigma_\upsilon = var(\upsilon) = 1$ is necessary for identifability reasons .
(Fahrmeir L 2007; Khatab and Fahrmeir 2009).
Continuous variables are observed directly, hence the underlying variable is obsolete.

3.2.2 General geoadditive structural model

$$\upsilon_i = u_i'\alpha + f_1(x_{i1}) + ... + f(x_{iq}) + f_{geo}(s_i) + \delta_i, \tag{5}$$

with independent and identically distributed Gaussian errors $\delta_i\sim N(0,1)$. The restriction to
$\sigma_\upsilon =var(\upsilon) = 1$ is necessary for identifiability reasons.
RESULTS. We applied a geoadditive latent variable model, using the three types of
undernutrition as indicators of latent nutritional status. The decision which covariates
should be used in the measurement model, and which should be used in the structural
equation, is based on the same criteria that was used in (Khatab 2007; Khatab and
Fahrmeir 2009).

Our interest is in analyzing the three types of undernutrition of children using latent variable models, and in investigating how they can be established as indicators of the latent variable "undernutrition status". Based on the previous separate analyses (Khatab, 2007), we are able to determine which factors can have direct effects and which can have indirect effects on the indicators.

In order to choose the covariates used in the measurement model (which have direct effects on the disease indicators); or in the case of the structural model, those have indirect effects via their common impact on the latent variable "nutritional status," we used the following criteria: if the effects of covariates turned out to be significantly different (in terms of confidence intervals) for the three diseases, we decided to keep them in the measurement model, otherwise covariates were included in the geoadditive predictor of the structural equation for the latent variable (Khatab and Fahrmeir 2009).

We started by using the easiest model possible, a classic factor analysis for continuous indicators. The predictor of the structural equation of the model yields LMV0:

$$\eta = 0 \tag{6}$$

Estimates of factor loadings are depicted in Table 2. The estimated mean factor loadings show that indicator 2 (*weight-for-age*) has the highest factor loading. That means the most effect on the z-scores is on underweight for age and is followed by the indicator of stunting. The classic factor analysis model has been extended by introducing direct and indirect parametric covariates, which modified the latent construct.

Parameter	Mean	Std	2.5%	97.5%
Factor Loadings				
1. stunting λ_{11}	1.244	0.02	1.206	1.28
2. underweight λ_{21}	1.36	0.08	1.353	1.38
3. wasting λ_{31}	0.770	0.015	0.739	0.801

Table 2. Results of Model LVM0 of Z-scores indicators with $\eta = 0$.

The next model was selected based on the previous separate analyses (reported in Khatab, 2007). This leads to the latent variable model.

In the fundamental analysis (LVM1), the vector a_j comprises the covariates urban, antenatal visits, educational level of mothers, access to flush toilet, and availability of electricity, with direct effects on y_j ; and u_i' comprises the remaining categorical covariates sex, work, treatment during pregnancy and access to controlled water and radio, having common effects on the latent variable υ . However, the results of model LVM1 (not reported here) have been extended or changed to model LVM2 by including some covariates that have direct effects on the parametric direct covariates in LVM2. The results of model LVM2 (Table 3) shows that most of the parametric direct covariates are significant and remained quite stable when including these covariates in the direct parametric effects. It demonstrates that the female children whose mothers are educated, had treatment during their pregnancy, had access to controlled water, had access to radio and working currently have higher Z-score of *weight-for-age* and are better nourished. However, males whose mothers are currently working are associated with a higher level of (*weight-for-height*)(at 97%). Although working status has a slight effect on the indicator of stunting, it is associated with other indicators. According to the covariate of radio, it has mostly a non-significant effect. Moreover, the results of LVM2 indicate a negative effect of the education on the indicator 2.

Parameter	Mean	Std	2.5%	10%	90%	97.5%
Factor Loadings						
stunting λ_{11}	1.041^{**}	0.021	1.00	1.02	1.079	1.095
underweight λ_{21}	1.191^{**}	0.007	1.178	1.187	1.208	1.210
Wasting λ_{31}	0.673^{**}	0.017	0.644	0.656	0.703	0.714
Parametric indirect Effects						
urban	-0.057	0.049	-0.153	-0.119	0.011	0.044
anvis	0.054	0.065	-0.058	-0.013	0.153	0.198
toilet	0.142^{**}	0.059	0.017	0.060	0.212	0.250
elect	0.0683^{*}	0.056	-0.026	0.010	0.151	0.186
Parametric Direct Effects						
male (a_{11})	-0.238^{**}	0.0518	-0.321	-0.285	-0.153	-0.119
work (a_{12})	0.09	0.055	-0.042	-0.007	0.134	0.168
trepr (a_{13})	0.155^{*}	0.069	-0.004	0.041	0.226	0.274
water (a_{14})	0.083^{**}	0.035	0.0148	0.0384	0.127	0.153
educ (a_{15})	0.216^{**}	0.039	0.143	0.167	0.265	0.291
radio (a_{16})	0.062	0.0300	-0.029	-0.0095	0.0711	0.093
male (a_{21})	-0.064^{**}	0.0138	-0.082	-0.067	-0.032	-0.030
work (a_{22})	0.109^{**}	0.0176	0.051	0.056	0.085	0.107
trepr (a_{23})	0.072^{**}	0.023	0.024	0.026	0.085	0.117
water (a_{24})	0.048^{**}	0.007	0.039	0.043	0.057	0.065
educ (a_{25})	0.067^{**}	0.013	0.0507	0.058	0.074	0.076
radio (a_{26})	0.047^{**}	0.0056	0.004	0.005	0.020	0.039
male (a_{31})	0.051^{*}	0.042	-0.015	0.010	0.119	0.148
work (a_{32})	0.096^{*}	0.0453	-0.006	0.021	0.135	0.163
trepr (a_{33})	-0.056	0.056	-0.182	-0.141	0.005	0.045
water (a_{34})	0.001	0.028	-0.054	-0.036	0.037	0.056
educ (a_{35})	-0.076^{**}	0.032	-0.135	-0.115	-0.035	-0.015
radio (a_{36})	0.0018	0.0248	-0.068	-0.050	0.013	0.032
Smoothing Parameters						
Chage	0.035^{**}	0.028	0.008	0.01	0.065	0.107
BMI	0.004^{**}	0.0056	0.0006	0.001	0.010	0.018
Mageb	0.003^{**}	0.0045	0.0004	0.0006	0.007	0.015
reg	0.121^{**}	0.045	0.055	0.071	0.175	0.227

Table 3. Results of LVM2, including direct and indirect effects. (**: Statistically significant at 2.5% and 10%)

The reason for this is that in the analysis of latent models, we used three indicators (which were assumed to have high level of correlations among each other) instead of one indicator, which was used by the separate analysis.

It is observed that the indicators have a higher correlation which can affect the results, so we have made a further analysis excluding the indicator of wasting (*weight-for-hight*) to examine the effects of various factors on the other indicators (underweight and stunting), and results are compared (LVM3) with analysis when all three indicators (LVM2) are present.

The results of LVM3 (Table 4) indicate that the antenatal visits and the availability of electricity are associated positively with nutritional status. With regard to the direct covariates, the females and the education level of mothers have a positive significant effect on the indicator of stunting. While, only the work status is associated positively with the indicator of underweight. The factor loadings estimates show that the *weight-for-height* is seen to be more serious in Nigeria (its higher factor loading of 1.14).

Parameter	Mean	Std	2.5%	97.5%
Factor Loadongs				
stunting λ_{11}	1.147^*	0.028	1.097	1.203
underweight λ_{21}	0.987^*	0.0274	0.934	1.040
Parametric Indirect Effects				
urban	0.0357	0.060	-0.357	0.152
anvis	0.346^*	0.075	0.205	0.492
toilet	0.156	0.082	-0.013	0.313
elect	0.153^*	0.058	0.033	0.269
Parametric Direct Effects				
male (a_{11})	-0.242^*	0.059	-0.357	-0.1372
work (a_{12})	0.087	0.064	-0.028	0.211
trepr (a_{13})	0.124	0.083	-0.044	0.290
water (a_{14})	0.065	0.086	-0.1033	0.241
educ (a_{15})	0.184^*	0.067	0.055	0.330
radio (a_{16})	0.019	0.0365	-0.049	0.088
male (a_{21})	-0.057	0.045	-0.150	0.026
work (a_{22})	0.118^*	0.053	0.0155	0.224
trepr (a_{23})	0.022	0.060	-0.090	0.137
water (a_{24})	0.0079	0.069	-0.124	0.139
educ (a_{25})	0.046	0.0529	-0.051	0.154
radio (a_{26})	0.028	0.029	-0.027	0.089
Smoothing Parameters				
Chage	0.016^*	0.018	0.064	0.143
BMI	0.004^*	0.011	0.075	0.319
Mageb	0.135^*	0.085	0.0003	0.009
reg	0.159^*	0.054	0.081	0.291
Chage	0.016^*	0.018	0.064	0.143

Table 4. Estimates of factor loadings of the LVM3 with only two indicators in Niegria.

Figure 1 shows the non-linear effect of the child's age to be associated with a malnutrition status in Nigeria for LVM1 and LVM2, respectively. It shows that the rates of malnutrition of children increase sharply from about 5 to around 20 months of age. The rates of malnutrition are at low level between 20 and 30 months of age, then rise again through the

remainder of the third year. This pattern highlights the first two years of life as the most
nutritionally vulnerable for children in Nigeria.

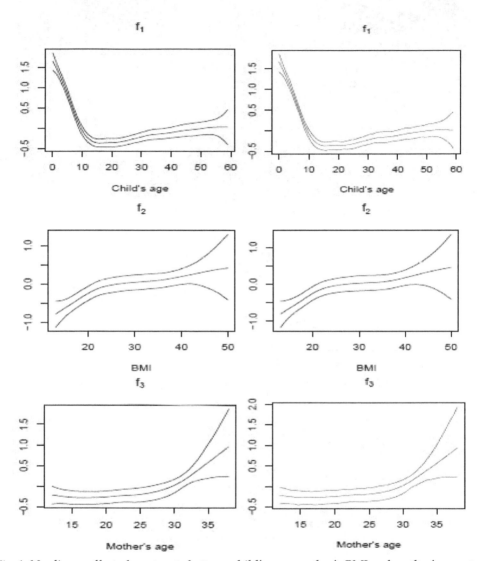

Fig. 1. Nonlinear effects from top to bottom: child's age, mother's BMI and mother's age at
birth for LVM1 (left) and LVM2 (right) of "malnutrition status" of children for Nigeria,
using latent varaible model for continuous responses

The nonlinear effect of the BMI of the mother shows that obesity of the mother probably
poses less of a risk for the child's nutritional status, due to the fact that a very low BMI
suggested acute undernutrition of the mother. The Z-score is highest (and thus stunting
lowest) at a BMI of around 30-40 months.

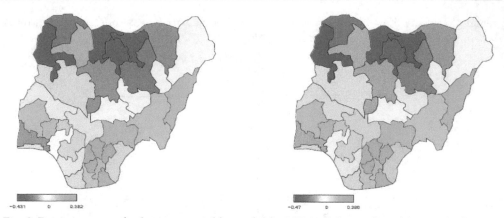

Fig. 2. Posterior mean for leatent varaiable model for LVM1 (left panel) and LVM2 (right panel) on malnutrion status for Nigeria

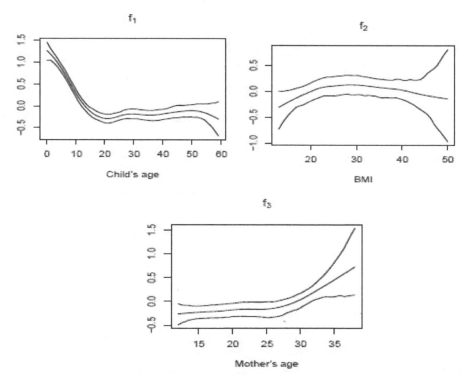

Fig. 3. Nonlinear effects from top to bottom: child's age, mother's BMI and mother's age at birth using only two indicators of latent varaible "malnutrition status" of children for Nigeria, using latent varaible model for continuous responses.

The effect of the mother's age seems to be slight on the Z-scores of children up till about the age of 25 months; thereafter, there is a strong effect shown.

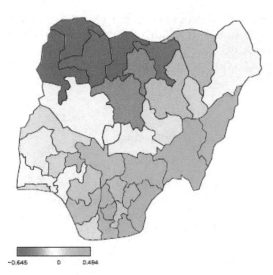

Fig. 4. Posterior mean for Latent varaible model, using only two idicators of latent varaible
"Malnutrion status" for Nigeria

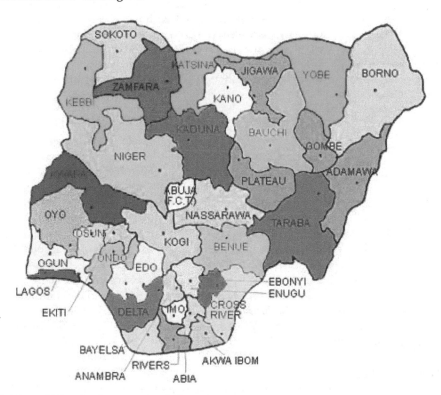

Fig. 5. Map of Nigeria showing the different states

In addition, the patterns of the nonlinear effect in LVM3 (Figure 3) are similar to the patterns of LVM1 and LVM2. The same is true with regard to the spatial effects of LVM3 (Figure 4). Figure 2 shows that the districts in the southeastern through the southern part of the country are associated with better nutrition of children in Nigeria.

4. Discussion

The results of estimating the geoadditive latent variable models with continuous response variables are indicated and suggest the following:

4.1 Child's sex
The likelihood of being stunted and underweight was lower for girls than for boys; a finding consistent with .(Klasen 1996; Lavy, Strauss et al. 1996; Svedberg 1996; Gibson 2001; Kandala 2001; Borooah 2002; S.B 2003); on the other hand, Gibson (2001) did not find any significant gender difference between the *height-for-age* and the *weight-for-age* in Papua, New Guinea.

4.2 Malnutrition among residences
Although, rural living was expected to have many problems, such as, poor health, use of unprotected water supplies, lack of charcoal as fuel, lack of milk consumption, and lack of personal hygiene (which assumed to be the risk factors of nutritional status), the results indicate that the place of residence is not associated with significant effects on wasting, underweight, and for stunting. This is consistent with some studies, but not with others: Adebayo (2003) found that where the mother lives (rural/urban) has no statistical significance for child's *weight-for-height*, and a similar impact of where the mother lives, as in *height-for-age*, is observed in *weight-for-age*, though Kandala found that urban areas have a statistical significance for a child's *height-for-age* in Tanzania and Malawi (Lavy, Strauss et al. 1996; Gibson 2001; Borooah 2002)

4.3 Mother's education
Maternal education, which is related to household wealth, is a determinant of good child-care knowledge and practices. The education attainment of mothers is mostly significant in the analysis of LVM.
The results with two indicators are quite similar to the results with three indicators with regard to this variable. This result supports the suggestion that an educated mother assumes the responsibility of taking a sick child to receive health care. Further, the time that mothers spend discussing their child's illness with a doctor is almost directly proportional to their level of education: consequently, illiterate women (with sick children) get much less out of visiting a doctor than literate women do. These findings are consistent with many studies in the context of developing countries (Africa Nutrition chartbooks 1996, Borooah 2002), which reported that maternal education has a strong and significant effect on stunting. They found that at primary levels of education,, effects on stunting are small or negligible, and they increase only at secondary or higher levels.(Chartbooks 1996; Borooah 2002).

4.4 Working mothers
Work has a non significant effect on the malnutrition status of children in Nigeria. The results are consistent with some previous studies and not consistent with others. Some

studies reported that when mothers are working, the household income is increased and the access to better food will be increased, as well as the access to a quality level of medical care. On the other hand, when mothers are employed outside the home, the duration of full breastfeeding is shortened and necessitates supplementary feeding. This is usually preformed by illiterate care-takers, which might affect the health of children negatively.

4.5 Drinking water
A household's source of drinking water has been shown to be associated with the nutritional status of a child in Nigeria (*weight-for-age*) in separate analysis (Khatab, 2007), and it seems to be mostly significant in the results of LVM. In other words, the source of water is associated with the nutritional status of a child through its impact on the risk of childhood diseases such as diarrhea, and is affected indirectly as a measure of wealth and availability of water.

4.6 Access to toilet
The type of toilet used by a household is an indicator of household wealth and a determinant of environmental sanitation. This means that poor households, which are mostly located in rural areas, are less likely to have sanitary toilet facilities. Consequently, this results in an increased risk of childhood diseases, which contributes to malnutrition.
The results indicate that in households where a flush toilet exits, stunting and underweight (separate analysis) are significantly lower and the nutritional status of children (analysis with LVM) is better.

4.7 Availability of electricity and radio in household
Despite access to electricity and radio, which facilitates the acquisition of nutritional information allowing more successful allocation of resources to produce child health (Kandala, 2001), only the availability of electricity was significant and had a positive effect on reducing stunting, and underweight with separate analysis, and it seems to be significant on the LVM "nutritional status". This may be because mothers allocate their leisure time to radio or television, but it doesn't help improve the level of nutrition of their children. At the same time, it reduces the length of time spent engaging in their children's affairs.(Kandala 2001)

4.8 Antenatal visits
The variables that deal with access to health care, such as children of mothers who obtained clinical visits during pregnancy and had vaccines and treatment, have a positive and significant effect on malnutrition status. Therefore, health service investments are more effective in reducing stunting, wasting and underweight among indigenous communities. Our results indicate that children of mothers who had clinical visits and got medical care during pregnancy are less likely to be stunted and to be underweight than their counterparts in Nigeria. The results with two indicators also indicate that the *anvis* has a positive effect.

4.9 Child's age
In the analysis, it was discovered that the situation among children who are stunted is quite similar; however, the deterioration in nutritional status is set between 5-20 months of age.

Similarly, deterioration in child's *weight-for-height* sets during the first 4-5 months of age, as reported in much of the literature, is due to supplementation. However, it reaches its minimum level between ages 13 and 15 months, then rises again and reaches its minimum level between 16 and18 months of age; which is earlier than the case of stunting. A sudden pick-up effect is noticeable from age 18 months until about 45 months, where it attains its maximum level.

An improvement commenced after age 20 or 25 months and rose gradually until age 50 months. Previous studies assumed that it is an average effect of low *height-for-age* and *weight-for-height* during this period of life (Adebayo, 2003)

The level of wasting suggests that insufficient food intake may be an important factor in the rise of malnutrition in both countries. In addition, the implication of this finding is that wasting is not clearly noticeable in the first four months of life. As soon as a child is fed with other supplementation such as liquids or other forms of diet, which due to the unhygienic source of preparation of such supplementation, may facilitate infections and diseases such as diarrhoea, then acute malnutrition may set in.

4.10 Mother's BMI

A mother's nutritional status affects her ability to successfully carry, deliver, and care for her children and is of great concern in its own right. The BMI pattern shows linear trends with positive slopes. Malnutrition in women is assessed using BMI. When the BMI of non-pregnant women falls below the suggested cut-off point, which is around $18.5kg/m2$, malnutrition is indicated. Women who are malnourished (thinness or obesity) may have complications during childbirth and may deliver a child who can be wasted, stunted or underweight. The results indicate that there is an association between the thinness of the mother and the nutritional status of the child.

4.11 Mother's age at birth

The results show that the influence of mothers who are younger than 20 years is higher on the nutritional status of children.

A possible cause for this is childbirth among very young girls, whose bodies are not physically ready to endure the processes of childbirth. The problem is compounded by the fact that some African countries have poor obstetric care. Furthermore, these mothers could not reach health facilities, or, when they do, it is too late. Effective ways must be devised to delay age at first marriage and first birth. These two factors will almost certainly determine the number of children she will have in her lifetime. While early age at first birth has health implications, it also has economic implications.

In addition, one study obtained in Nigeria reported that younger mothers (teenagers) are less likely in comparison to older mothers to breastfeed their children after birth, which means that the age of the mother at birth of a child influences whether the child will receive colostrum or not, which might   affect the nutritional status of children (Adebayo and Fahrmeir 2005).

Moreover, previous studies which were obtained in some developing countries have shown that some African countries do not allow girls back to go back school after they give birth. As a consequence, a girl who drops out of school will continue the cycle of poverty(Alderman H 1997; Wasao; 1999).

4.12 Malnutrition in region

As reported in the 2003 NDHS, the trend in the nutritional status of Nigerian children has worsened with regard to stunting and wasting (from 36% in 1990 to 46% in 1999 for stunting and 11% in 1990 to 12% in 1999 for wasting). The results, based on our analysis, indicate that mostly districts in the northeast and southeast and northwest are more likely to be associated with *nutritional problems,* providing a more complete picture of the situation. The result also revealed striking regional variations, with the northeast, south and southeast in much worse situations in terms of stunting and underweight than the northwest and southwest For more information about the different states in Nigeria, see figure 5 . On the other hand, the children who live in the northwest part of the country are more likely to be wasted than their counterparts in other parts of the country. These regional and zonal disparities may reflect the contribution of other factors, such as socio-cultural conditions and morbidity of children, in determining the nutritional status of children under the age of five. The high prevalence of stunting observed in the 2003 NDHS survey is in the context of large-scale deepening poverty and household food insecurity. Severe rural poverty appears to be found in the southwest of Nigeria, in the north-center, and in the extreme northeast.

These results are consistent with some previous studies which discuss the relation between poverty and malnutrition as persistent problems in Nigeria.

4.13 Summary

The results showed that the place of residence, mother's working, type of toilet and availability of electricity and radio in households have negligible effects on the undernutrition of children.

We find that the analysis identify the association of child's age, mother's age at birth and mother's BMI as effecting undernutrition. It was found that children are at a high risk during the first 15-20 months of life and that the risk rises again between ages 25-50 months. The effect of BMI on the child's nutritional status is approximately linear with positive slope, which means that there is an association between the thinness condition of mothers and nutritional status. According to the mother's age at birth, it shows that younger mothers are less likely to affect their children's nutritional status positively.

It is found that children living in some provinces in the southeast regions and some regions in the southern part of the country are associated with undernutrition.

4.14 Policy implications

Affected areas should improve socioeconomic conditions. Because, if living standards are improved, there will be better health care and a reduction in infant and child diseases, child malnutrition and child mortality.

The policymakers need to give more attention to some areas which have high rates of poverty, such as the southern part of Nigeria. These areas are more likely to have a higher proportion of undernutrition compared to other areas, due to poor health facilities and complications during childbirth or even carelessness and misdiagnosis during hospital care. Therefore, the most important issues to address in these areas are health care, proper food, and raising the educational level of parents.

5. Appendix

As presented in this paper, LVMs are based on the results of the separate models which were presented in Khatab, 2007. At that stage, we have used separate geoadditive probit models with the binary target variables for diarrhea, cough, and fever using covariate information from the 2003NDHS. The computations for the separate models were carried out using BayesX program (Brezger A, Kneib T, Lang S, 2005). We are showing here the results of Model 3, which was selected from a long hierarchal analysis based on its DIC (the value of deviance information criterion).

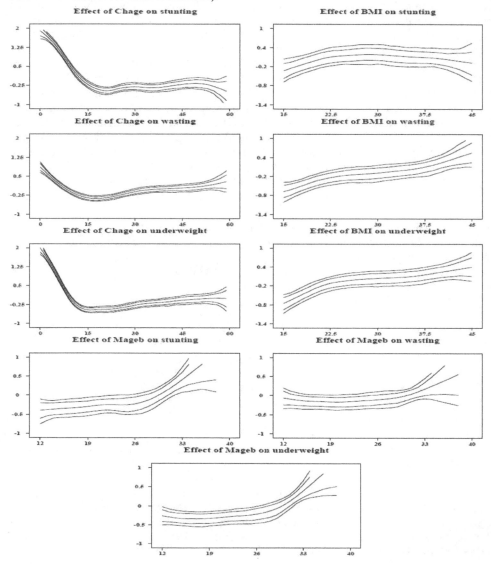

Source:Khatab, 2007

Fig. A1. Nonlinear effects of child's age, BMI, and Mother's age at birth using separate Bayesian Gaussian Model children for Nigeria using Bayesian latent variable model for continuous responses.

Variable	Mean	S.dv	10%	median	90%
const	−1.133*	0.154	-1.33	-1.133	-0.94
male	−0.117*	0.030	-0.156	-0.117	-0.077
urban	0.032	0.039	-0.020	0.032	0.083
work	0.027	0.033	-0.016	0.025	0.070
trepr	0.075*	0.039	0.026	0.074	0.128
anvis	0.147*	0.039	0.095	0.147	0.199
radio	0.017	0.037	-0.030	0.017	0.063
elect	0.131*	0.039	0.077	0.129	0.180
water	0.044	0.044	-0.008	0.043	0.106
educ	-0.543	0.943	-1.766	-0.509	0.606
toilet	0.078*	0.048	0.013	0.078	0.140

Table A1. Fixed effects of separate model using Bayesian geoadditive model on Stuniting

Variable	Mean	S.dv	10%	median	90%
const	−0.710*	0.121	-0.863	-0.718	-0.551
male	−0.032*	0.022	-0.061	-0.033	-0.004
urban	-0.022	0.030	-0.059	-0.023	0.016
work	0.044*	0.026	0.009	0.043	0.077
trepr	0.014	0.031	-0.027	0.014	0.053
anvis	0.079*	0.030	0.040	0.080	0.116
radio	0.035*	0.028	0.0007	0.034	0.072
elect	0.065*	0.029	0.024	0.067	0.101
water	0.046*	0.033	0.001	0.047	0.089
educ	0.063*	0.038	0.013	0.064	0.111
toilet	0.105*	0.044	0.051	0.106	0.159

Table A2. Fixed effects of separate model using Bayesian geoadditive model on underweight

Variable	Mean	S.dv	10%	median	90%
const	−0.041*	0.127	-0.214	-0.032	0.116
male	0.026	0.024	-0.005	0.025	0.058
urban	-0.051	0.030	-0.111	-0.050	0.006
work	0.049*	0.027	0.011	0.050	0.083
trepr	-0.046	0.034	-0.116	-0.045	0.022
anvis	-0.038	0.030	-0.076	-0.039	0.0004
radio	0.018	0.032	-0.023	0.020	0.060
elect	-0.019	0.031	-0.060	-0.019	0.020
water	0.028	0.036	-0.016	0.026	0.075
educ	0.030	0.041	-0.022	0.030	0.0847
toilet	0.0037	0.048	-0.055	0.0006	0.068

Table A3. Fixed effects of separate model using Bayesian geoadditive model on wasting

6. References

[http://hdr.undp.org/docs/events/Berlin/Background_paper.pdf] webcite, U. N. U. S.-S. A. t. h. c. o. t. b.-a.-u. s.

Adebayo, S. B. and L. Fahrmeir (2005). "Analysing child mortality in Nigeria with geoadditive discrete-time survival models." *Stat Med* 24(5): 709-28.

Alderman H, J. B., V Lavy and R Menon (1997). "Child Nutrition, Child health and School Enrollment:A longitudinal Analysis." *The World Bank* Policy research Working (Papwe.1700).

Borooah, V. (2002). "The Role of Maternal Literacy in Reducing the Risk of Child Malnutrition in India." *ICER - International Centre for Economic Research*.

Brezger A, K. T., Lang S (2005). "BayesX - Software for Bayesian Inference based on Markov Chain Monte Carlo simulation Techniques." *Available at: http://www.stat.uni-uenchen.de/lang/BayesX* 1.4.

Chartbooks, A. N. (1996). "Nutrition of Infants and young Children in Mali. Macro international Inc." *Calverton, Maryland, U.S.A.*

Fahrmeir L, a. L. S. (2001). "Bayesian Inference for Generalized Additive Mixed Models Based on Markov Random Field Priors." *Applied Statistics* 50: 201-220.

Fahrmeir, L., Kneib, T.and Lang, S (2004). "Penalized structured additive regression of space-time data:a Bayesian perspective." *Statistica Sinica* 14: 731-761.

Fahrmeir L , R. A. (2007). "A Bayesian semiparametric latent variable model for mixed responses " *Psychometrika* 72: 327– 346.

Gibson, J. (2001). "Literacy and Intra-household externalities." *World Development* 29(155-66).

Kandala, N. B., C. Ji, et al. (2007). "Spatial analysis of risk factors for childhood morbidity in
    Nigeria." *Am J Trop Med Hyg* 77(4): 770-9.

Kandala, N. B., Lang, S., Klasen, S. and Fahrmeir, L (2001). "Semiparametric Analysis of the
    Socio-Demographic Determinants of Undernutrition in Two African Countries."
    Research in Official Statistics 4(1): 81-100.

Kandala, N. B., M. A. Magadi, et al. (2006). "An investigation of district spatial variations of
    childhood diarrhoea and fever morbidity in Malawi." *Soc Sci Med* 62(5): 1138-52.

Khatab, K. (2007). "Analysis of childhood diseases and malnutrition in developing countries
    of Africa." *Dr.Hut Verlag -Munich, Germany.*

Khatab, K. and L. Fahrmeir (2009). "Analysis of childhood morbidity with geoadditive
    probit and latent variable model: a case study for Egypt." *Am J Trop Med Hyg* 81(1):
    116-28.

Klasen, S. (1996). "Nutrition, Health, and Mortality in Sub-Saharan Africa: Is there a Gender
    Bias?" *Journal of Development Studies* 32: 913-932.

Lavy, V., J. Strauss, et al. (1996). "Quality of health care, survival and health outcomes in
    Ghana." *J Health Econ* 15(3): 333-57.

Pelletier DL, F. E. (1995). "The effects of malnutrition on child mortality in developing
    countries." *Bulletin of the World Health Organization* 73: 443-448.

Pelletier, D. L., E. A. Frongillo, Jr., et al. (1995). "The effects of malnutrition on child
    mortality in developing countries." *Bull World Health Organ* 73(4): 443-8.

Pelletier, D. L. a. E. A. F. (2003). "Changes in Child Survival Are Strongly
Associated with Changes in Malnutrition in Developing Countries." *Journal of Nutrition* 133:
    107-119.

Raach, A. W. (2005). "A Bayesian semiparametric latent variable model for binary, ordinal
    and continuous response." *Dissertation, available from edoc.ub.uni-muenchen.de.*

S.B, A. (2003). "Semiparametric Bayesian Regression for Multivariate Responses." *Ph.D
    Thesis, Hieronymus Verlag, Munich, Germany.*

Sen, A. (1999). "Development as Freedom." *Oxford: Oxford University Press.*

Smith LC, H. L. (2000). "Explaining child malnutrition in developing countries: a cross
    country analysis. International Food Policy Research Institute, Food Consumption
    and Nutrition Division discussion paper." 60.

Smith LC, O. A., Jensen HH (2000). "The geography and causes of food insecurity in
    developing countries." *Agricultural Economics* 22: 199-215.

Survey, D. a. H. (2003). "Demographic and Health Survey for Nigeria." *DHS.*

Svedberg, P. (1996). "Gender Bias in Sub-Saharan Africa: Reply and Further Evidence."
    Journal of Development Studies 32: 933-943.

UNICEF (1998). "The State of the World's Children." *New York: UNICEF.*

UNICEF (2008). "The State of the world children." *UNICEF.*

Vella, V., A. Tomkins, et al. (1992). "Determinants of child nutrition and mortality in north-
    west Uganda." *Bull World Health Organ* 70(5): 637-43.

Wasao., T.-R. C. a. S. (1999). "Factors Affecting Children's Nutritional and Health Status in
    Kenya: A District-Level Analysis." *Paper presented at the Population Association Of
    America annual meeting in New York Marriot Marquis Hotel on March*: 25-27.

WHO (1999). "Infant and Young Child Growth: The WHO Multicentre Growth Reference
    Study.Executive   Board:Implementation   of   Resolu-   tions   and   Decisions   "
    EB105/Inf.doc/1.Geneva:WHO.

Permissions

The contributors of this book come from diverse backgrounds, making this book a truly international effort. This book will bring forth new frontiers with its revolutionizing research information and detailed analysis of the nascent developments around the world.

We would like to thank Prof. Alfonso J. Rodriguez-Morales, for lending his expertise to make the book truly unique. He has played a crucial role in the development of this book. Without his invaluable contribution this book wouldn't have been possible. He has made vital efforts to compile up to date information on the varied aspects of this subject to make this book a valuable addition to the collection of many professionals and students.

This book was conceptualized with the vision of imparting up-to-date information and advanced data in this field. To ensure the same, a matchless editorial board was set up. Every individual on the board went through rigorous rounds of assessment to prove their worth. After which they invested a large part of their time researching and compiling the most relevant data for our readers. Conferences and sessions were held from time to time between the editorial board and the contributing authors to present the data in the most comprehensible form. The editorial team has worked tirelessly to provide valuable and valid information to help people across the globe.

Every chapter published in this book has been scrutinized by our experts. Their significance has been extensively debated. The topics covered herein carry significant findings which will fuel the growth of the discipline. They may even be implemented as practical applications or may be referred to as a beginning point for another development. Chapters in this book were first published by InTech; hereby published with permission under the Creative Commons Attribution License or equivalent.

The editorial board has been involved in producing this book since its inception. They have spent rigorous hours researching and exploring the diverse topics which have resulted in the successful publishing of this book. They have passed on their knowledge of decades through this book. To expedite this challenging task, the publisher supported the team at every step. A small team of assistant editors was also appointed to further simplify the editing procedure and attain best results for the readers.

Our editorial team has been hand-picked from every corner of the world. Their multi-ethnicity adds dynamic inputs to the discussions which result in innovative outcomes. These outcomes are then further discussed with the researchers and contributors who give their valuable feedback and opinion regarding the same. The feedback is then collaborated with the researches and they are edited in a comprehensive manner to aid the understanding of the subject.

Apart from the editorial board, the designing team has also invested a significant amount of their time in understanding the subject and creating the most relevant covers. They scrutinized every image to scout for the most suitable representation of the subject and create an appropriate cover for the book.

The publishing team has been involved in this book since its early stages. They were actively engaged in every process, be it collecting the data, connecting with the contributors or procuring relevant information. The team has been an ardent support to the editorial, designing and production team. Their endless efforts to recruit the best for this project, has resulted in the accomplishment of this book. They are a veteran in the field of academics and their pool of knowledge is as vast as their experience in printing. Their expertise and guidance has proved useful at every step. Their uncompromising quality standards have made this book an exceptional effort. Their encouragement from time to time has been an inspiration for everyone.

The publisher and the editorial board hope that this book will prove to be a valuable piece of knowledge for researchers, students, practitioners and scholars across the globe.

List of Contributors

Regina Maria Pinto de Figueiredo
Foundation for Tropical Medicine Dr. Hector Vieira Dourado (FMT/HVD), Brazil

E. Khan, R. Hasan, J. Mehraj and S. Mahmood
Department of Pathology and Microbilogy, Aga Khan University, Stadium Road, Karachi, Pakistan

Bordi Licia
Laboratory of Virology, National Institute for Infectious Diseases "L. Spallanzani", Rome, Italy

Meschi Silvia, Selleri Marina, Lalle Eleonora, Castilletti Concetta and Capobianchi Maria Rosaria
Laboratory of Virology, National Institute for Infectious Diseases "L. Spallanzani", Rome, Italy

Carletti Fabrizio and Di Caro Antonino
Laboratory of Microbiology and Infectious Disease Biorepository, National Institute for Infectious Diseases "L. Spallanzani", Rome, Italy

Aránzazu Portillo and José A. Oteo
Hospital San Pedro-Centre of Biomedical Research (CIBIR), Spain

Lucy Ndip and Roland Ndip
University of Buea, Cameroon

David Walker and Jere McBride
University of Texas Medical Branch, Galveston, USA

Ying Bai and Michael Kosoy
Division of Vector-Borne Diseases, National Center for Emerging and Zoonotic Infectious Diseases, Centers for Disease Control and Prevention, USA

Marcia Marinho
Laboratory of Microbiology, Department of Support, Animal Production and Health Course for Veterinary Medicine of UNESP, Campus Araçatuba, São Paulo, Brazil

Diana M. Castañeda-Hernández
Tuberculosis Control Program, Health and Social Security Secretary, Pereira and Fundación Universitaria del Área Andina, Pereira, Columbia

Alfonso J. Rodriguez-Morales
Instituto José Witremundo Torrealba, Universidad de Los Andes, Trujillo; Faculty of Health Sciences, Universidad Tecnológica de Pereira, Pereira and Office of Scientific Research, Cooperativa de Entidades de Salud de Risaralda (COODESURIS), Pereira, Venezuela

Ute Inegbenebor
Department of Physiology, College of Medicine, Ambrose Alli University, Ekpoma, Nigeria

Yasuyoshi Mori, Norihiro Tomita, Hidetoshi Kanda and Tsugunori Notomi
Eiken Chemical Co., Ltd., Japan

Hippolite O. Amadi
Imperial College London, United Kingdom

John C. Meade and Denise C. Cornelius
University of Mississippi Medical Center, Department of Microbiology, Jackson, MS, USA

Rubén Bueno Marí and Ricardo Jiménez Peydró
Laboratorio de Entomología y Control de Plagas, Inst. Cavanilles de Biodiversidad y Biología Evolutiva, Universitat de València, Spain

Khaled Khatab
Institute of Occupational and Social Medicine, Medical School, RWTH Aachen University, Germany